Practical
Orthopaedic Trauma Surgery

A Trainee's Companion

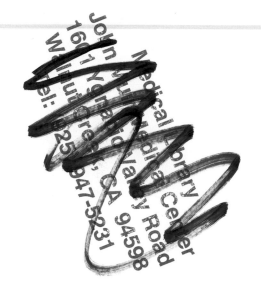

This highly illustrated textbook provides an essential guide for surgeons in training. It follows a step-by-step approach to performing a surgical procedure. It includes details of positioning the patient, the approach and reduction technique, the implant to be inserted, protocols for post-operative mobilisation, complications to look for, when the patient should be seen in the outpatient clinic and whether the implant should be removed. Intraoperative pictures have been incorpoated to make the surgeon aware of all the important issues involved. It covers the most common trauma procedures that surgeons in training are expected to perform during their residency. Each procedure has been written by an expert. This will be an invaluble resource for the resident in training during the long on-call nights in the hospital while preparing for the operations necessary to help trauma patients.

Peter V. Giannoudis is Professor of Trauma and Orthopaedic Surgery at St James' University Hospital, Leeds, UK.

Hans-Christoph Pape is Professor of Trauma and Orthopaedic Surgery at Pittsburgh School of Medicine.

Practical Procedures in Orthopaedic Trauma Surgery

A Trainee's Companion

Edited by

Peter V. Giannoudis

Academic Department of Orthopaedic and Trauma Surgery, School of Medicine, University of Leeds, St James' University Hospital, Leeds, UK

and

Hans-Christoph Pape

Department of Orthopaedic Surgery, Pittsburgh Medical School, Pittsburgh, USA

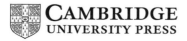

CAMBRIDGE
UNIVERSITY PRESS

CAMBRIDGE UNIVERSITY PRESS
Cambridge, New York, Melbourne, Madrid, Cape Town, Singapore, São Paulo

Cambridge University Press
The Edinburgh Building, Cambridge CB2 2RU, UK

Published in the United States of America by Cambridge University Press, New York

www.cambridge.org
Information on this title: www.cambridge.org/9780521678599

© Cambridge university Press 2006

First published 2006

Printed in the United Kingdom at the University Press, Cambridge

A catalogue record for this publication is available from the British Library

ISBN-13 978-0-521-67859-9 paperback
ISBN-10 0-521-67859-5 paperback

To my wife Rania and my children Marilena and Vasilis,
whose love and support made this book a reality

PVG

To Claudia and Julia, who missed me while I was on call

HCP

Contents

List of contributors   *page* xi
Preface   xiii
Acknowledgments   xiv

Part I Upper extremity

1   Fractures of the clavicle   3

   1.1 Open reduction and internal
   fixation of midshaft fractures   3
   Peter V. Giannoudis

**2   Section I: Fractures of the proximal
   humerus   8**

   2.1 General considerations   8
   David Limb

   2.2 Tension band wiring for displaced
   greater tuberosity fractures   10
   David Limb

   2.3 Open reduction and internal
   fixation of 3- and 4-part fractures (using
   a Philos plate)   14
   David Limb

   2.4 Hemiarthroplasty for fracture
   dislocation   17
   David Limb

   Section II: Fractures of the humeral shaft   22

   2.5 Open reduction and internal
   fixation: posterior approach   22
   Peter V. Giannoudis

   2.6 Antegrade intramedullary nailing of
   the humerus   26
   Paige T. Kendrick, Craig S. Roberts, David
   Seligson

**Section III: Fractures of the distal
humerus   30**

   2.7 Open reduction and internal
   fixation of supracondylar fractures   30
   Paige T. Kendrick, Craig S. Roberts, David
   Seligson

   2.8 Open reduction internal fixation:
   capitellum   35
   Paige T. Kendrick, Craig S. Roberts, David
   Seligson

   2.9 Retrograde intramedullary nailing   38
   Paige T. Kendrick, Craig S. Roberts, David
   Seligson

   2.10 Paediatric supracondylar
   fractures: MUA/percutaneous fixation
   of distal humerus fractures   40
   Paige T. Kendrick, Craig S. Roberts, David
   Seligson

**3   Section I: Fractures of the proximal
   ulna   45**

   3.1 Tension band wiring of olecranon
   fractures   45
   Gregoris Kambouroglou

   3.2 Open reduction and internal
   fixation of olecranon fractures   48
   Gregoris Kambouroglou

   **Section II: Fractures of the ulnar
   shaft   51**

   3.3 Open reduction and internal
   fixation: plating   51
   Gregoris Kambouroglou

3.4 Elastic nails for ulnar shaft fractures   53
Gregoris Kambouroglou

Section III: Fractures of the distal ulna   56

3.5 Open reduction and internal
fixation for distal ulnar fractures   56
Gregoris Kambouroglou

**4 Section I: Fractures of the proximal
radius   60**

4.1 Open reduction and internal
fixation of radial head fractures   60
Reinhard Meier

4.2 Excision of radial head   62
Reinhard Meier

**Section II: Fractures of the radial
shaft   65**

4.3 Open reduction and internal
fixation: anterior approach   65
Christopher C. Tzioupis, Peter V. Giannoudis

4.4 Elastic intramedullary nailing for
diaphyseal forearm fractures in children   71
Brian W. Scott

Section III: Fractures of the distal radius   77

4.5 Open reduction and internal
fixation for distal radius fractures: volar
approach   77
Peter V. Giannoudis

4.6 Open reduction and internal
fixation for distal radius fractures: dorsal
approach   81
Doug Campbell

4.7 Closed reduction and K-wire
fixation of distal radius fractures   85
Reinhard Meier

4.8 Closed reduction and application of
an external fixator in distal radius
fractures   87
Reinhard Meier

5 Fractures of wrist   90

5.1 Percutaneous fixation of scaphoid
fractures   90
Doug Campbell

5.2 Open reduction and internal
fixation of acute scapholunate
dissociation   93
Doug Campbell

**6 Section I: Fractures of the first
metacarpal   98**

6.1 Kirschner wire fixation
of basal fractures of the first
metacarpal   98
Reinhard Meier

6.2 Open reduction and internal
fixation of basal fractures of the first
metacarpal   99
Reinhard Meier

6.3 Ulnar collateral ligament
repair   101
Reinhard Meier

**Section II: Fractures of the
metacarpals II–V   104**

6.4 Open reduction and internal
fixation of midshaft fractures of the
metacarpals   104
Reinhard Meier

6.5 Closed reduction and
intramedullary fixation of distal
third fractures of the metacarpals II-V   106
Reinhard Meier

**Section III: Fractures of the
phalanx   109**

6.6 Open reduction and internal
fixation of condylar fractures   109
Reinhard Meier

6.7 Open reduction and internal
fixation of midshaft fractures   110
Reinhard Meier

Part II Pelvis and acetabulum

7 Fractures of the pelvic ring   117

7.1 Application of anterior frame   117
Peter V. Giannoudis

7.2 Plating of the pubic symphysis   120
Peter V. Giannoudis

7.3 Sacroiliac screw insertion   125
Peter V. Giannoudis

7.4 Open reduction and internal
fixation of Sacro-iliac joint anteriorly   130
Peter V. Giannoudis

8 Fractures of the acetabulum   133

8.1 Open reduction and internal
fixation of posterior wall fractures –
Kocher–Langenbeck approach   133
Peter V. Giannoudis

8.2 Open reduction and internal
fixation via the ilioinguinal approach   142
Peter V. Giannoudis

Part III Lower extremity

**9 Section I: Extracapsular fractures
of the hip   151**

9.1 Dynamic compression hip screw   151
Raghu Raman, Peter V. Giannoudis

**Section II: Intracapsular fractures
of the hip   158**

9.2 Cannulated screw fixation   158
Christopher C. Tzioupis, Peter V. Giannoudis

9.3 Hemiarthroplasty for intracapsular
hip fractures: Austin Moore uncemented
arthroplasty and Thompson's cemented
hemiarthroplasty   163
David A. Macdonald

**10 Section I: Subtrochanteric fractures
of the femur   168**

10.1 Intramedullary fixation for
subtrochanteric fractures using a
proximal femoral nail   168
Peter V. Giannoudis

Section II: Fractures of the femoral shaft   177

10.2 General aspects   177
Hans-Christoph Pape, Stefan Hankemeier,
Thomas Gosling

10.3 Open reduction and internal
fixation: plating   180
Stefan Hankemeier, Thomas Gosling,
Hans-Christoph Pape

10.4 Intramedullary nailing   183
Stefan Hankemeier, Thomas Gosling,
Hans-Christoph Pape

10.5 Flexible intramedullary nails
in children   188
Brian W. Scott

10.6 Application of an external
fixator   192
Stefan Hankemeier, Thomas Gosling,
Hans-Christoph Pape

**Section III: Fractures of the
distal femur   198**

10.7 General aspects   198
Stefan Hankemeier, Thomas Gosling,
Hans-Christoph Pape

10.8 Minimally invasive plate
osteosynthesis   198
Stefan Hankemeier, Thomas Gosling,
Hans-Christoph Pape

10.9 Retrograde nailing   202
Stefan Hankemeier, Thomas Gosling,
Hans-Christoph Pape

11 Fractures of the patella   206

11.1 Tension band wiring   206
Stefan Hankemeier, Thomas Gosling,
Hans-Christoph Pape

**12 Section I: Fractures of the
proximal tibia   210**

12.1 Open reduction and internal
fixation of a lateral tibial plateau
fracture   210
John F. Keating

12.2 Open reduction and internal
fixation of a bicondylar tibial plateau
fracture   214
John F. Keating

12.3 External fixation of bicondylar
tibial plateau fractures   216
John F. Keating

12.4 Open reduction and internal
fixation of anterior tibial spine
fractures   219
John F. Keating

Section II: Fractures of the tibial shaft   **222**

12.5 Intramedullary nailing   222
Charles M. Court-Brown

12.6 Plating of the tibia   230
Charles M. Court-Brown

Section III: Fractures of the distal tibia   **236**

12.7 Open reduction and internal fixation: plating pilon   236
Peter V. Giannoudis

12.8 Circular frame fixation for distal tibial fractures   241
Toby Branfoot

13   Fractures of the ankle   **246**

13.1 Open reduction and internal fixation of bimalleolar ankle fractures   246
Christopher C. Tzioupis, Peter V. Giannoudis

14   Fractures of the foot   **254**

14.1 Open reduction and internal screw fixation for talar neck fractures   254
Martinus Richter

14.2 Open reduction and internal plate fixation for os calcis fractures   258
Martinus Richter

14.3 Open reduction and internal screw and K-wire fixation for Lisfranc fracture dislocations   262
Martinus Richter

Part IV Spine

15   Fractures of the cerrical spine   **269**

15.1 Application of a halo and halo-vest for cervical spine trauma   269
Peter Millner

15.2 Operative posterior stabilization of thoraco-lumbar burst fractures   272
Peter Millner

15.3 Anterior stabilization of complex thoraco-lumbar burst fractures   278
Peter Millner

Part V Tendon injuries

16   Reconstruction of tendons   **285**

16.1 Achilles tendon repair   285
Peter V. Giannoudis

16.2 Repair of tendon injuries in the hand   288
Caroline McGuiness, Simon Knight

Part VI Compartments

17   Decompression fasciotomies   **295**

17.1 Fasciotomy for acute compartment syndromes of the upper and lower limbs   295
Roderick Dunn, Simon Kay

References   304
Index   315

Contributors

Toby Branfoot, M.B. B.S., F.R.C.S., Ed. (Tr. & Orth.), M.Sc.
Consultant Trauma Surgeon
Department of Trauma and Orthopaedics
St James's University Hospital
Leeds, L59 7TF, UK

Doug Campbell, F.R.C.S. (Orth.)
Consultant Orthopaedic Surgeon
Department of Hand Surgery
St James's University Hospital
Leeds, LS9 7TF, UK

Charles M. Court-Brown, M.D., F.R.C.S., Ed. (Orth.)
Professor of Orthopaedic Trauma
Orthopaedic Trauma Unit
Royal Infirmary of Edinburgh
Edinburgh, EH3 9YW, UK

Roderick Dunn, M.B. B.S., D.M.C.C., F.R.C.S. (Plast.)
Senior Fellow in Hand and Microsurgery
Department of Plastic and Reconstructive Surgery
St James's University Hospital
Leeds, LS9 7TF, UK

Peter V. Giannoudis, B.Sc., M.B. B.S., M.D., E.E.C.(Ortho.)
Professor Trauma and Orthopaedic Surgery
School of Medicine
University of Leeds
St James's University Hospital
Leeds, LS9 7TF, UK

Thomas Gosling, M.D.
Orthopaedic Trauma Fellow
Department of Trauma Surgery
Hannover Medical School
Hannover, GERMANY, 30625

Stefan Hankemeier, M.D.
Orthopaedic Trauma Fellow
Department of Trauma Surgery
Hannover Medical School
Hannover, GERMANY, 30625

Gregoris Kambouroglou, M.D.
Consultant Trauma and Orthopaedic Surgeon
Oxford Trauma Unit
John Radcliffe Hospital
Oxford, OX3 9DU, UK

Simon Kay, F.R.C.S., F.R.C.S. (Plast.), F.R.C.S.E.
Professor of Hand Surgery
Consultant in Plastic Surgery and Surgery of the Hand
Department of Plastic and Reconstructive Surgery
St James's University Hospital
Leeds, LS9 7TF, UK

John F. Keating, M.Phil., F.R.C.S., Ed. (Orth.)
Consultant Orthopaedic Surgeon
Orthopaedic Trauma Unit
Royal Infirmary of Edinburgh
Edinburgh, EH3 9YW, UK

Paige T. Kendrick, B.A.
Orthopaedic Trauma Fellow
Department of Orthopaedic Surgery
University of Louisville School of Medicine
Louisville, Kentucky, USA

Simon Knight, M.B. B.S., F.R.C.S.
Consultant Orthopaedic Surgeon
Department of Trauma and Orthopaedics
St James's University Hospital
Leeds, LS9 7TF, UK

David Limb, B.Sc., F.R.C.S., Ed. (Orth.)
Senior Lecturer
School of Medicine
University of Leeds
St James's University Hospital
Leeds, LS9 7TF, UK

David A. Macdonald, F.R.C.S. (Orth.)
Consultant Orthopaedic Surgeon
Department of Trauma and Orthopaedics
St James's University Hospital
Leeds, LS9 7TF, UK

Caroline McGuiness F.R.S.C. (Plas. Surg.)
Consultant Plastic Surgeon
Department of Plastic Surgery
St James' University Hospital
Leeds, LS9 7TF, UK

Reinhard Meier, M.D.
Orthopaedic Trauma Fellow
Department of Trauma Surgery
Hannover Medical School
Hannover, GERMANY, 30625

Peter Millner, F.R.C.S., (Orth.)
Consultant Spinal Surgeon
Department of Trauma and Orthopaedics
St James's University Hospital
Leeds, LS9 7TF, UK

Hans-Christoph Pape, M.D.
Professor of Trauma and Orthopaedic Surgery
Division of Trauma
University of Pittsburgh School of Medicine
3471 Forbes Avenue
Kaufmann Building, Suite 911, 15215
Pittsburgh, USA

Raghu Raman, M.R.C.S.,
Trauma Fellow
Department of Trauma and Orthopaedics
St James's University Hospital
Leeds, LS9 7TF, UK

Martinus Richter, M.D.
Head of the Orthopaedic Foot Service
Coburg Hospital
Coburg, GERMANY

Craig S. Roberts, M.D.
Associate Professor
Department of Orthopaedic Surgery
University of Louisville School of Medicine
Louisville, Kentucky, USA

Brian W. Scott, F.R.C.S. (Orth.)
Consultant Paediatric Orthopaedic Surgeon
Department of Trauma and Orthopaedics
Leeds Teaching Hospital
Leeds, LS9 7TF, UK

David Seligson, M.D.
Professor of Orthopaedic Surgery and
Vice Chairman
Department of Orthopaedic Surgery
University of Louisville School of Medicine
Louisville, Kentucky, USA

Christopher C. Tzioupis, M.D.
Trauma Fellow
Department of Trauma and Orthopaedics
St James's University Hospital
Leeds, LS9 7TF, UK

Preface

Over the years the evolution of orthopaedic surgical techniques led to the development of a plethora of orthopaedic textbooks aiming to present the principles of modern orthopaedic surgical practice in order to contribute to the continuing medical education of all the orthopaedic surgeons in training.

The notion of this book arose during the first years of our training. It was difficult to find a book to refer to as a quick yet thorough reference, prior to performing a surgical procedure.

Our aim was therefore to develop a book that would contain a step-wise approach to performing a surgical procedure. Details have been included such as positioning of the patient, the approach and reduction technique, the implant to be inserted, the protocol of post-operative mobilization, complications to look for, when the patient should be seen in the outpatient clinic and whether the implant should be removed. Intraoperative pictures have been incorporated to allow the surgeon to be aware of all the important issues involved.

The most common trauma procedures that a surgeon in training is expected to perform during his residency have been included. Each procedure has been written by an expert or under the supervision of an expert.

This book is expected to be the companion for the resident in training during the long on-call nights in the hospital while preparing for the operations necessary to help our trauma patients.

Acknowledgments

During the preparation of this book we had the pleasure of working together with people whose efforts and contribution made possible the birth of this edition. We particularly wish to acknowledge Cambridge University Press, and our publishing directors Geoffrey Nuttall and Peter Silver for their commitment to this project and the maintenance of this level of excellence.

Without the dedication and the hard work of our hospital staffs we would not have been able to accomplish this project.

We would also like to thank all the contributors who have shared with us their expertise.

We also appreciate the continuing support of our colleagues at our university hospitals and especially the daily stimulus of our registrars, whose quest for knowledge remains the major motivation and encouragement for our efforts.

Part I

Upper extremity

Fractures of the clavicle

Peter V. Giannoudis

1.1 OPEN REDUCTION AND INTERNAL FIXATION (ORIF) OF MIDSHAFT FRACTURES

Indications

(a) Open fractures.
(b) Painful non-union.
(c) Associated injury to the brachial plexus and/or sub-clavian artery.
(d) Floating shoulder.
(e) Bilateral fractures.
(f) Multiple-injured patient.
(g) Soft tissue interposition between the fragments.
(h) Impending skin necrosis or penetration from a prominent fragment.

Pre-operative planning

Clinical assessment

- Mechanism of injury: motor vehicle accident, sports injury, fall on outstretched hand, direct trauma.
- Deformity, ecchymosis, swelling, tenderness, crepitation.
- Look for pneumothorax or haemothorax, especially in presence of associated injuries.
- Assess and document vascular status of the upper arm and any difference in peripheral pulses between the injured and contralateral extremity.
- Assess neurological status (usually brachial plexus injury presents as an upper roots traction injury).

Radiological assessment

- Anteroposterior view of the clavicle, including sternoclavicular and acromioclavicular joints (Fig. 1.1).
- Oblique views.
- Lordotic view (usually after surgery for ORIF evaluation).

Operative treatment

Anaesthesia

- General anaesthesia at induction.
- Administration of prophylactic antibiotics as per local hospital protocol (usually second generation of cephalosporin is administered).

Table and equipment

- AO small fragment (3.5 mm) set.
- Ensure availability of the pre-planned plate length. A 3.5 DCP plate or a reconstruction plate can be used (Fig. 1.2a,b).
- Standard osteosynthesis set as per local hospital protocol.

Table set up

- The instrumentation is set up on the side of the operation.
- Image intensifier is from the ipsilateral side.
- Position the table diagonally across the operating room so that the operating area lies in the clean air field.

Practical Procedures in Orthopaedic Trauma Surgery: A Trainee's Companion, ed. Peter V. Giannoudis and Hans-Christoph Pape.
Published by Cambridge University Press. © Cambridge University Press 2006.

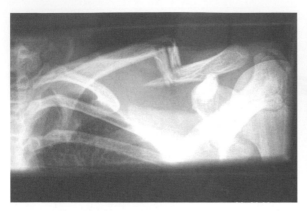

Fig. 1.1 Anteroposterior view of the clavicle, including sternoclavicular and acromioclavicular joints.

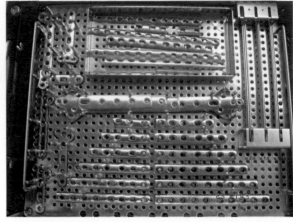

(a)

Draping and surgical approach

- Skin preparation is carried out using usual antiseptic solutions (aqueous/alcoholic povidone-iodine).
- Prepare the skin of the chest to the medial border of the scapula. Clean up to the anterior and lateral surface of the neck and down to below the level of the nipple.
- Use single U-drapes (Fig. 1.3 a,b).
- Make an incision over the clavicle (Fig. 1.4 a,b).
- Using the cutting diathermy bring down the incision through the skin to the periosteum (Fig. 1.5).
- Identify the clavicle and the fracture fragments.
- Perform a subperiosteal dissection on the clavicular edge and circumferentially only at the fracture site (Fig. 1.6).
- Drill a hole to the bone through a plate hole above the distal fragment and affix the plate to the distal fragment (Fig. 1.7).
- Then reduce the proximal fragment and secure the plate positioning over the bone by using a clamp.
- Place one screw at the proximal fragment and ensure reduction maintenance with fluoroscopic control (Fig. 1.8).
- Place the rest of the screws in the same manner (Fig. 1.9).
- Cancellous bone grafting is performed for bone defects or devitalized bone.
- Ensure fracture reduction, adequate screw length with fluoroscopic Lordotic views.

Closure

- Closure is performed as a full-thickness layer over the plate using 2/0 Vicryl and 3/0 subcuticular sutures for the skin (Fig. 1.10 a,b).

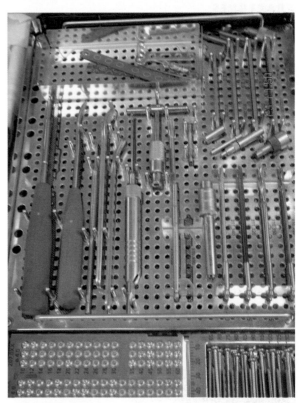

(b)

Fig. 1.2 a,b A 3.5 DCP plate or a reconstruction plate can be used.

Post-operative treatment

- Assess and document the neurovascular status of the extremity.
- Obtain post-operative radiographs (Fig. 1.11).
- Use a sling for the initial 10 post-operative days (Fig. 1.12).

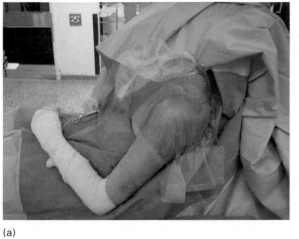

(a)

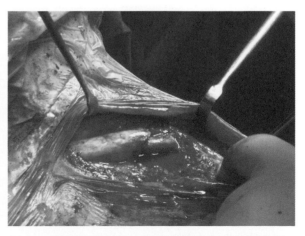

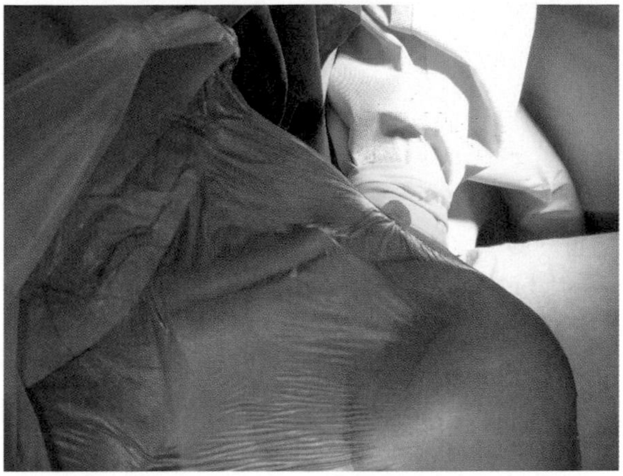

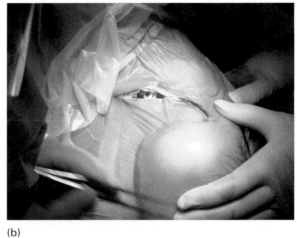

(b)

Fig. 1.3 a,b Positioning and draping of the patient.

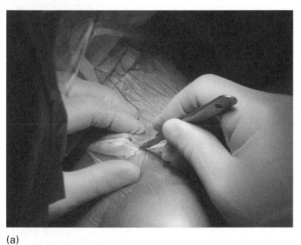

(a)

(b)

Fig. 1.4 a,b Make an incision over the clavicle.

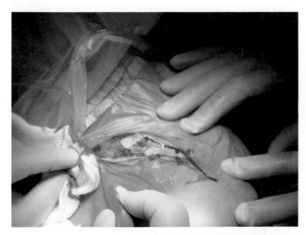

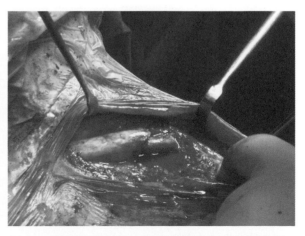

Fig. 1.5 Using the cutting diathermy bring down the incision through the skin to the periosteum.

Fig. 1.6 Perform a subperiosteal dissection on the clavicular edge and circumferentially only at the fracture site.

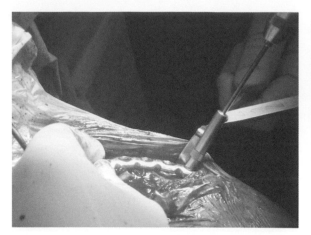

Fig. 1.7 Drill a hole to the bone through a plate hole above the distal fragment and affix the plate to the distal fragment.

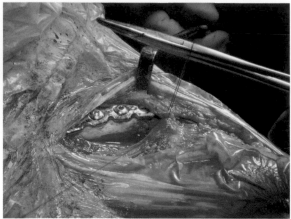

Fig. 1.10 (a)

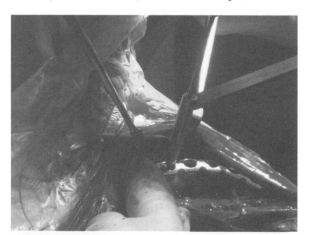

Fig. 1.8 Place one screw at the proximal fragment and ensure reduction maintenance with fluoroscopic control.

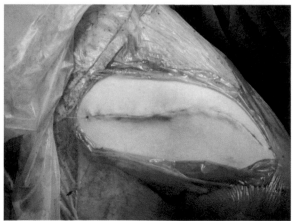

Fig. 1.10 (b)

Fig. 1.10 a,b Closure is performed as a full-thickness layer over the plate using 2/0 Vicryl and 3/0 subcuticular sutures for the skin

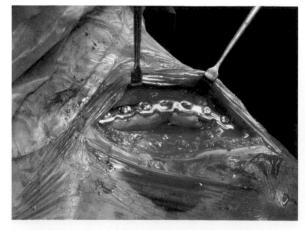

Fig. 1.9 Place the rest of the screws in the same manner.

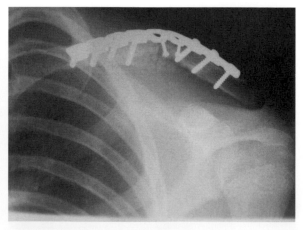

Fig. 1.11 Post-operative radiograph.

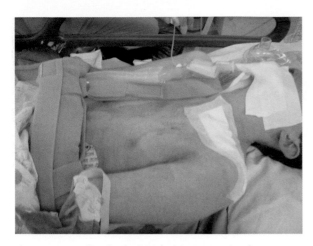

Fig. 1.12 Use a sling for the initial 10 post-operative days.

- Initiate active flexion and abduction 6 weeks after injury.
- Return to prior activities is possible 3 months after operative treatment.

Outpatient follow up

- Review at clinic in 3, 6 and 12 months with X-rays on arrival to consider plate removal.
- Beware of late vascular complications (thrombosis, pseudoaneurysm).

Implant removal

- Plate can be removed after 12 months.

2

Section I: Fractures of the proximal humerus

David Limb

2.1 GENERAL CONSIDERATIONS

The practicalities of surgical management of proximal humeral fractures are common to the various injuries treated. A generic description of the investigations required and practical set-up of the operating room will therefore be presented before discussing specific injuries.

Radiological assessment

- It is essential that all shoulder fractures be assessed with a minimum of two shoulder views – the antero-posterior (AP) and axial views.
- A scapular lateral completes the trauma series but is not always essential.
- The axial view can be obtained successfully in most cases – in the rare instances where the patient will not permit sufficient movement of the injured limb away from the side, angled views (modified axial) should be obtained. Never miss a dislocation (too many are missed, and most of these have not had an axial view taken).
- In complex cases a CT scan might assist, particularly in assessing whether the humeral head is intact and has any tuberosity attachments remaining. A humeral head fragment with an attached tuberosity is much less likely to suffer avascular necrosis than one with no remaining tuberosity attachments. Three-dimensional CT is particularly useful for assessing glenoid fossa fractures.

Anaesthesia

- General anaesthesia or scalene blocks can be used. Even if general anaesthesia is selected, a scalene block can add useful analgesia.

- The risk of phrenic nerve palsy and pneumothorax should be considered if a scalene block is to be used, particularly if there is already chest trauma (which not infrequently accompanies shoulder trauma).
- Great care has to be taken to avoid interference with anaesthetic tubes and pipes by the surgeon or assistant in general anaesthetic cases.

Table and positioning

- The table should allow the patient to be sat up at the hips into the beach chair position (Fig. 2.1). Usually the torso is raised 30 to 45° from the horizontal, but if access is needed to the front and back of the shoulder then a more upright position is necessary, supporting the spine and head but allowing access to the whole shoulder girdle.
- To avoid the patient sliding down the table, the table is tilted 'feet up' below the hips. The knees are flexed by lowering the end of the table or by placing a pillow behind the knees.
- Any part of the table that could intervene between the ends of a C-arm during X-ray screening of the shoulder should be radiolucent.
- Shoulder table attachments are available that convert normal operating tables to permit patient positioning as described above (e.g. Schlein table attachment).

Operating room set up

- Shoulder surgery requires the surgeon to stand in the axilla of the patient on the side of the injury. Either the C-arm is positioned, or an assistant stands, above the patient's shoulder.

Practical Procedures in Orthopaedic Trauma Surgery: A Trainee's Companion, ed. Peter V. Giannoudis and Hans-Christoph Pape.
Published by Cambridge University Press. © Cambridge University Press 2006.

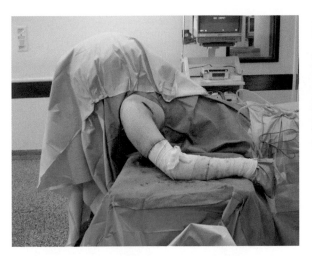

Fig. 2.1 The beach chair position.

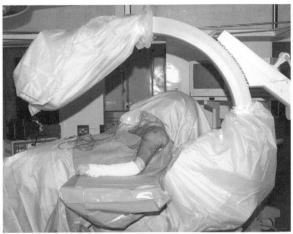

Fig. 2.2 C-arm draping and positioning for X-ray control during surgical fixation of shoulder fractures.

- The hand and forearm are draped and rested on a small table. The height of the table should be adjustable.
- It is preferable for the head of the table to be furthest away from the anaesthetic machine. The anaesthetist should be aware of this, as extension tubes may be needed for the gas lines.
- Alternatively the anaesthetist can work from the side of the patient opposite to the operated shoulder, with a suitable exclusion drape.
- An experienced radiographer is required to obtain good X-ray views of the shoulder during surgery.
- If the anaesthetist is working at the foot end of the patient, the scrub nurse can work across the patient's chest, provided great care is taken with anaesthetic pipes beneath the drapes. Alternatively the nurse can stand adjacent to the small table upon which the patient's arm rests.
- If no X-ray screening is necessary the scrub nurse can work from above the head end of the table or on the same side as the surgeon. If X-ray screening is used, the nurse works across the chest (see above) or from the same side as the surgeon.

Draping and approach

- Skin preparation is carried out using locally approved antiseptics. Prepare the forequarter from the midline of the chest to the medial border of the scapula. Clean up to the root of the neck and down to below the level of the nipple. The arm is prepared down to wrist level.
- A U-drape is used to shut off the forequarter and a separate impervious stocking is rolled up the arm to

above the level of the elbow. This leaves the draped arm free for manipulation during surgery. It is rested on the arm table and raising this relaxes the deltoid by abduction of the arm. This facilitates exposure of the humeral head.

- A deltopectoral approach is preferred for management of all proximal humerus fractures. It is possible to reduce and stabilize a greater tuberosity fracture through a deltoid split. If unexpected comminution is discovered or later surgery is required for complications, a deltoid split cannot be safely extended without risking injury to the axillary nerve.
- If X-ray screening is to be used, both ends of the image intensifier C-arm are covered with sterile drapes. The intensifier is positioned above the affected shoulder and angled in towards the midline by 20–30°. This will correct for the angulation of the scapula on the chest wall and give good views of the joint line.
- The C-arm passes over the shoulder, with the source anterior and the collimator behind the shoulder (Fig. 2.2). This gives good AP views during surgery and permits the C-arm to be rolled into a vertical position for axial views.

Surgical approach

- The incision for a deltopectoral approach extends from the clavicle across the lateral edge of the palpated coracoid process and down to the arm into the interval palpable between the anterior edge of the deltoid muscle

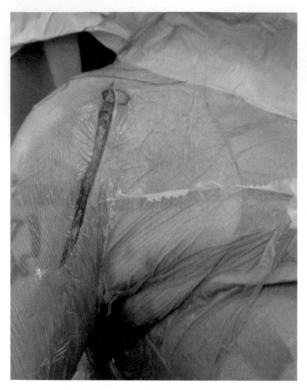

Fig. 2.3 The deltopectoral incision.

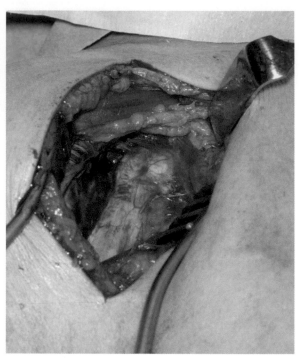

Fig. 2.4 Retraction to expose the subscapularis and proximal humerus.

and the adjacent biceps muscle (Fig. 2.3). The length of the incision is determined by the extent of exposure required.

- The deltoid and pectoralis major are separated digitally, retracting the cephalic vein (which marks the interval) laterally – cutting muscle fibres is not necessary. The interval can often be located by a fat stripe if the cephalic vein is not immediately apparent.
- Once fascia is exposed deep in the deltopectoral interval it is opened vertically, adjacent to the lateral border of the conjoint tendon as far up as the tip of the coracoid process.
- Sweep a finger under the conjoint tendon to ensure the axillary nerve is not in close proximity. Sweep a finger under the deltoid to ensure the subdeltoid bursa is opened – these two spaces are placements for the two blades of a self-retaining retractor (Fig. 2.4).
- The proximal humerus is now as visible as it is ever is – clothed in the thick rotator cuff tendons. The long head of biceps tendon can be identified at the lower part of the incision and followed in to the interval between subscapularis medially and the greater

tuberosity with supraspinatus attachment laterally and above.

2.2 TENSION BAND WIRING (TBW) FOR DISPLACED GREATER TUBEROSITY FRACTURES

Indications

Fractures of the greater tuberosity displaced by 5 mm or more.

Note

- Many consider this recommendation, commonly quoted in the literature, to be excessively conservative and would offer surgery for fractures displaced by as little as 2 mm.
- Displacement cannot always be judged on an anteroposterior (AP) film, as the infraspinatus and teres muscles will displace the tuberosity posteriorly and medially behind the humeral head. It is essential that at least an axial view of the shoulder is also taken to properly assess displacement.

Pre-operative planning

Clinical assessment

- Shoulder pain is often felt in the region of the deltoid insertion, on the lateral aspect of the arm.
- Look for any history suggestive of dislocation – greater tuberosity fractures are not uncommonly associated with anterior shoulder dislocation. Often repair of the tuberosity fracture (if displaced after reduction) will stabilise the shoulder, but be aware that soft tissue procedures such as labral repair could be necessary either at the time of tuberosity repair, or later.
- Assess and document the neurovascular status of the arm. It is particularly important to examine the axillary nerve. Since deltoid function can be severely compromised by pain, skin sensation in the 'regimental badge' area should be carefully recorded.

Radiological assessment

- Anteroposterior (Fig. 2.5) and axillary views are essential. A scapular lateral view completes the trauma series, though is not essential in the assessment of isolated greater tuberosity fractures.
- Pre-operative X-ray screening should be available, particularly in multifragmentary greater tuberosity fractures. The fragments can be impossible to see at surgery, being hidden from view by the thick rotator cuff tendons.

Operative treatment

Anaesthesia

- General anaesthesia with prophylactic antibiotics according to local protocols.
- Scalene block according to anaesthetic skills available.

Table and equipment

- The table must allow the patient to be sat up in the 'beach chair' position and allow access to the shoulder by a C-arm.
- A table attachment allowing the same position, supporting the torso and head, is equally acceptable (e. g. Schlein table attachment).
- A small Mayo table, suitably padded and covered, can be used to support the arm.

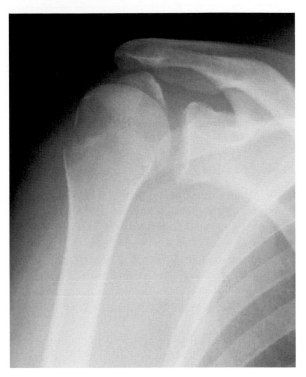

Fig. 2.5 Displacement of the greater tuberosity into the subacromial space.

- Drill with 2–2.5 mm bit.
- Heavy non-absorbable suture material (e. g. No. 5 Ethibond®) – stainless steel wire can be used, but because it is used around a tendon insertion it will fragment and migrate once shoulder function is restored.

Table set up and patient positioning

- The patient is sat up approximately 45° (beach chair position).
- Arrange the table in theatre so that the surgical team have access to the head and affected side of the body.
- The affected arm is draped free and rested on a padded Mayo table. The height of the table is adjusted to hold the arm in 30–45° of abduction, thus relaxing the deltoid muscle and facilitating access to the proximal humerus.
- Image intensifier access is in line with the body, from the head end of the table. Both ends of the C-arm are covered in sterile drapes.

Draping and surgical approach

- Skin preparation is carried out as described above.
- A deltopectoral approach is preferred for the management of all proximal humerus fractures, as it can readily be used for any later procedures that become necessary. It is possible to reduce and stabilise a greater tuberosity fracture through a deltoid split.

Surgical fixation

- The deltopectoral approach or deltoid split takes the surgeon down to the bed of the greater tuberosity – exposed cancellous bone is found (Fig. 2.6 a,b), but the tuberosity itself often has to be sought.
- The direction of displacement should be apparent on pre-operative X rays and anticipated in planning. It depends upon the fracture configuration and what are the dominant tendon attachments on the displaced fragments.
- If the fragment contains principally the supraspinatus tendon insertion then the tuberosity will displace into the subacromial space. Retrieval from here is usually easy, by grasping with tissue forceps.
- If the fragment includes principally the attachments on infraspinatus and teres (and this might be because of a chronic supraspinatus tear) then the fragment will displace behind the humeral head and can be more difficult to identify and retrieve.
- If the fragment is not easily palpable and cannot be grasped, it is still usually possible to identify the posterior rotator cuff by pulling the humeral head downwards. Place a heavy suture in the visible edge of the rotator cuff and pull – if the first tug does not deliver the tubcrosity it can be retrieved by placing a further traction suture in the cuff tendon brought into view by the first traction suture.
- Once the tuberosity is identified assess the quality of the bone of the tuberosity and the head.
- If the tuberosity is a large single fragment with good bone quality then fixation can be obtained by lag screw fixation. If not, then a tension band technique is more appropriate.
- The material usually selected for tension band fixation is a No. 5 non-absorbable suture such as Ethibond. It is unlikely that the bone quality will be good enough for this to be placed through drill holes in the tuberosity for fixation – the best grip on the tuberosity is achieved by placing the suture to take a broad bite of the insertion of the rotator cuff onto the tuberosity fragment. For large

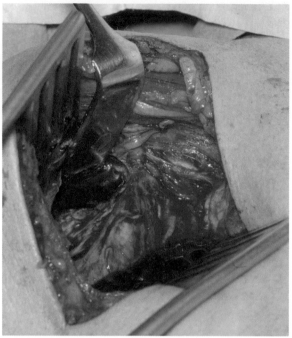

(a)

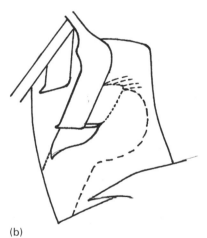

(b)

Fig. 2.6 a,b The bed of the greater tuberosity.

fragments two sutures can be placed side-by-side in the cuff.
- The tuberosity fragment can be pulled into a reduced position using these sutures (Fig. 2.7 a,b) – the direction in which traction is exerted to bring about anatomical reduction (checked on a C-arm if necessary) determines where the suture material should be fixed to the proximal humerus. The tension suture can be fixed to a screw and washer or through drill holes in bone. The latter avoids any concern about later implant removal.

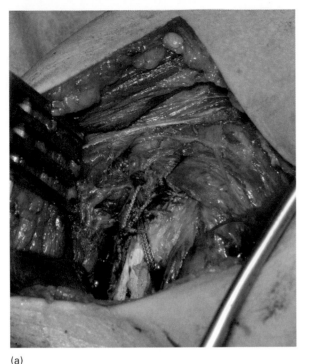

(a)

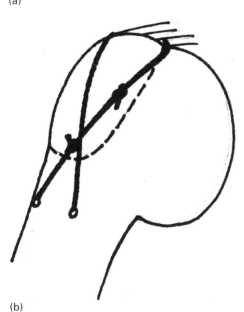

(b)

Fig. 2.7 a,b The greater tuberosity held in its bed by heavy tension band sutures.

• For posterior tuberosity fragments that displace in a posterior direction, it is often the case that traction has to be applied in an anterior direction to reduce the tuberosity. If this is the case, then a bite of the subscapularis insertion on the lesser tuberosity holds the tuberosity that was reduced by the tension band principle.

• For fragments that displaced in a superior or posterio-superior direction it is observed that the reduction is held by pulling the Ethibond sutures down onto the lateral or anterolateral humeral shaft. Two drill holes are created using a 2.5 mm drill through which the needle is passed to create a tension band holding the tuberosity in a reduced position.

• Often the tuberosity is very fragmented – remember the important role of surgery is not to anatomically replace every small bony fragment, but to secure the rotator cuff back onto the proximal humerus and allow it to function. The reduction of bony fragments is checked and a search is made for any substantial fragments that remain displaced and might have a significant rotator cuff attachment. Occasionally fragments also have to be pursued if they are displaced into the subacromial space and might cause impingement.

• After fixation the field is washed out. It is not necessary to suture the deltopectoral interval, which falls back together. Drains are not usually necessary. Routine fat and skin closure follows and the patient is fitted with a collar and cuff sling.

Post-operative treatment

• Post-operative X rays confirm that a satisfactory reduction has been achieved (Fig. 2.8).

• The point of fixation is to allow early mobilization. Passive physiotherapy can commence immediately.

• The duration of sling use, return to active use and resistive exercises depend to an extent on operative findings. If the tuberosity was a substantial fragment and has been replaced in its bed, then fixation is usually secure enough to allow the sling to be discarded as soon as initial pain settles. Active use for activities of daily living can also begin immediately, though resistive exercises and lifting should be deferred until time has been allowed for bony union – often an empirical 6 weeks.

• If the tuberosity fragments were small and the repair were more akin to repair of the rotator cuff edge into the bony bed, then a more cautious approach to mobilization is indicated.

• In the latter case it is reasonable to allow immediate passive and active-assisted physiotherapy but also to continue with arm support for 6 weeks or so. Work against resistance is introduced cautiously at 6 weeks and built up over the next 6 weeks. Heavy lifting might

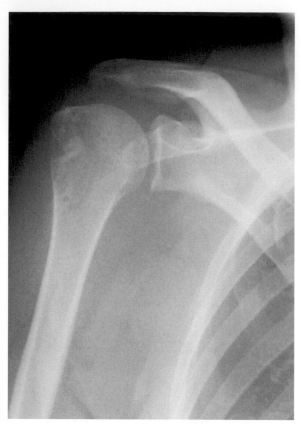

Fig. 2.8 Post-operative films demonstrating adequate reduction of the greater tuberosity.

be deferred by 3 months and in extreme cases, where a poor quality cuff was found and repaired into the tuberosity bed, then this might even be delayed until 6 months.

2.3 OPEN REDUCTION AND INTERNAL FIXATION (ORIF) OF 3- AND 4-PART FRACTURES (USING A PHILOS PLATE®)

The decision to treat a 3- or 4-part fracture by internal fixation or by prosthetic hemiarthroplasty can be very difficult. Patients fare much better if they can keep their own humeral head, restored to a reasonable anatomical configuration with an effective rotator cuff.

The best functioning joint replacements however are those that are carried out as a primary procedure – the results are far poorer if hemiarthroplasty is carried out because of failed fixation or for complications of the fracture and its treatment. Sadly we cannot often predict which of our patients will be unlucky enough to follow a complicated course.

This section assumes that a decision has been made to treat a fracture surgically. The range of surgical options is wide. The underlying principle, as with any periarticular fracture, is that the joint surface is reconstructed to articulate anatomically with the glenoid and is then secured with the correct length, alignment and rotation onto the shaft. A prerequisite of regaining a near-anatomical articulation, however, is that the tuberosities have to be restored to their correct locations in order for proper articulation to occur. The surgical option described here uses a specially designed plate to fulfil these criteria, though the principles described can be applied using alternative devices.

Anaesthesia, table and patient positioning and the surgical approach (deltopectoral) have already been described. The principles of tuberosity fixation described above will also be followed.

Equipment

- General set for the surgical approach, including adequate retractors. A Norfolk and Norwich self-retaining retractor is usually sufficient but specially designed shoulder retractors improve exposure. Unfortunately they also interfere with radiological screening and are more difficult to remove and replace when checking progress on X ray.
- Philos plate set – plates of different lengths are available and the set includes a jig for correct aiming of locking screws.
- Small fragment set including locking screws.
- No. 5 ethibond (or similar) sutures.

Surgical approach

- As already noted, the deltopectoral approach is used to expose the proximal humerus. This should be extended far enough down the arm so that the tendon insertions of the pectoralis major muscle and deltoid can be located. This determines where the plate will lie on the shaft – sufficient anterior deltoid is elevated only to allow the plate to sit down to touch bone – do not detach either tendon.
- At this point the fracture is almost invisible! If only we could see all the fragments that are visible on X rays

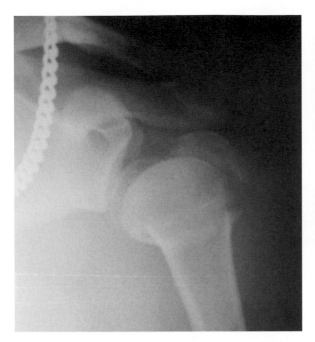

Fig. 2.9 Displaced proximal humerus fracture to be treated by plate fixation.

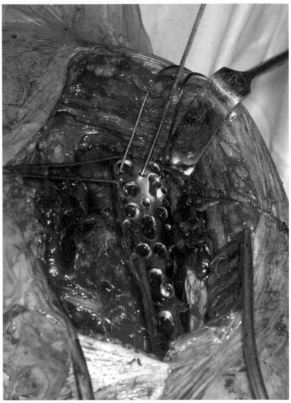

Fig. 2.10 Sutures placed in the cuff insertions onto tuberosities are passed through holes in the plate for secure tuberosity fixation.

(Fig. 2.9), these fractures would be so much easier to fix.

- It is important that the reduction process does not further compromise the blood supply to the humeral head. Detachment of cuff tendons and capsule is *not permitted* – X rays are essential to check reduction.
- Any fracture line splitting the tuberosities is identified. Heavy No. 5 Ethibond sutures are placed in the insertion of the subscapularis onto the lesser tuberosity and supraspinatus/infraspinatus on the greater tuberosity. If necessary traction can be applied to these to pull the tuberosities back to their expected positions – don't worry if the humeral head still appears displaced on X ray.
- An instrument such as a small fragment periosteal elevator is inserted through the fracture line and is used to push the humeral head up into the coracoacromial arch.
- As the humeral head is restored towards its anatomic location the tuberosities fall, or can be pulled, back into their beds around the head fragment. By temporarily clipping the Ethibond sutures together, holding the tuberosities beneath the humeral head, the reduction of the head and tuberosities can be gauged with the arm held in neutral rotation.

- Once a satisfactory reduction has been achieved it is held using the tension band sutures. Since the shaft is fractured, however, the tension sutures can be passed through appropriately positioned holes on the Philos plate (Fig. 2.10). It is very difficult to pass heavy sutures through these holes once the plate has been fixed to bone. The plate is slid down the sutures, pressed against the reconstructed head and the tension sutures can be tied after checking plate height (Fig. 2.11).
- The plate height on the humerus is such that it should reach almost to the cuff insertion on the greater tuberosity. Any higher and it can cause impingement afterwards. If there is a tendency for the plate to be pulled out of position as the tension sutures are tied through the plate its position can be fixed by a temporary K-wire through one of the small holes in the plate.
- The plate is then attached to the shaft of the humerus. A slotted hole allows some adjustment of the plate height

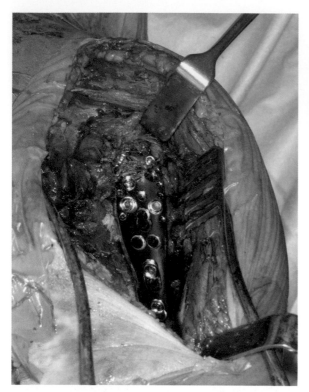

Fig. 2.11 Preplaced sutures are tied for secure fixation of tuberosity fragments that may not be captured by screws.

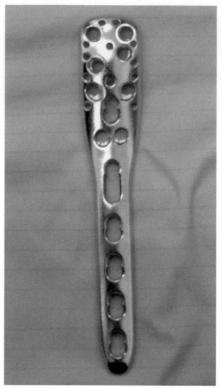

Fig. 2.12 The Philos plate®. Note the broad, low-profile upper segment for locking screws into the head and a lower plate for fixation to the shaft. The uppermost hole of the shaft segment is a slot to allow fine tuning of plate height so that it does not project above the tuberosity and impinge.

or shaft impaction into the head after the screw hole is drilled (Fig. 2.12).

- Once the plate is in a satisfactory position and the tuberosities are controlled by tension sutures, the whole proximal humerus can be stabilized in this position by the placement of locking screws through the plate into the head and tuberosities.
- Check films in both AP and axial planes are obtained from the image intensifier.
- Routine closure of fat and skin layers after a washout.
- Temporary shoulder immobilizer until post-operative pain has settled.

Post-operative care

- The aim of fixation is to allow early mobilization.
- Check X rays in AP and axial planes (Fig. 2.13).
- Immediate passive and active assisted mobilization – care has to be taken in passive stretching of internal and external rotation for the first 6 weeks, as some

tuberosity fragments might be held only by tension band sutures.
- Implant removal is not usually necessary.

Complications

- Fixed angle devices such as this give an excellent hold even in osteoporotic bone. The fact that the implant is a fixed device also causes problems if avascular necrosis develops.
- Avascular necrosis results in collapse of the humeral head. The implant remains fixed, however, and the screws do not back out as they do with T-plates. Consequently the screws can perforate the humeral head. This should be anticipated and if necessary appropriate action taken by either removing the screws or revising the implant to a hemiarthroplasty.

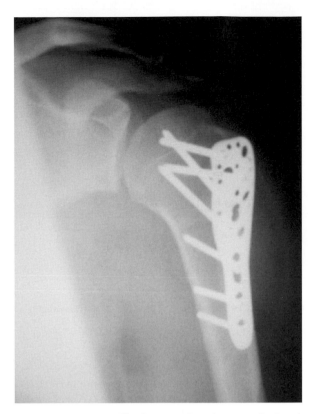

Fig. 2.13 Postoperative film demonstrating adequate reduction of the fracture.

2.4 HEMIARTHROPLASTY FOR FRACTURE DISLOCATION

Indications

- Debatable!
- Fracture dislocations in which the humeral articular surface has no remaining soft tissue attachments, which have a very high incidence of avascular necrosis.
- Head splitting fractures, which have a high incidence of necrosis of at least one of the head fragments or involve comminution of the head and crushing of articular cartilage with inevitable post-traumatic arthritis
- Chronic fracture dislocations (usually posterior) with destruction of 50% or more of the humeral head (Figs. 2.14 a,b).
- Severe 3- or 4-part fractures in which it is assessed, and agreed with the patient, that immediate hemiarthroplasty is likely to give a better outcome on balance than fixation with the attendant risks (Fig. 2.15). This

requires an assessment of the personality of the fracture and an appraisal of how well reconstruction could restore normal mechanics, the risks of re-displacement or avascular necrosis (AVN) and the various patient-dependent factors that affect rehabilitation and outcome.

Patient positioning

- The beach chair position is used, though the torso is only angled upright by 30–45° – this allows the humerus to be dropped into a vertical position and from there allows slight adduction of the humerus behind the patient to improve access to the shaft.
- The side table is used at a low height in order that the arm can be dropped to a vertical and extended position, allowing access to the humeral shaft for preparation and prosthesis insertion.

Equipment

- Dedicated instruments are necessary for shoulder hemiarthroplasty. These have become more sophisticated as jigs have been developed to allow implant placement at a preselected depth within the humeral shaft and with correct rotational alignment within the shaft.
- Dedicated fracture implants are also emerging on the market. Whilst Neer's original prosthesis gave few choices of head or stem size, current modular systems allow a wide variety of stem sizes and head configurations (depth, radius of curvature, offset, head-stem angle). Fracture-specific stems have more space for bone graft and tuberosity placement beneath the humeral head. It is vital therefore that the surgeon checks that a full set of instruments and a full inventory of fracture implants is available.
- Fixation is obtained only through the distal stem in the shaft of the humerus. Although uncemented prostheses are available, which press-fit distally sufficiently well for use in trauma, most surgeons prefer to cement components to give the good initial rotational control of the stem in the shaft that is necessary for mobilization. Cement mixing chambers and a cement gun are therefore needed.
- The canal can be plugged with bone from the humeral head, but alternatively a cement restrictor might be used.

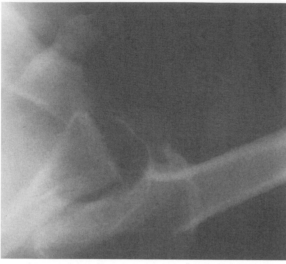

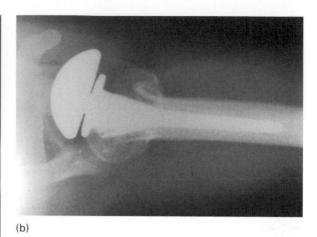

(b)

(a)

Fig. 2.14 (a) Axial view of a chronic locked posterior fracture dislocation; (b) axial view of same patient after prosthetic replacement, restoring stability.

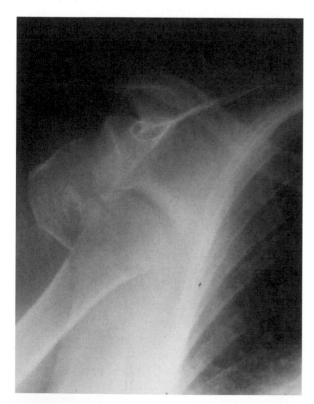

Fig. 2.15 Fracture dislocation: for treatment by hemiarthroplasty.

Pre-operative planning

- Generally, X rays and CT scans have been used to determine if reconstruction is possible. These images can be used for planning purposes.
- The canal width is measured from X rays, allowing for radiological magnification or digital resizing. With conventional radiographs templates might be available from the manufacturer to estimate stem size (allow for a cement mantle by subtracting up to 2 mm from the measured minimum canal width).
- The humeral head diameter and depth can be measured to give an indication of where to start when doing a trial reduction. Measurements are often inaccurate, however, due to tilting of the displaced head fragment.
- If hemiarthroplasty is being carried out for chronic posterior fracture dislocation a brace will be necessary to maintain reduction after hemiarthroplsty. A suitable external rotation +/− abduction brace should be measured and tested before surgery.

Surgical technique

- The greater and lesser tuberosities are identified and a heavy No. 5 Ethibond suture is placed in the region of the rotator cuff insertion of each (Fig. 2.16). These sutures can be used to control the tuberosities and later can be used as tension band sutures for definitive tuberosity fixation.

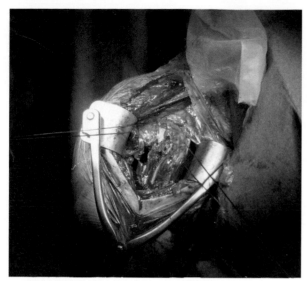

Fig. 2.16 Heavy non-absorbable sutures are placed in the insertions of the cuff tendons into the tuberosities and are used to retract the tuberosities at this stage.

- The humeral head is located and gently retrieved. Often it has displaced beneath subscapularis and if it has gone a long way inferiorly then great care has to be taken not to damage neurovascular structures, particularly the axillary vein, during retrieval.
- The humeral head is retained for estimating prosthetic head size and for use as bone graft.
- The shoulder is washed out and the glenoid fossa is checked for signs of unsuspected damage.
- The humeral canal is gently reamed and washed. The purpose of this is to determine the appropriate stem size for the largest reamer that fits easily down the canal to the depth of the intended stem.
- An appropriate trial stem is inserted – it will be too loose at this stage, but this allows it to be freely moved when judging the correct placement.
- A trial head is fitted that is as close as possible in size to the removed natural head. The joint is provisionally reduced.
- Tension is applied to the sutures in the tuberosities to restore the greater tuberosity to its anatomical location. The trial prosthesis gently pushed up from below and in front until it snugly fits into the coracoacromial arch and faces the glenoid fossa. It is important during this procedure that the forearm is placed pointing forwards so that the humeral shaft is in neutral rotation.

- Usually the rotation of the component is correct when the anterior fin of the prosthesis sits just behind the biceps groove – if it is still visible.
- The tuberosities are used to gauge the height of the prosthesis. If they do not fit around the humeral stem (and they do not have excess inherent bulk) then a smaller head size should be tried. If the tuberosities seem too large and loose then a larger head size should be tried.
- At the end of the procedure it should be possible to bring the tuberosities around the prosthesis until they meet, but still allow the humeral prosthesis to be translated backwards and forwards in the joint by about 50% of the width of the glenoid fossa.
- Once happy with the size of the head, the humeral stem height and rotation should be checked once more. The shaft fragment is then marked with diathermy to indicate the position of the fin on the prosthesis, and reference marks on the fins are used to identify how far above the shaft the fins have to be left at the end of cementation. The trial prosthesis is then removed.
- The canal is washed out. Two No. 5 Ethibond sutures are preplaced through drill holes in the humeral shaft. The humeral head is used to make a bone block to restrict cement in the humeral canal and the block is placed at the depth of the stem tip. Remaining bone from the humeral head is gathered for use as bone graft.
- The humeral stem is cemented in the shaft according to the markings for rotation and the reference points for height. Some systems have special jigs to reproduce the best position identified at trial reduction. As the cement sets, the prosthesis often looks disconcertingly prominent in the shaft (Fig. 2.17). Resist the temptation to push the implant deeper as this will defunction the deltoid afterwards.
- Leave a small trough between the stem and the cortex of the humerus by pushing down or removing cement. Bone graft will later be placed in this trough to facilitate union between the shaft and tuberosities. The tuberosities will never bond to a bare prosthesis!
- Slide the Ethibond sutures through the shaft drill holes as the cement sets to prevent the sutures becoming locked in the cement mantle.
- Impact the head onto the stem if a modular system is being used (Fig. 2.18).
- Once the cement has cured the joint is washed out. The tuberosities are reduced and bone graft is packed between the tuberosities (Fig. 2.19) and stem and down into the shallow gutter at the upper shaft. The intention is to get the tuberosities to unite to each other and to

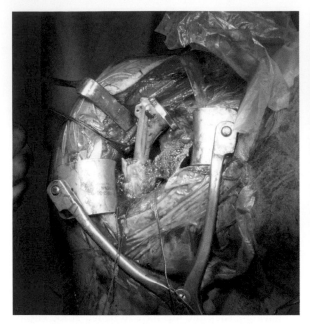

Fig. 2.17 Stem cemented at correct height, leaving space for tuberosity reattachment below the head.

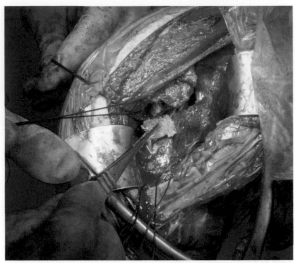

Fig. 2.19 Bone graft from the humeral head fragment is packed beneath the tuberosities and between the shaft and tuberosity, fragments, before preplaced retraction sutures are tied.

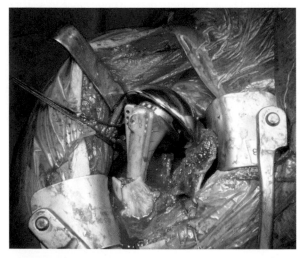

Fig. 2.18 Trial reduction determines the correct head size and the head is connected before the tuberosities are reconstructed.

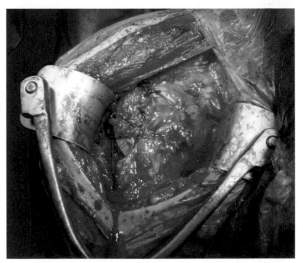

Fig. 2.20 Retraction sutures and sutures placed through drill holes in the shaft before cementing are used in tension band mode to reconstruct the proximal humerus around the prosthesis.

the shaft around the correctly placed head. Holes in the fins of the prosthesis are a distraction – the tuberosities should be primarily fixed to each other and the shaft, not to the fins of the prosthesis, though the holes in the fins provide a supplementary way of achieving this.

• Using the principles of tuberosity tension band fixation discussed in the two preceding sections the tuberosi-

ties are fixed anatomically around the prosthesis, over bone graft, using a combination of the sutures placed at the cuff insertions and those sutures preplaced in the shaft (Fig. 2.20).

• Many favour adding a further suture which loops around both tuberosities beneath the cuff insertion, perforates the cuff insertion towards the bottom of the cuff tendons and passes through a hole drilled in the

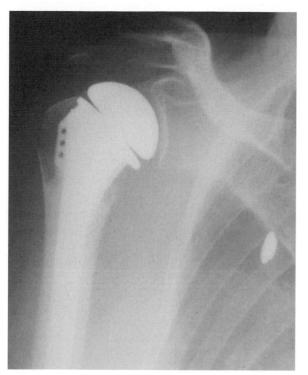

Fig. 2.21 Postoperative X ray demonstrating correct reattachment of tuberosities.

medial part of the neck of the prosthesis. This suture therefore forms a loop around the neck of the prosthesis just below the margins of the head component. The incidence of greater tuberosity migration is said to be less if this suture is placed.

- After secure tuberosity fixation the range of movement is checked – hopefully the physiotherapist can be instructed that no restrictions will be placed on range of movement because of limitation found at this stage.
- A drain is placed.
- The deltopectoral interval is allowed to fall back together and routine fat and skin closure follows.

Post-operative care

- Check X rays in AP and axial views (Fig. 2.21).
- Routine antibiotic regimen for joint replacement – e.g. two doses of cephalosporin post-operatively after a single dose on induction of anaesthesia.
- Shoulder immobilizer for comfort – exchange for collar and cuff as physiotherapy begins.
- The post-operative rehabilitation programme is controversial. Recent enthusiasm for immediate aggress-

ive mobilization has been curbed by an observed increased risk of tuberosity dehiscence. The stiffness that is perceived to be a huge problem is now thought to be less so if good, secure and stable tuberosity fixation is obtained, and this can be facilitated by immobilization for up to 6 weeks. The jury is still out and there is a lot of variation in practice.

Complications

- If only shoulders could be used as freely and easily as hips and knees after lower limb joint replacement! However, although the initial rehabilitation requirements are high, ultimately good pain relief and function can be obtained, equivalent to what is seen after lower limb arthroplasty.
- Discomfort and stiffness are not so much complications as expected events that can be overcome with effective rehabilitation. The patient must be aware that surgery gives them the opportunity to regain their shoulder function. It is only actually achieved however after following a proper rehabilitation programme.
- Infection and neurovascular injury are rare, as they are after any joint replacement, but can be catastrophic.
- The main problem that can be identified on early review is dehiscence of the tuberosities. If detected it is worth reoperating and attempting to regraft and fix the offending tuberosity. Shoulder function is very poor if the tuberosity retracts and does not unite, because associated cuff function is lost.
- If all goes well the patient should be reassured that the shoulder will ache at night and with use for at least six months. It will ache after heavy use and in cold weather for more than a year. This should not prevent the patient following the recommended mobilization exercises, as stiffness and persistent discomfort can otherwise become chronic.
- Since the results of shoulder replacement depend critically on the patient's participation in an effective rehabilitation programme, patient selection is paramount in achieving the good results that are possible after shoulder replacement. As with any joint replacement, however, patients will always consider an artificial joint put in for trauma to be less good than their natural, normal joint before injury. This contrasts with the patients having joint replacements for arthritis where the artificial joint is an immediate improvement on the joint the patient had before surgery.

Section II: Fractures of the humeral shaft

Peter V. Giannoudis (2.5), Paige T. Kendrick, Craig S. Roberts and David Seligson (2.6)

2.5 OPEN REDUCTION AND INTERNAL FIXATION (ORIF): POSTERIOR APPROACH

Indications

The majority of humeral shaft fractures can be treated non-operatively with high rates of union and excellent functional outcomes. Based on the fracture personality as well as the concominant injuries, indications for ORIF are:

(a) Open fractures.
(b) Failure of closed treatment.
(c) Non-union.
(d) Periprosthetic fractures.
(e) Pathologic fractures.
(f) Intra-articular extension.
(g) Segmental fractures.
(h) Polytrauma patient with multiple injuries.
(i) Ipsilateral forearm and elbow fractures.
(j) Neurovascular compromise.
(k) Long spiral fractures.
(l) Brachial plexus injuries.

Pre-operative planning

Clinical assessment

- Obtain a careful history of the injury (direct trauma, application of torsional force).
- Identify and assess associated injuries.
- Physical examination should include: chest, neck, shoulder, arm, elbow, forearm, wrist and hand examination.

- Proceed to a thorough neurologic examination. Radial nerve injury is the most common, but any peripheral nerve and the brachial plexus can be injured.
- Vascular assessment
  - Palpate the axillary, brachial, radial pulses.
  - Assess the tissue perfusion of the hand.
- Evaluate the soft tissue compartments of arm and forearm.

Radiological assessment

Good quality AP and lateral radiographs are essential, including the shoulder and elbow joints (Fig. 2.22 a,b).

Timing of surgery

- Most operative treatment of closed fractures can be delayed and then treated electively within 3–5 days of injury.
- Open fractures require emergent irrigation and debridement, and possible immediate internal fixation if the conditions of the soft tissues and the patient's overall status are satisfactory.

Operative treatment

Anaesthesia

- General anaesthesia and/or regional (block).
- Administration of prophylactic antibiotics as per local hospital protocol.

Table and equipment

- AO large fragment (4.5 mm) set.
- Implant choice:
  - A narrow 4.5 mm dynamic compression plate.

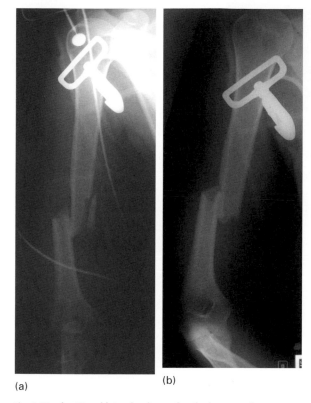

(a)   (b)

Fig. 2.22 a,b AP and lateral radiographs of a humerus fracture.

- Standard osteosynthesis set as per local hospital protocol.
- Fluoroscopy is necessary for intraoperative imaging.

Table set up

- The instrumentation is set up on the side of the operation.
- Image intensifier is from the ipsilateral side.
- Position the table diagonally across the operating room so that the operating area lies in the clean air field.

Patient positioning

- The patient is positioned in a lateral decubitus position with the upper arm supported by a padded post (Fig. 2.23).
- Prior to draping, the surgeon needs to confirm that good quality, fluoroscopic imaging intraoperatively can be obtained.

Draping and surgical approach

- Prepare the skin of the whole arm including the shoulder.
- Skin preparation is carried out using usual antiseptic solutions (aqueous/alcoholic povidone–iodine).
- The arm is draped free with single use U-drapes over the side of the table with the elbow flexed. The hand and forearm is draped with a stockinette.
- Skin landmarks: from the distal border of the deltoid to the tip of olecranon on the skin before the incision.
- Incise the skin, subcutaneous tissue and fascia.
- Identify the thick white triceps tendon (Fig. 2.24).
- Proximally identify the interval between the lateral and long head of the triceps and dissect bluntly.
- Distally, sharply dissect these superficial heads by division of the triceps tendon.
- Identify and preserve the lateral cutaneous brachial nerve.
- Retract the long and lateral heads of triceps to reveal the radial nerve (accompanied by the profunda branchii artery in the spiral groove and the medial head of the triceps) (Fig. 2.25).
- Divide the medial head vertically between the two branches of the radial nerve that supply it and expose the humeral shaft.
- Mobilization of the radial nerve (Fig. 2.26):
  - It must be done from below upwards.
  - Retract it out of the way with a ribbon gauze soaked in saline, or with a rubber sling, and protect it.
  - Avoid damage to the accompanying profunda artery.
- Now the exposure can be continued distally to the elbow.
- Strip the medial head of triceps from the posterior aspect of the humerus in a lateral direction.
- Using a retractor, expose the intermuscular septum.
- Split the septum vertically, keeping close to bone to expose the radial nerve.
- The wound is irrigated and the fracture haematoma is evacuated.
- The major fracture lines are defined and the fracture fragments identified.

Fracture reduction and implant positioning

- Reduction must be atraumatic and can be achieved by careful traction to restore length, which is then maintained with pointed reduction forceps in oblique or spiral fractures.

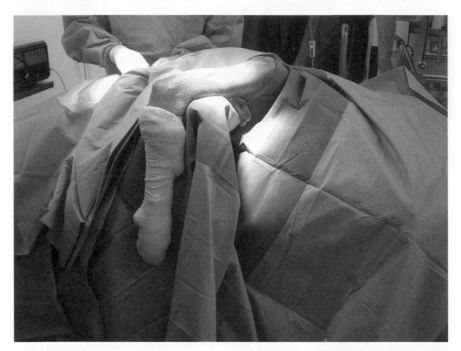

Fig. 2.23 Positioning of the patient in a lateral decubitus position.

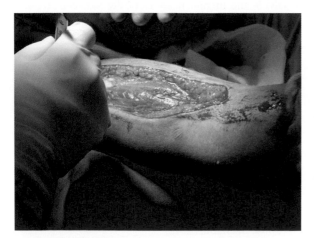

Fig. 2.24 Incision through the skin, subcutaneous layer and identification of the triceps tendon.

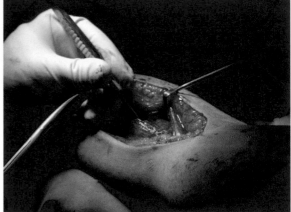

Fig. 2.25 Proximal dissection of the lateral and long head of the triceps.

- Stabilize the fragments using reduction clamps.
- In transverse fractures prebend the plate to prevent a fracture gap during screw insertion (Fig. 2.27).
- In spiral or oblique fractures a lag screw fixation must be inserted whenever possible (Fig. 2.28).
- The screws should engage 6 to 8 cortices both above and below the fracture (Fig. 2.29).

- The screws must be inserted in an offset pattern rather than in parallel sequence, to reduce the risk of fatigue fractures through rotational load.
- Inspect the nerve and make sure it is not under the plate, especially at the ends of the plate.
- The stability of the construct is tested using gentle manual stress.

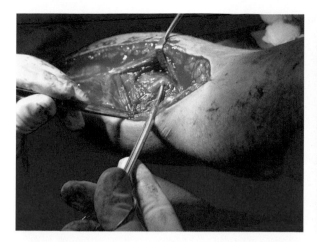

Fig. 2.26 Mobilization of the radial nerve.

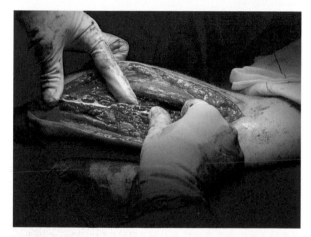

Fig. 2.27 Prebend the plate to prevent a fracture gap during screw insertion.

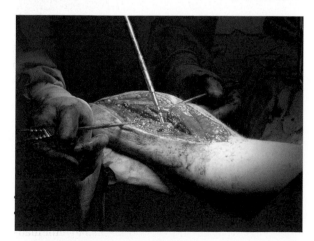

Fig. 2.28 A lag screw fixation must be inserted whenever possible.

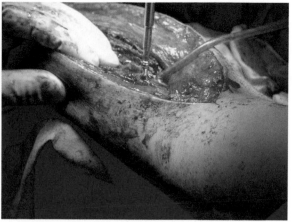

Fig. 2.29 The screws should engage 6 to 8 cortices both above and below the fracture.

- Implant position and fracture reduction is confirmed using fluoroscopic imaging.

Closure

- Irrigate the wound thoroughly and achieve haemostasis.
- Closure in layers using 1/0, 2/0 Vicryl for the triceps aponeurosis and the fat layer and a subcuticular (3/0 PDS) material for the skin (Fig. 2.30 a,b).

Post-operative care and rehabilitation

- Two further doses of prophylactic antibiotics.
- Meticulous assessment and documentation of neurovascular status.
- Radiographs in 24 hours (Fig. 2.31).
- Patients are placed in a sling, which is removed to permit an active range of motion exercises of the shoulder and elbow within a day or two of surgery.

Outpatient follow up

- Review in clinic two weeks after surgery with radiographs on arrival.
- Carefully assess for shoulder, elbow, wrist and hand function.
- Then on a monthly basis until the fracture unites and the patient returns to normal activities, with radiographs at each visit.
- Full elbow and shoulder motion should be obtained within one month of surgery.

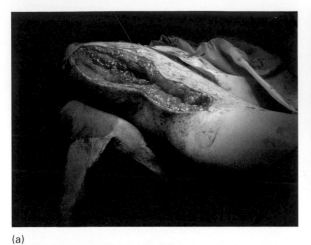

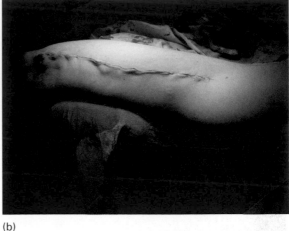

(a)   (b)

Fig. 2.30 a,b closure in two layers using a subcuticular (3/0 PDS) material for the skin.

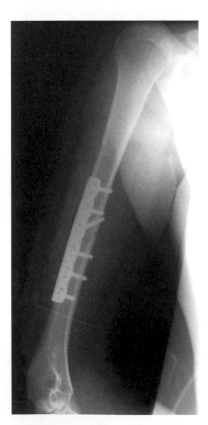

Fig. 2.31 Post-operative radiograph of humerus plating.

- Regular weight lifting is allowed at 12 weeks provided that reduction is maintained and there are evident radiographical signs of healing with no evidence of implant failure.

Complications

- Failure of fixation.
- Non-union.
- Loss of motion of shoulder or elbow.
- Infection.
- Radial nerve palsy.

Implant removeal

- Removal is not routinely indicated.

2.6 ANTEGRADE INTRAMEDULLARY NAILING OF THE HUMERUS

Indications

- Antegrade intramedullary nails can be used to stabilize most closed midshaft and distal diaphyseal fractures. Nailing generally is contraindicated in open humerus fractures, unless it can be confirmed directly that there is no radial nerve interposition in the fracture site.

Pre-operative planning

Clinical assessment

- The arm is shortened and floppy.
- Assess the neurologic condition of the extremity, particularly the axillary nerve and the radial nerve.

Radiographic assessment

- Anteroposterior and lateral radiographs of the humerus to assess fracture pattern (Fig. 2.32).

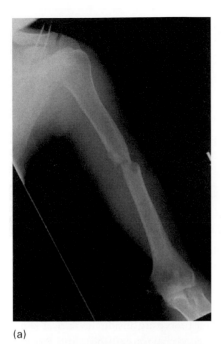

(a)

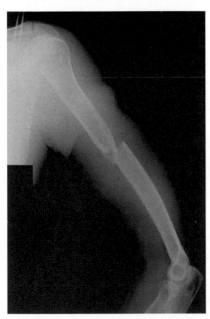

(b)

Fig. 2.32 (a) Pre-operative AP and (b) lateral radiographs show a displaced humeral shaft fracture.

- Medullary canal size and the overall length of the canal up to the proximal aspect of the olecranon fossa are assessed to ensure feasibility of nailing and availability of appropriate implants.

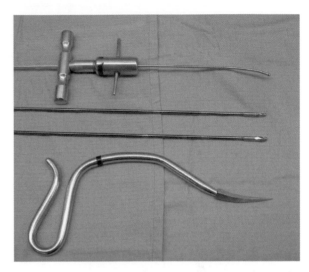

Fig. 2.33 Instrumentation for intramedullary nailing of humeral shaft fracture involves a curved awl, a ball-tipped guide wire and a t-handle chuck.

Timing of surgery

- Most closed fractures can be treated semi-urgently in the first 10 days from injury.
- Open fractures are a surgical emergency.

Operative treatment

Anaesthesia

- General anesthesia in the supine position through an endotracheal tube with the endotracheal tube oriented away from the affected arm.
- Administer prophylactic antibiotics.

Table and equipment

- A curved awl, ball-tipped guide wire, and a t-handle chuck is needed (Fig. 2.33), in addition to flexible reamers and nail instruments.
- A radiolucent operating room table.
- An image intensifier.

Table set up

- The instrumentation is set on the side of the operation.
- The image intensifier is at the foot of the table on the same side as the surgeon.

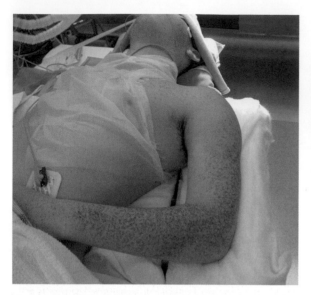

Fig. 2.34 Operative set up involves draping the arm free over the side of the table with the ability to extend the shoulder and rotate the arm.

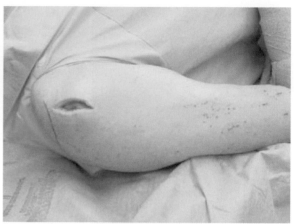

Fig. 2.35 Lateral skin incision is used, the deltoid is split in line with its fibres, and the rotator cuff is incised.

Patient positioning

- Supine flat position with the patient's arm over the side of the table (Fig. 2.34). Tilt the head slightly to the contralateral side, provided that the cervical spine has been cleared. The ability to extend the arm is also important.
- Before draping, one needs to ensure that both AP and axillary views are possible and are not blocked by metal components of the operating room table.

Fracture reduction

- Longitudinal traction, adduction of the arm, and slight internal rotation usually reduces the fracture.

Draping and surgical approach

- The arm should be draped free with a stockingette over the forearm.
- Lateral incision over the superior and anterior aspect of the greater tuberosity (Fig. 2.35). May need to adduct and extend the shoulder.
- Deep dissection – incise the deltoid in line with its fibres. Incise the rotator cuff in line with its fibres.

- Identify entry site to the intramedullary canal just inside the greater tuberosity, inside the critical zone, after confirming good position with the C-arm. Be careful not to make the starting point too anterior, causing anterior cortical blowout.
- Pass the guide wire, while holding the fracture reduced.
- Enlarge the canal by reaming until there is 1.0–1.5 mm of cortical shatter.
- Select a nail 1.0–1.5 mm smaller than the largest reamer size. Common nail lengths are 20–26 cm.

Implant positioning

- Introduce the nail gently, by hand, under fluoroscopic control without using a mallet. The humerus needs to be stabilized whilst the nail is introduced.
- Check the nail height. The nail needs to be under the articular surface in order to avoid impingement.
- Proximal interlocking – use the jig, make percutaneous incisions, and spread the soft tissues down to bone. Avoid the region of the axillary nerve and brachial plexus.
- Check fracture reduction and alignment, especially rotation. Shoulder position should be neutral or in slight internal rotation. Transverse fractures can be impacted if necessary.
- Anteroposterior distal interlocking is safest. Make an incision over the distal hole(s). Retract the medial neurovascular bundle.
- Need to image perfect circle(s) with the C-arm.

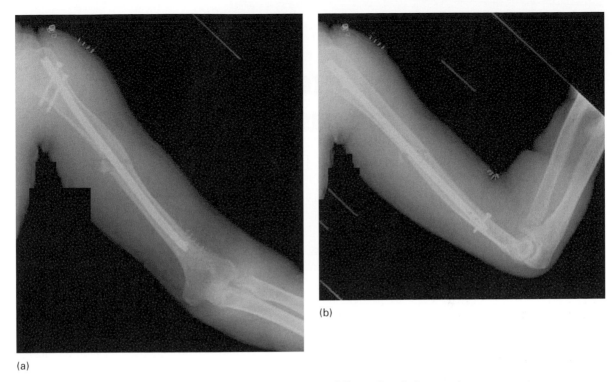

(a)

(b)

Fig. 2.36 (a) Final AP and (b) lateral radiographs after antegrade intramedullary nailing of a humerus fracture.

- Obtain final radiographs in both the AP and lateral planes (Fig. 2.36).

Closure

- Anatomic repair of the rotator cuff with a non-absorbable suture and anatomic repair of the deltoid are both necessary.
- Perform skin closure in the routine fashion.
- A shoulder sling is usually applied.

Post-operative rehabilitation/care

- Two additional doses of prophylactic antibiotics.
- Codman exercises and elbow and wrist range of motion exercises are allowed when awake and alert.
- Shoulder motion and weightbearing on the arm are restricted initially.

Outpatient follow up

- Post-operative radiographs including AP and axillary views need to be performed at 2-week, 4-week, and 6-week intervals and then on a monthly basis.
- A sling is usually continued until good fracture healing is demonstrated.
- Avoid physical therapy immediately after surgery.

Post-operative complications

- Shoulder pain is likely secondary to rotator cuff dysfunction, or failure of the rotator cuff to heal completely is common.

Implant removal

- Removal is often advised in patients with evidence of rotator cuff dysfunction/irritation.

Section III: Fractures of the distal humerus

Paige T. Kendrick; Craig S. Roberts; David Seligson

2.7 OPEN REDUCTION AND INTERNAL FIXATION (ORIF) OF SUPRACONDYLAR FRACTURES

Indications

- Most adult fractures fit into one of the following categories:
  (a) Extra-articular (supracondylar fracture without intercondylar fracture).
  (b) Intra-articular (supracondylar fracture plus inter-condylar extension/articular involvement).
- Both intra-articular and extra-articular supracondylar fractures of the humerus in the adult usually require open reduction and internal fixation.
- Periarticular fractures with dislocation may also have ligamentous instability.

Pre-operative planning

Clinical assessment

- Pain is localized to the posterior elbow and lower part of the humerus.
- The arm is shortened, floppy, and flexed.
- Assess the condition and integrity of the skin and the extent of the tissue injury.
- A thorough neurovascular examination is important, with special attention to radial nerve, posterior interosseous nerve, and ulnar nerve function.

Radiological assessment

- Good quality AP and lateral radiographs are essential (Fig. 2.37).
- If adequate radiographs cannot be obtained, a CT should be obtained.

- The fracture fragments should be drawn out on paper to ensure a three-dimensional (3-D) understanding of the fracture pattern.
- A primary surgical plan should also be developed on paper, as well as a backup plan if the initial plan does not work out.

Timing of surgery

- Most operative treatment of closed fractures can be delayed and then treated electively within 3–5 days of injury.
- Open fractures require emergent irrigation and debridement, and possible immediate internal fixation if the conditions of the soft tissues about the elbow and the patient's overall status are satisfactory.

Operative treatment

Anaesthesia

- General anesthesia is used.
- Prophylactic perioperative antibiotics should be administered.
- A Foley catheter is usually necessary.

Table and equipment

- A full set of all surgical instrument including large self-retaining retractors (Beckman's), bone clamps, anatomic plates or contour plates with templates, small fragment instruments and implants, cannulated small screws up to 60 mm in length, Kirschner wires, cerclage wire (fixation of a possible olecranon osteotomy), power drill, and a sagittal saw (for osteotomy) (Fig. 2.38).
- Fluoroscopy is necessary for intraoperative imaging.

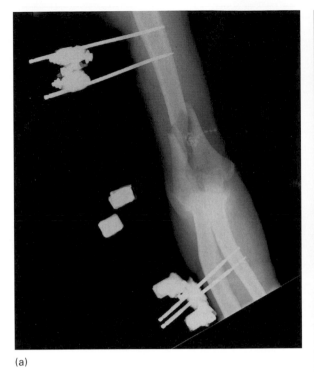

(a)

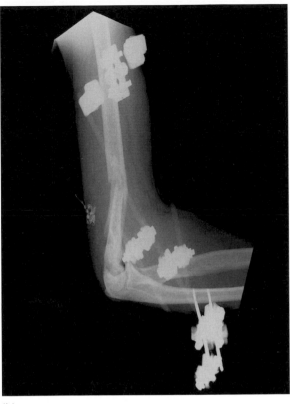

(b)

Fig. 2.37 (a) Pre-operative AP and (b) lateral radiographs of an adult supracondylar humerus fracture. In this case, the fracture has been grossly realigned with an external fixator.

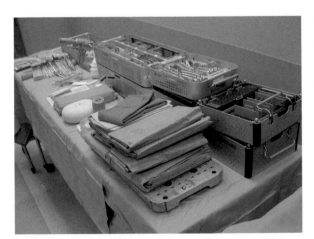

Fig. 2.38 Instrumentation for fixation of supracondylar fracture involves small fragment implants, reconstruction plates, and precontoured anatomic plates.

Table set up

- The instrumentation is set up on the side of the operation.
- The image intensifier is on the same side with its base at the foot of the operating table.

Patient positioning

- Chest rolls and adequate padding at all areas including face (Fig. 2.39).
- Prone positioning is preferred with adequate padding, with avoidance of shoulder extension or abduction greater than 90° in order to avoid stretching of the brachial plexus (Fig. 2.40). An alternative lateral position is with the arm flexed over a paint-roller type arm cast.
- Prior to draping, the surgeon needs to confirm that good-quality, fluoroscopic imaging intraoperatively can be obtained. Several fluoroscopic images should be obtained prior to formal draping.

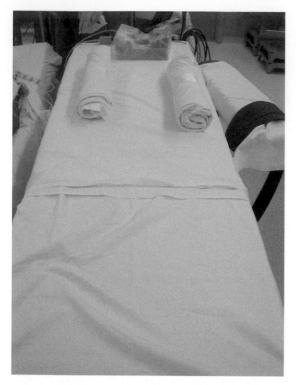

Fig. 2.39 Operative set up involves prone positioning with chest rolls.

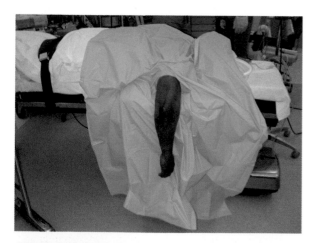

Fig. 2.40 The arm is draped free over the side of the table with the elbow flexed.

Fracture reduction

- Exact reduction of all components may not be possible.
- Elbow flexion and gentle longitudinal traction usually help.

Draping and surgical approach

- The skin of the whole arm including the shoulder should be prepared with the antiseptic solution.
- If it is anticipated that an autologous bone gaft might be needed, the respective iliac crest should also be prepped and draped.
- The arm is usually placed in 80° of abduction with the humerus supported by a bump of 4 rolled sheets and the elbow flexed over the side of the table and the arm in a pocket made from a sheet.
- Posterior incision is made from 5 cm distal to the olecranon to a point 10–12 cm proximal to the major fracture line.
- The incision should have a gentle medial curve around the olecranon.
- Ulnar nerve is isolated proximally at the level of the elbow joint, traced proximally, and then isolated using a Penrose drain or vascular loop.
- The trochlear joint capsule is pierced from the medial side and a sponge is brought through the joint and out the other side and left in place to protect the underlying joint.
- A Beckman self-retaining retractor is useful for ensuring exposure.
- Various olecranon osteotomies are possible: none, an extra-articular osteotomy, an intra-articular osteotomy.
- Various osteotomy-cut configurations can be utilized (straight or Chevron type).
- The osteotomy level is marked on the olecranon using electrocautery.
- The method of fixation of the osteotomy needs to be decided prior to making an osteotomy.
- If an intramedullary screw is planned for lateral fixation of the olecranon osteotomy. The screw path should be predrilled prior to making the osteotomy.
- The olecranon is scored with an osteotome and then the osteotome is completed with the sagittal saw. Avoid plunging with the saw and touching the articular cartilage of the humerus.
- The triceps is reflected proximally with the olecranon fragment.
- Medial and lateral triceps dissection is usually required for mobilization.
- Palpation followed by visualization of the radial nerve in the spiral groove is necessary when the proximal dissection is performed.
- The wound is irrigated and the fracture haematoma is evacuated.

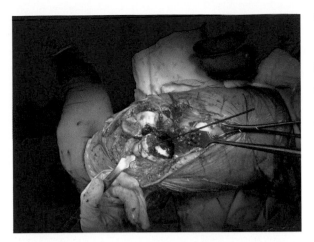

Fig. 2.41 Operative exposure involves a posterior incision, often with an olecranon osteotomy for exposure of the articular fracture.

- The major fracture lines are defined and the fracture fragments identified.
- The articular fragments need to be inspected first.
- The trochlear and the capitellar fragments, and the olecranon fossa need to be carefully evaluated.
- If there is no intercondylar split and the articular segment is intact, then proceed to identify the radial nerve proximally, although this step is not necessary for a distal fracture.
- Anatomic reduction of the articular segment is performed under direct visualization of the posterior aspect of the distal humerus in the coronal and axial planes, and fluoroscopic evaluation of the reduction in the lateral view (Fig. 2.41).
- Provisional fixations are achieved using a guidepin placed from a lateral to medial direction for a small cannulated screw (4.0 mm or 5.0 mm cannulated screw).
- After an articular block is established, the supracondylar/metaphyseal component of the fracture is inspected.
- The metaphyseal/supracondylar component of the fracture is inspected to understand the planes and extent of major fracture lines and the degree of comminution.
- The metaphyseal, supracondylar fracture is reduced and the articular block is reduced to the proximal shaft usually by a combination of arm manipulation, reduction forceps and bone clamps, and manual pressure.
- Reduction is confirmed by direct visualization of the posterior aspect of the humerus in the coronal and axial planes, and then fluoroscopic evaluation of the lateral reduction (sagittal plane).

- Provisional fixation is achieved using Kirschner wires to cage the fracture.

Implant positioning

- The goal is to place two plates at a 90° orientation ('90–90 plating') whenever possible.
- One plate (either a 3.5 reconstruction plate or a 3.5 dynamic reconstruction plate) can be placed on the lateral column on the posterior aspect of the humerus with preferably 6 cortices of fixation distally and 6 cortices of fixation proximally.
- The second plate, usually a 3.5 reconstruction plate, is contoured using the bending irons, and is then usually placed on the medial aspect of the humerus (90° to the lateral plate) with 6 cortices of fixation proximally and 6 cortices of fixation distally (Fig. 2.42).
- Extra care should be taken to ensure that implants are not protruding anteriorly with impingement into the radiocapitellar joint.
- The stability of the construct is tested using gentle manual stress.
- The need for bone grafting is determined based on the presence of fracture-significant comminution, bone loss, or a persistent fracture gap.
- The wound is copiously irrigated prior to insertion of the bone graft.
- Implant position and fracture reduction is confirmed using first fluoroscopic imaging and then intraoperative plain AP and lateral radiographs (Fig. 2.43).

Closure

- After the wound is irrigated and haemostasis is achieved, the osteotomy is repaired.
- Two main fixation options exist: intramedullary screw fixation or a tension band (Kirschner wires preferably into the region of the coronoid with a figure-of-eight. In addition, composite fixation can also be used (figure-of-eight wire in addition to intramedulary screw) if the bone is soft and screw purchase is suboptimal.
- The ulnar nerve should be inspected for impingement and proximity to the medial plate to determine the need for ulnar nerve transposition.
- The main options for ulnar nerve transposition are submuscular or subcutaneous transposition.
- The triceps tendon usually requires some side-to-side repair proximally.
- Routine subcutaneous closure and skin closure are performed.

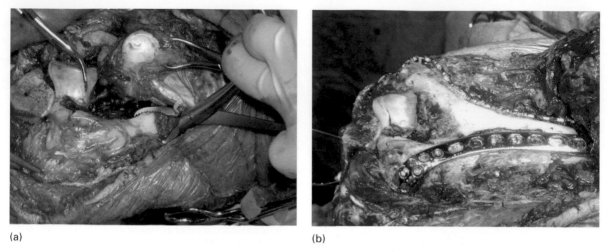

(a)   (b)

Fig. 2.42 The operative strategy involves reduction of the articular surface (a) followed by reduction and fixation of the lateral and medial columns (b).

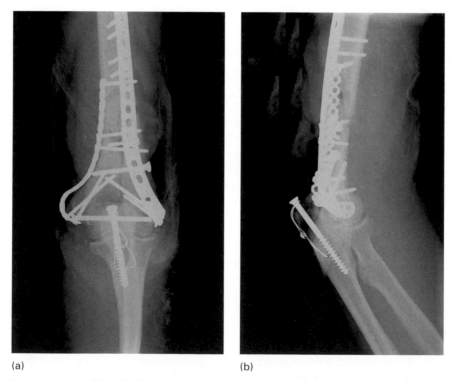

(a)   (b)

Fig. 2.43 a,b AP and lateral radiographs show satisfactory restoration of length and the articular surface. Olecranon osteotomy has been stabilized with an intramedullary screw and tension band wire.

- Self-suction drains are usually required and brought out through a separate stab incision.

Post-operative rehabilitation

- Prophylactic perioperative antibiotics are utilized for 24 hours.
- Use long posterior splint extending the length of the arm and forearm.
- Splint should hold arm with the arm flexed at 90°.
- Patient should be seen in clinic 10–14 days after surgery.

Post-operative complications

- Watch 'hardware' symptoms such as pain and tenderness.
- About 30% of patients need the tension band wire removed.
- Watch for infection and nerve damage.

Outpatient follow up

- One week after surgery, if the incision is healing, the splint may be taken off for short periods of time to allow motion of the elbow area.
- At 3 weeks, the splint is removed and elbow therapy can be started.
- Radiographs are usually obtained at each post-operative visit (2 weeks, 6 weeks, 10–12 weeks, 16–20 weeks, etc.).

Implant removal

- Implants are not routinely removed unless they are causing symptoms. Olecranon osteotomy hardware can sometimes be quite irritating because of its subcutaneous location and can usually be safely removed after 6 months.

2.8 OPEN REDUCTION AND INTERNAL FIXATION (ORIF): CAPITELLUM

Indications

- Fractures are treated depending on their fracture pattern. Most capitellar fractures fit into one of the following categories :
  - (a) Type I: large bone fragment with articular cartilage.
  - (b) Type II: small bone fragment with articular cartilage (the more superficial lesions of Kocher–Lorenz).
  - (c) Type III: comminuted.
  - (d) Type IV: coronal shear fracture.
- Open reduction and internal fixation (ORIF) is indicated for a displaced fracture.

Pre-operative planning

Clinical assessment

- More common in middle-aged or elderly patients.
- Pain is localized to the lateral elbow and during attempted extension.
- Elbow swelling is not as pronounced.
- Assess the condition and degree to which the skin is contused.
- Carefully assess radial nerve function, particularly the ability of the patient to extend the thumb, fingers and wrist.
- Understand the fracture pattern.

Radiological assessment

- Standard AP and lateral radiographs demonstrate the fracture in most cases (Fig. 2.44).
- Type III fractures sometimes require a CT for evaluation because comminution and subchondral bony involvement may be difficult to assess on plain films.
- A traction radiographic view under anesthesia is often helpful.

Timing of surgery

- Most closed fractures can be treated electively within 3–5 days of injury.
- Open fractures require emergent irrigation and debridement, and possible immediate internal fixation.
- Some capitellar fractures are also best treated by excision of fragments.

Operative treatment

Anaesthesia

- Prophylactic perioperative antibiotics are given.
- General anesthesia in the supine position is required.

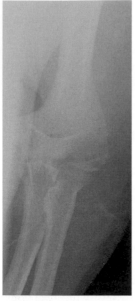

(a)

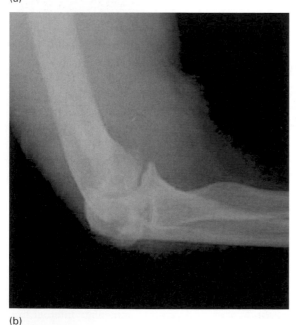

(b)

Fig. 2.44 AP (a) and lateral radiographs (b) show a comminuted capitellar fracture.

Table and equipment

- Instrumentation includes a mini-fragment set, 3.5 reconstruction plates, a small-fragment set, self-compressing screws (Herbert screws, Acutrac screws, etc.), and small cannulated screws (Fig. 2.45).
- An image intensifier.

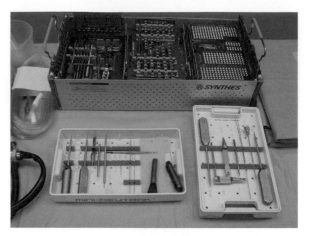

Fig. 2.45 Instrumentation for fixation includes small fragment implants and self-compressing screws.

Table set up

- The instrumentation is set up on the side of the operation.
- The image intensifier is on the same side as the operation with the base at the foot of the operating table.

Patient positioning

- The patient can be positioned supine in most cases.
- A tourniquet is placed about the upper arm.

Fracture reduction

- Closed reduction is usually a waste of time.
- Longitudinal traction, elbow flexion, and supination can be attempted.

Draping and surgical approach

- Prepare the skin and drape the patient in the usual fashion, but check the ability to image the elbow with fluoroscopy before the prepping and draping are started.
- A lateral incision over the supracondylar ridge can be used in most cases from a point 2 cm proximal to the lateral epicondyle to 4 cm distal to the radial head (Fig. 2.46). The radial nerve is at risk both proximally and distally.
- After going through the deep fascia, locate the extensor muscles attaching to the lateral epicondyle, and detach and reflect these.

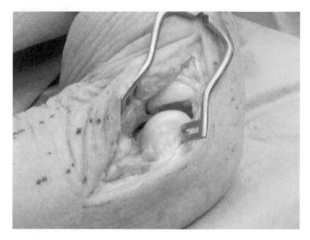

Fig. 2.46 The operative approach to capitellar fractures involves a lateral incision.

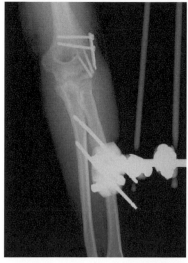

(a)

- The capitellar fracture is inspected.
- The fracture pattern and the size of the fracture fragment(s) should be determined.
- The articular cartilage is inspected.
- Loose articular cartilaginous fragments are removed from the joint.
- The capitellar fracture is reduced anatomically and provisionally held with reduction forceps and the dental pick.
- The fracture is then provisionally pinned with K-wires.

Implant positioning

- A large fracture fragment (s) can be affixed with 2.7 mm or 3.5 mm screws.
- Smaller fracture fragments require smaller implants such as 2.0 mm screws.
- If screws must be placed through the articular cartilage, then the screw(s) should be countersunk, if this can be done without splitting the fracture fragment. Alternatively, self-compressing screws (e.g., Herbert screws, Acutrac screws, etc.) can be used.
- Generally, implants will be directed retrogradely from distal to proximal and angled anteriorly for type 1–3 fractures, and from anterior to posterior for a type 4 fracture.
- Obtain final radiographs of the elbow (Fig. 2.47).

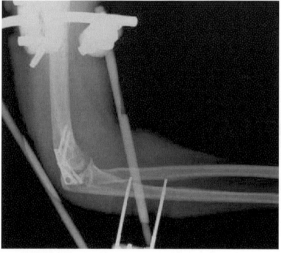

(b)

Fig. 2.47 (a) Final AP and (b) lateral radiographs of a capitellar fracture. In this case, self-compressing screws, a lateral buttress plate, and spanning external fixator were required.

Closure

- Irrigate the wound thoroughly and achieve haemostasis.
- The wound is closed in a routine fashion after repair of the extensor attachment.
- A posterior splint is usually applied initially. The period of immobilization is dependent on the rigidity of the internal fixation but usually less than 2 weeks because of the risk of permanent stiffness.

Post-operative complications

- The major complication is loss of elbow motion, which is seen more frequently after fragment excision than after ORIF.
- Avascular necrosis of the capitellar fragment is a less common complication.
- Malunion is rare.
- Non-union does occur and is usually treated with fragment excision and soft tissue release.

Outpatient follow up

- Radiographs are taken at 2 weeks, 4 weeks, and 6 weeks after surgery, and then monthly until the fracture is healed.

Implant removal

- Implant removal is indicated for radio-capitellar joint impingement or soft tissue irritation.

2.9 RETROGRADE INTRAMEDULLARY NAILING

Indications

- Indicated for distal one-third and shaft humeral fractures.
- Retrograde nailing of the humerus is rarely indicated for a closed proximal or midshaft diaphyseal fracture in polytrauma. Nailing is generally contraindicated for open humerus fractures.

Pre-operative planning

Clinical assessment

- The proximal nature of the humerus fracture makes the arm feel floppy and unstable.

Radiological assessment

- Anteroposterior and lateral views of the humerus (Fig. 2.48).
- Measure the size of the medullary canal and the overall length of the canal from the superior articular surface of the humeral head to the proximal aspect of the olecranon fossa.
- The canal width has to be adequate with no cracks.

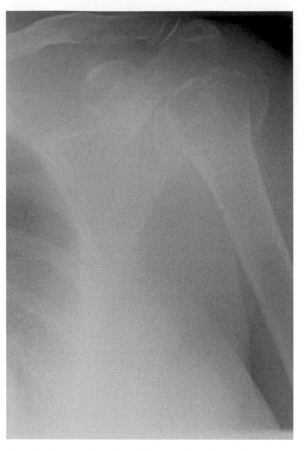

Fig. 2.48 Pre-operative AP and lateral radiographs of a humerus fracture.

Timing of surgery

- Surgery can be performed on a semi-urgent or elective basis.

Operative treatment

Anaesthesia

- General anesthesia via an endotracheal tube.
- The endotracheal tube should be oriented away from the affected extremity.

Table and equipment

- The image intensifier is on the same side as the surgeon, with the base of the machine at the foot of the table.
- Instrumentation includes drill bits and routers to open the intramedullary canal (Fig. 2.49), flexible reamers, and a self-retaining retractor are necessary.

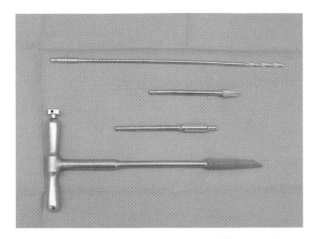

Fig. 2.49 Instrumentation for retrograde humeral nailing includes drill bits and rooters to open the intramedullary canal, in addition to standard flexible reamers.

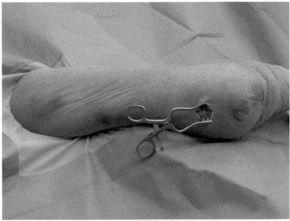

Fig. 2.50 The arm is draped free. The incision is made centred over a point just proximal to the olecranon fossa. The triceps is split in order to expose the posterior cortex of the humerus.

- A regular fracture table.
- An image intensifier.

Table set up

- Instrumentation is set up on the side of the operation.

Patient positioning

- Positioning can be either supine, prone, or in a lateral decubitus position on a regular operating room table with the arm free (Fig. 2.50).
- The prone and lateral decubitus positions make the procedure easier for the surgeon but harder physiologically for the patient.
- Before draping, one should ensure that you are able to obtain AP and lateral views.

Fracture reduction

- The proximal fragment is usually abducted and internally rotated.
- Gentle lateral pressure with a Myerding mallet can be used to neutralize the abduction forces. Gentle longitudinal traction is usually necessary.
- Pass the guide wire while holding the fracture reduced.

Draping and surgical approach

- Make a posterior incision over the proximal half of the olecranon fossa.

- Deep dissection – split the triceps in line with its fibres.
- Identify the proximal aspect of the olecranon fossa.
- Avoid the region of the radial nerve proximally.
- Identify entry point into medullary canal 1.5–2.0 cm proximal to the olecranon fossa.
- Start the entry portal with a 4.5 mm drill bit.
- The entry portal is enlarged with a router. Avoid the thin bone of the olecranon fossa because of the risk of cortical blowout.
- Enlarge the canal by reaming.
- Avoid comminution of the entry portal into the intramedullary canal by staying parallel to the humeral shaft, especially when introducing the reamer into the intramedullary canal of the humerus.
- Select a nail 1.0–1.5 mm smaller than the largest reamer size. Common nail lengths are 20–24 cm.

Implant positioning

- Introduce the nail gently by hand under fluoroscopic control. Do not use a mallet.
- Check nail depth – the tip of the nail should be solidly in the humeral head and should stop short of the subchondral bone.
- Distal interlocking (elbow end of the nail) – make percutaneous incisions, spread the soft tissues down to bone. The radial nerve is at risk from lateral–medial screws and the musculocutaneous nerve/brachial artery from anterior–posterior screws.

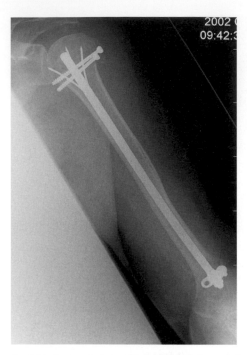

Fig. 2.51 Post operative radiograph after retrograde humeral nailing.

- Check fracture reduction and alignment, especially rotation. The arm should be in neutral or slight internal rotation. Compress the fracture if necessary.
- Proximal interlocking (around the shoulder) involves percutaneous incisions, or larger incisions can be made, and soft tissues are spread down to bone.
- Need to image perfect circle(s) with the C-arm. The axillary nerve is at risk from over-penetration of anterior-to-posterior screws.
- Obtain final radiographs in both the anterior and lateral planes (Fig. 2.51).

Closure

- Irrigate the wound and achieve haemostasis.
- Repair of the distal aspect of the triceps tendon is necessary.
- Skin closure is performed in the routine fashion.

Post-operative rehabilitation

- Two further doses of prophylactic antibiotics.
- Post-operative radiographs including AP and axillary views need to be performed.
- A sling is necessary.
- Avoidance of weight bearing on the arm is necessary.

- Elbow range-of-motion is limited and protected.
- Formal physical therapy is usually avoided immediately post-operatively.

Outpatient follow up

- The patient is seen at 2-week, 4-week, and 6-week intervals, and then monthly until the fracture is healed.

Implant removal

- Implant removal is usually performed for soft tissue irritation.

Complications

- Post-operative exercises and activities should not create torsional stresses on the humerus.

2.10 PAEDIATRIC SUPRACONDYLAR FRACTURES: MANIPULATION UNDER ANAESTHETIC (MUA)/PERCUTANEOUS FIXATION OF DISTAL HUMERAL FRACTURES

Indications

- Supracondylar fractures are classified according to the mechanism of injury which reflects the position of the elbow on which the child fell, as well as the displacement of the distal fragment.
- Extension-type fractures are the most common, representing about 95% or more of these fractures.
- Closed reduction/percutaneous fixation is indicated for displaced fractures.

Pre-operative planning

Clinical assessment

- There are three types of fractures
  (a) Type I: This type is a non-displaced fracture. The fracture line is usually well visualized on AP and lateral views; however, a posterior fat pad ('sail sign') may be the only sign of a fracture when it is otherwise radiographically occult.
  (b) Type II: This type is an angulated fracture with an intact posterior cortex.
  (c) Type III: This type is completely displaced, with the relationship between the two bony fragments completely lost.

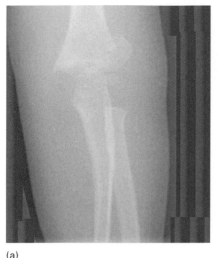
(a)

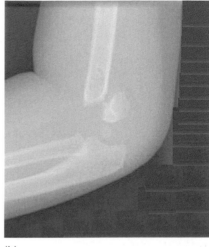
(b)

Fig. 2.52 Pre-operative AP (a) and lateral radiographs (b) show a displaced Type II supracondylar fracture of the right humerus.

- The most important component of the pre-operative assessment is the neurovascular assessment. The presence or absence of a radial pulse needs to be documented as soon as possible.
- It is also important to assess for compartment syndrome, and the function of the median nerve (including the anterior interosseous nerve), the radial nerve and the ulnar nerve.

Radiological assessment

- Good quality AP and lateral radiographs are necessary in order to differentiate between types (Fig. 2.52).
- The lateral radiograph may show a posterior fat pad sign which in some cases may be the only sign of a fracture.

Timing of surgery

- Surgery should be done on an urgent or semi-urgent basis largely based on the neurovascular status.
- Timing should be determined on a case-by-case basis by an experienced orthopaedic surgeon.

Operative treatment

Anaesthesia

- General anaesthesia is necessary.
- Administer prophylactic antibiotics.

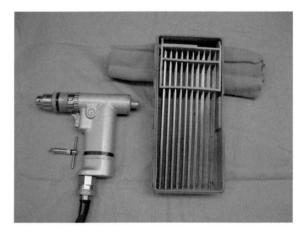

Fig. 2.53 Instrumentation for supracondylar fracture pinning includes smooth pins and a drill.

Table and equipment

- End-threaded or smooth wires, a power drill, wire cutters, wire caps, pliers, and intraoperative fluoroscopy are necessary (Fig. 2.53).
- Additional soft tissue instruments such as small retractors ought to be available because of the possibility of the need for open reduction.
- A cast cart needs to be available at the end of the case.

Patient positioning

- The child is positioned supine on the operating room table with the arm completely free (Fig. 2.54).

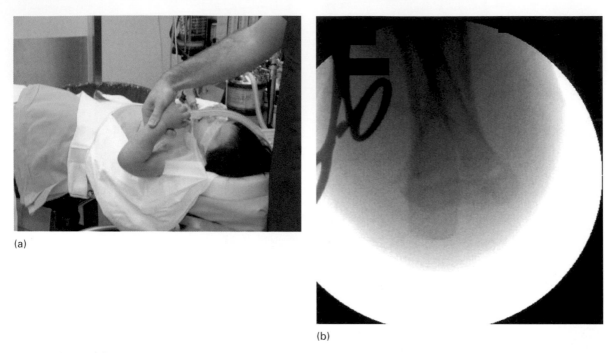

(a)

(b)

Fig. 2.54 Set up involves arm over the side of the table (a) with the ability to obtain intraoperative images (b).

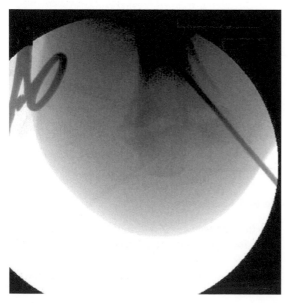

Fig. 2.55 The first pin is across the fracture site from a lateral to medial direction.

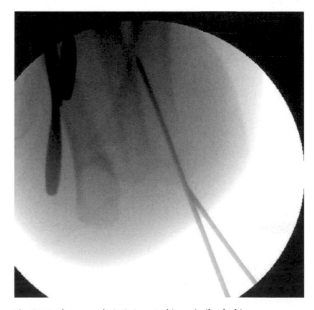

Fig. 2.56 The second pin is inserted in a similar fashion.

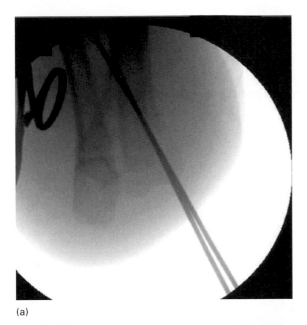

(a)

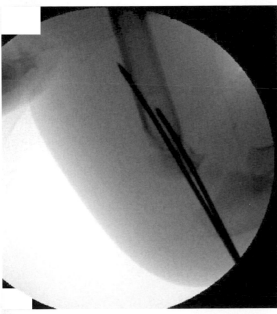

(b)

Fig. 2.57 Final AP (a) and lateral (b) radiographs of two pins inserted from a lateral to medial direction.

Fracture reduction

- Manual longitudinal traction is placed on the foream and countertraction is applied on the upper arm.
- Medial or lateral displacement is then corrected with manual pressure, and then the forearm is externally rotated to correct the internal rotation deformity.

- The elbow is hyperflexed and manual pressure, usually with the surgeon's thumb, is placed on the olecranon. The elbow is held with the arm maximally rotated and the elbow flexed.
- If these manoeuvres do not reduce the fracture, then there are several other considerations. The posterior periosteum is probably torn and the distal fragment cannot be controlled easily. The sharp bony spike of the proximal fragment may also be buttonholed through the brachialis.
- One can attempt to dislodge the fragment by milking the muscle out from proximal to distal. When doing so, pressure is carefully applied laterally only, in order to avoid injuring the medial neurovascular structures.
- Satisfactory reduction needs to be confirmed on fluoroscopy.
- The image intensifier should be moved around the arm. If the arm is rotated the reduction is lost.
- The AP view is nearly impossible with the elbow flexed. A transcondylar view can be obtained.
- If that view is impossible but the reduction is good on the lateral radiograph, the surgeon should proceed with percutaneous pinning and then recheck the AP view after fixation is achieved.
- If the reduction is inadequate, open reduction should be strongly considered.

Draping and surgical approach

- Prepare the skin using antiseptic solution.
- Use end-threaded smooth pins and a power drill for insertion.
- Palpate the ulnar nerve.
- A lateral pin is inserted first (Fig. 2.55). It is inserted through the lateral epicondyle and is directed medially at an angle of 35–45° on the AP view and in line with the humeral shaft on the lateral view. The pin needs to engage the medial cortex in order to have good purchase for Type 2 fractures. A second lateral pin can be used instead of a medial pin (Fig. 2.56).
- The forearm can either be maintained in full external rotation or neutral rotation with the elbow fully flexed whilst the wire is inserted. Place the palm under (dorsal to) the elbow to determine the plane of the humerus and drive the pins parallel to the arm.
- The medial pin is inserted next through the medial epicondyle and anterior to the ulnar nerve. The pin is directed laterally on the AP view and in line with the humeral shaft on the lateral view.

- The elbow can also be extended to 80° of flexion to maintain the ulnar nerve in a posterior position. The foream is held externally rotated.
- The pin needs to engage the lateral cortex in order to achieve good purchase.
- After the second pin is in position, the elbow can then be extended and a standard AP view obtained.
- Obtain final radiographs in the operating room (Fig. 2.57).
- The pins are bent outside of the skin. Pin caps are placed atop the pins.

Closure

- Incisions (if present) are thoroughly irrigated and haemostasis is achieved.
- Routine wound closure.

Post-operative rehabilitation

- Two further doses of prophylactic antibiotics.
- The child usually needs to be hospitalized and kept in overnight in order to observe for neurovascular compromise.
- The elbow is splinted in 80–90° of flexion and a sling is applied.

Post-operative complications

- The greatest complication with supracondylar fractures in children is neurovascular compromise.

Outpatient follow up

- Radiograph approximately 1 week post surgery to ensure reduction, then 2, 4 and 6 weeks later, and then monthly.
- The posterior splint and sling are usually contained for 3 to 4 weeks.

Implant removal

- Pins can usually be removed between 3 to 6 weeks after surgery.

3

Section I: Fractures of the proximal ulna

Gregoris Kambouroglou

3.1 TENSION BAND WIRING OF OLECRANON FRACTURES

Indications

- Displaced transverse fracture of the olecranon with disruption of the extensor mechanism.
- The technique can be used with caution in oblique or fragmented fractures once issues related to these fracture patterns are addressed.

Pre-operative planning

Clinical assessment

- Mechanism of injury: forced extension usually following a fall. **Beware** of the high-energy fracture patterns that may suggest that the fracture is only a portion of the injury.
- Findings: pain, swelling and occasionally impressive ecchymosis over the elbow region. **Beware** of injury to the soft tissue envelope that may interfere or preclude surgical intervention.
- Findings: loss of active extension associated with displaced fractures. **Beware** of examination pitfall where passive gravity-assisted extension leads to the assumption of an intact extensor mechanism.
- Findings: check for ulnar nerve impairment and ensure the injury is in isolation.

Radiological assessment

- Anteroposterior and lateral radiographs of the elbow are the absolute minimum imaging requirement.

Beware of more complex injuries that may need further imaging, most commonly in the form of a CT scan (Fig. 3.1).

Operative treatment

Anaesthesia

- Regional/general.
- Pre-operative administration of antibiotics (cephalosporin).
- Prescrub and drying of the limb.
- Tourniquet application, if there are no contraindications. **Ensure** the tourniquet does not interfere with the operative field and that no preparation solution leaks underneath. Inflate the tourniquet once the limb has been elevated for approximately 3 minutes.

Equipment and patient positioning

- Tension band set (TBW) set: size 18 G wire, 2.0 mm Kirschner wires, wire tighteners and cutters, small punch and toffee mallet, power instruments, pointed reduction forceps, 14G IV cannula.
- Patient lies supine on the operating table with an ipsilateral scapular raise, usually covered one-litre bag of IV fluids. If the patient is obese be careful with the padding and use appropriate side protection. **Beware**: once patient is positioned, ensure adequate radiographic control is possible (Fig. 3.2).
- Radiographic control: an image intensifier is preferable, although plain films at the end of the procedure are possible and occasionally easier to obtain.

Practical Procedures in Orthopaedic Trauma Surgery: A Trainee's Companion, ed. Peter V. Giannoudis and Hans-Christoph Pape.
Published by Cambridge University Press. © Cambridge University Press 2006.

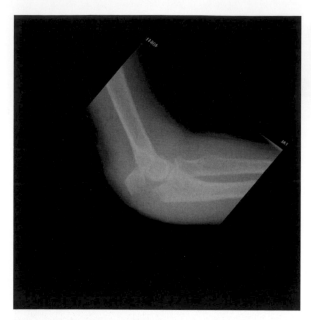

Fig. 3.1 Displaced olecranon fracture.

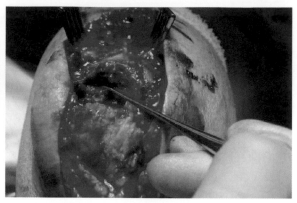

Fig. 3.3 Elevation of depressed fragment.

- Use a direct approach to the posterior surface of the ulna. It is easier to locate the distal part of the ulna and work proximally.
- Expose the fracture with minimal stripping of just the bone edges using a No. 15 scalpel blade. Evacuate the fracture haematoma. Take care of undisplaced fracture lines, often encountered and not visible on plain films.

Fracture reduction

- Inspect the articular surfaces and remove any osteo-chondral fragments. Irrigate the joint thoroughly and reduce any depressed articular fragments using a Mac-Donald's or Watson–Cheyne elevator by gently teasing the depressed fragment (Fig. 3.3). Once this is accomplished, the void under the depressed fragment needs grafting either with bone from the proximal part of the olecranon or using bone substitute material. The latter, in the form of dry hydroxyapatite, is preferable.
- The proximal ulna fragment is controlled with the bone reduction forceps and the forearm extended. Posterior cortical interdigitation usually indicates the accuracy of the reduction. One **must pay attention** to the exact fracture pattern since oblique fractures must be firstly stabilized with an intrafragmentary 3.5 mm lag screw and then neutralized with a TBW.
- The fracture is held reduced with direct pressure or with the medium-size bone reduction forceps. A drill hole through the distal fragment may be required to facilitate this manoeuvre (Fig. 3.4).

Implant insertion

- Using the AO triple 2 mm guide, two 2 mm Kirschner wires are inserted. Subchondral placement of the wires

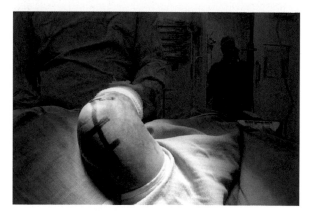

Fig. 3.2 Patient positioning and incision.

Draping and approach

- Paint the hand and, using stockinet, hold the hand and paint the rest of the arm. Single-use drapes are preferable; if not available, use shut-off and traditional draping methods.
- The arm is held over the chest and the assistant/scrub nurse is on the opposite side. A towel clip may be used initially to hold the arm in position.
- Make a linear incision, curved slightly laterally over the apex at the elbow. Occasionally the soft tissue conditions may dictate positioning of the incision.

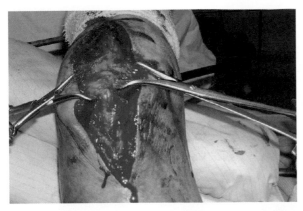

Fig. 3.4 Fracture reduction.

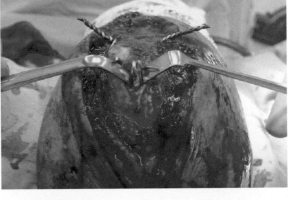

Fig. 3.6 Wire burial.

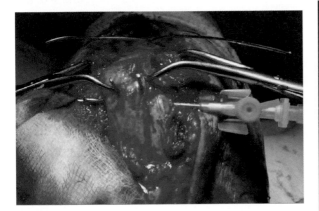

Fig. 3.5 Wire passage.

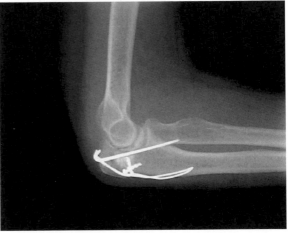

Fig. 3.7 Post-operative radiograph.

through the anterior cortex of the ulna is preferable. Once through the cortex the wires are backed by approximately 1.5 cm.

- Using the 2 mm drill bit a hole is drilled in the distal fragment 3–4 cms from the fracture line and a piece of 18 G wire is passed through and crossed over the ulna, away from the fracture site.
- Using the 14 G IV cannula as a guide, another piece of wire is threaded through, **under the triceps tendon and over the Kirschner wires** (Fig. 3.5). The two ends of the wires are twisted at opposite directions by pulling and twisting. The helix must be symmetrical. Tightening the wires must stop once the wires commence changing colour or twist asymmetrically as they are about to fatigue and break.
- The Kirschner wires are cut with approximately 3–4 cm protruding, and are bent over and over 90°. Using a No. 15 scalpel the triceps tendon is split and the wires are driven home using the small punch and the

toffee mallet, with the cut end buried in the olecranon (Fig. 3.6).

Closure

- Once the implants are secure, take the elbow through the full range of motion of flexion/extension **and** supination/pronation.
- An anteroposterior and lateral radiograph of the elbow are obtained. **Ensure** that a straight lateral of the joint is checked for potential penetration of the joint if the subchondral position of the Kirschner wires is chosen (Fig. 3.7).
- Release the tourniquet and achieve haemostasis. Closure is preferable in two layers without the use of a drain, using a subcuticular (3/0 PDS) material for the skin.

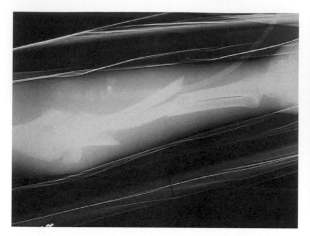

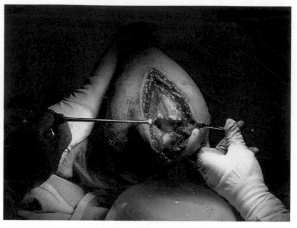

Fig. 3.8 Complex forearm injury with segmental ulna fracture and fracture/dislocation of the elbow.

Fig. 3.9 Boyd approach. Good visualization of the radial head and coronoid.

- Thick (2.5 cm) steristrips are used as dressings with dry gauze, cotton wool and bandage. Avoid Mepore-type dressings.

Post-operative instructions and rehabilitation

- The arm is elevated on pillows, avoiding pressure on the elbow apex.
- The wound is inspected at 48 hours post-operatively and active range motion of the joint commenced if it is healthy and dry.

Follow up

- Outpatient physiotherapy and fracture clinic appointments at 6 and 12 weeks with radiographs on arrival.
- Routine removal of the hardware is not recommended but accept that they are often symptomatic in terms of soft tissue irritation and/or that they impinge on the range of motion. In case of ongoing symptoms or loosening, the hardware can be removed.

3.2 OPEN REDUCTION AND INTERNAL FIXATION (ORIF) OF OLECRANON FRACTURES

Indications

- Fragmented proximal ulna fractures.
- Fractures distal to the coronoid process.

Pre-operative assessment

Clinical

- High-energy injuries: check for associated injuries: Monteggia equivalent injury, elbow dislocation.
- Osteopenic bone: potential fixation problems.

Radiological assessment

- Forearm radiographs: do not miss the distal radio-ulnar joint (DRUJ) (Fig. 3.8).
- CT of the elbow is occasionally helpful, especially to assess an associated fracture of the radial head.

Operative treatment

Anaesthesia

- General.
- Consider the risks of compartment syndrome prior to instituting regional anaesthetic.

Operative equipment

- AO small-fragment set.
- 3.5 mm reconstruction plates.

Set up and positioning

- Hand table.
- Prescrub the limb and antibiotic prophylaxis.
- Tourniquet at 275 mmHg.
- Image intensifier.

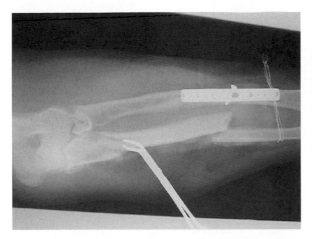

Fig. 3.10 Intraoperative radiograph of a complex forearm injury.

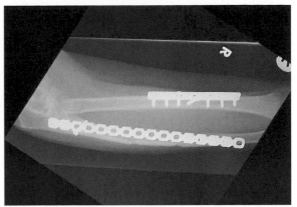

Fig. 3.12 Fracture union of a complex ulnar fracture using lag screws.

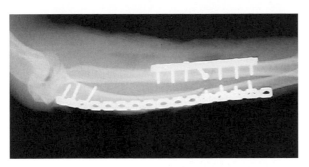

Fig. 3.11 Post-operative radiograph showing bridging plate.

Approach

- One vs. two incisions: for excision of the radial head, use the single (Boyd) approach (Fig. 3.9) with the curved limb of the incision over the radial head.
- For reconstruction of the radial head, two incisions are preferred. Caution regarding the skin bridge.
- Avoid thin skin flaps and devascularisation of bone fragments.

Fracture reduction

- If coronoid is on a large wedge fragment, reduction and fixation is relatively easy from the posterolateral surface of the ulna with intrafragmentary screws.
- Coronoid fractures associated with dislocation of the elbow joint are easier approached laterally, taking anconeus off the ulna. It is usually feasible to stabilize these fractures with an intrafragmentary screw through the plate.
- For complex fractures, an indirect reduction technique and a bridging plate are used (Figs. 3.10 and 3.11).

Implant positioning

- Steps in reduction and fixation follow the concept of turning a complex fracture into a more simple pattern, preferably with lag screws as described above (Fig. 3.12).
- The construct is neutralized with a 3.5 mm reconstruction plate contoured around the olecranon. Strive to achieve a 6-cortices fixation proximally and distally.
- Fragmentation and/or bone quality occasionally does not allow proximal cortical fixation; in this instance, use a long intramedullary screw with the most distal screws interlocked on to it.

Closure

- Prior to closure assess the stability of the construct and the joint in flexion/extension and pronation/supination of the forearm.
- Subcuticular absorbable material is used for skin closure, with wide steristrips as dressings.
- An above-elbow back slab is applied over generous padding. The elbow is flexed to a comfortable position that does not compromise the soft tissues and predispose to compartment syndrome.

Post-operative rehabilitation and follow up

- The intraoperative assessment dictates the post-operative regime. As a rule the wound is inspected at 48 hours and the back slab maintained until the soft tissue envelope recovers and the wound is dry. Physiotherapy is commenced.

- An elbow cast brace is provided and motion of the forearm and elbow commenced. It is common that the elbow is unstable beyond 150° of extension in which case the brace is locked at −30° for a period of 3 weeks.
- A radiograph is obtained at 3 weeks and the hinged brace unlocked to allow full extension. It is kept on for another 3 weeks, following which it is removed and radiographs obtained to check for fracture union.

- Further follow up is organized at 3 months with further radiographs. Patients are discharged if fracture union is evident clinically and radiologically and there are no ongoing problems with the hardware.

Hardware removal

- Hardware is not routinely removed.
- When hardware appears to impinge on motion (usually extension) early removal is recommended.

Section II: Fractures of the ulnar shaft

Gregoris Kambouroglou

3.3 OPEN REDUCTION AND INTERNAL FIXATION: PLATING

Indications

- Displaced fractures of the middle third of the ulna in adults.
- Monteggia fractures: fracture of the ulna shaft with fracture and/or dislocation of the proximal radius/radial head.
- Fractures of both forearm bones.

Pre-operative planning

Clinical assessment

- Mechanism of injury: Nightstick injury: direct blow; Monteggia fractures: axial compression; forearm fracture: any combination. Ensure adequate examination of the elbow and wrist joint for associated pathology.
- Low- vs. high-energy injury, ensure no open fractures are missed with ulna wound volarly and covered by splint when first examined.
- Arm at risk for compartment syndrome: document neurovascular status early and monitor changes.
- In multiple-injured patients treatment sequence follows the 'life-before-limb' protocol.
- Look for occult injuries in the rest of the arm, especially in the carpus/hand.

Radiological assessment

- Rule of 2: 2 views, 2 joints (and 2 visits). Radiographs may be incomplete initially as pain/splints may interfere with the result.

- Traction views in theatre may be necessary for valid pre-operative planning.

Operative treatment

Anaesthesia

- Timing of surgery essential: in low-energy injuries this is not an issue whilst in high-energy ones with displacement, shortening and/or dislocation, early intervention is preferable to avoid complications.
- General anesthesia preferable. Avoid regional anesthetic/blocks in acute injuries as they may mask symptoms indicating compartment syndrome in the immediate post-operative period.
- Pre-operative administration of antibiotics and pre-scrub the limb.
- Apply tourniquet if not contraindicated and inflate following elevation for 3 minutes once limb prepped and draped.

Equipment and patient positioning

- Supine with radiolucent hand table
- Tourniquet cylinder and diathermy in the opposite side.
- Table turned 45° away from the anaesthetic end to prevent contamination of the assistant.
- AO small fragment (3.5 mm) set. Ensure availability of the preplanned plate length in segmental fractures. Small laminar spreader for indirect reduction techniques.

Draping and approach

- Single use upper-limb drapes.
- Folded towels under the elbow/proximal forearm.

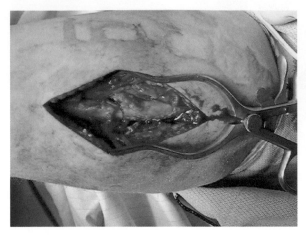

Fig. 3.13 Fracture exposure.

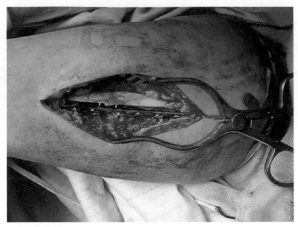

Fig. 3.14 Plate positioning and fracture fixation. Note the dorsal wedge.

- Direct approach over the ulna.
- Minimal exposure of the fracture ends. A No. 15 scalpel rather than a periosteal elevator is preferable.

Fracture reduction

- The aim of reduction in ulna fractures is to restore length, alignment and rotation.
- Once the fracture plane is identified and the interposed soft tissues cleared use a Macdonald's as a bone lever to reduce the fracture. Beware of the almost always present undisplaced bending wedge during this manoeuvre.
- In segmental fragmentation or fractures with extensive fragmentation use the indirect reduction technique with a long late-anchored screw distally and a push-pull screw proximally.

Implant insertion

- In fractures with a substantial wedge fragment attempts are made to reduce and hold it without de vascularising the fragment. The fragment size has occasionally dictated the use of the mini fragment 2.7 mm screws.
- A 3.5 mm AO DCP with purchase in 6 cortices is used.
- The fracture pattern dictates plate placement for middle-third fractures, whilst for segmental/proximal fracture the volar surface is used (Figs. 3.13, 3.14).
- For most middle-third fractures plate contouring is not necessary.

- Ensure the plate is flush with the ulna, as any eccentric positioning may result in subcutaneous and prominent hardware.
- Once the fracture is stabilized take the forearm through the range of motion. When there is a dislocation of the radial head, congruency and stability of the elbow are checked so that the post-operative mobilization regime can be decided.
- Plain radiographs of the forearm are obtained. It is important to check two views taken at 90° to each other. **This is not done** by simply rotating the wrist joint but by rotating the forearm from the shoulder with the elbow flexed.
- Ensure adequate films of the elbow joint are available when there is an injury to the radio-humeral joint.

Closure

- Release the tourniquet and perform haemostasis.
- Close in 2 layers without the use of a drain using a subcuticular (3/0 PDS) material for the skin.
- Thick (1 inch/2.54 cm) steristrips are used as dressings with dry gauze and cotton wool.
- In isolated fractures of the ulna shaft a simple wool and crepe bandage is used.
- In associated injuries of the elbow use an above-elbow back slab with the forearm in the position where the radial head is congruently reduced.

Post-operative treatment

- The arm is elevated using a Bradford sling set up in the recovery room.

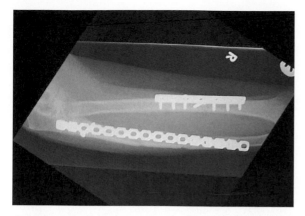

Fig. 3.15 Fracture union.

- Circulation and neurological observations are requested for the immediate post-operative period.
- The wound is inspected at 48 hours. If the radial head is stable throughout the range of pronation and supination, the slab is removed and active range of motion started.
- If there is concern regarding the stability of the radial head, a forearm splint is requested, which allows flexion extension at the elbow but prevents forearm rotation. This is maintained for 3 weeks.

Outpatient follow up

- Depends on the injury type: stable fractures at 6 and 12 weeks with radiographs on arrival. If there is clinical and radiological evidence of fracture union, patients are discharged from further follow up (Fig. 3.15).
- Fracture dislocations to be seen at 3 weeks for clinical and radiological assessment and referral to physiotherapy for forearm range of motion
- Routine removal of the hardware is not recommended.

3.4 ELASTIC NAILS FOR ULNAR SHAFT FRACTURES

Indications

- Displaced fractures of the ulnar diaphysis in children older than 6 years of age.

Pre-operative planning

Clinical assessment

- Assess neurovascular status of the limb.
- Ensure that there are no other associated injuries.

Radiological assessment

- Full-length forearm radiographs: ensure no associated wrist or elbow injury (Monteggia lesion).
- Fracture pattern indicative of the technical difficulty: transverse and shortened fractures are more difficult to reduce and hold with closed methods.
- Measure the diameter of the canal: the desired nail thickness is 0.4 of the canal diameter.

Operative treatment

Anaesthesia

- General anaesthesia.

Table and equipment

- Small basic orthopaedic set equipped with MacDonald or Watson–Cheyne elevators.
- Elastic nail set.
- Image intensifier.

Patient positioning

- Supine with the arm on the arm table.
- Prescrub the limb and set tourniquet at 100 mmHg above systolic blood pressure.
- Secure patient's head on the table as occasionally the head lies too close to the edge of the table and there is a risk of injury whilst manipulating the arm.

Draping and approach

- Upper limb drapes.
- Tourniquet not inflated routinely.
- Turn the table 45° away from the anaesthetic machine.
- Mark the subcutaneous border of the ulna 3 cm distal to the olecranon tip.
- Make a 2 cm incision to the bone (Fig. 3.16).

Fracture reduction

- In principle, increase the deformity and attempt to hitch the fragments to each other.
- In oblique/fragmented patterns of the middle-third, traction with the distal forearm in neutral is helpful.
- Under image intensification make the entry point in the proximal ulna and insert the appropriate size nail up to the fracture site. This allows some control of the proximal fragment to facilitate reduction (Fig. 3.17).

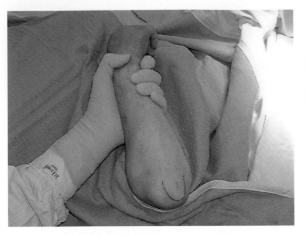

Fig. 3.16 Landmarks and entry point for ulnar flexible nails.

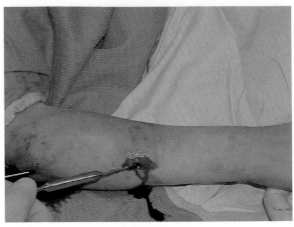

Fig. 3.18 Percutaneous fracture reduction.

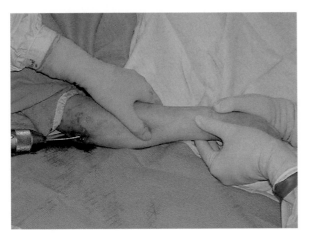

Fig. 3.17 Fracture reduction.

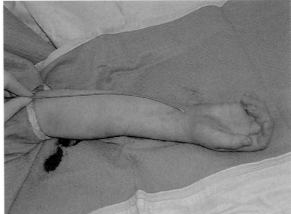

Fig. 3.19 Prebending the TENS.

- Decide early if closed reduction is feasible.
- It may be that closed methods are not adequate for the passage of the nail. Open reduction is performed with a limited direct approach over the fracture site. Insert a MacDonald in the fracture site and use it as a lever to reduce the fracture (Fig. 3.18).

Implant positioning

- Prior to the insertion, and under image intensification, the nail is prebent with the apex of the concavity at the level of the fracture site (Fig. 3.19).
- The nail is advanced with steady rotational movements. Avoid the use of the hammer as it may result in penetration of the opposite cortex.

- It is essential that the fragments be relatively opposed to each other for the nail passage to the distal fragment.
- The nail is advanced to the level of the metaphysis, 3 to 4 cm proximal to the physis. The protruding nail is cut and using the punch and the mallet is driven home. Ensure the nail does not cause damage to the distal physis.
- Leave the nail proud by 2 cm to facilitate removal.
- Ensure that there is no residual rotational deformity and obtain hard copies of the radiological images.

Closure

- Following irrigation the wound(s) is closed with absorbable material.
- An above-elbow back slab is applied.

Post-operative rehabilitation

- On day 1 the arm is placed in an above-elbow cast.
- The cast is maintained for 4 weeks (patient ≤ 10 years of age) to 6 weeks (≥10 years).

Follow up

- Following the 4 to 6 weeks, the cast is removed and a radiograph obtained.

- Do not routinely refer patients to physiotherapy.
- Parents and patients are advised to remain off contact or high-risk sports for a period of another 4 to 6 weeks.

Implant removal

- Routine removal of the nails no earlier than 6 and no later than 9 months from the time the fracture is healed.
- The procedure can be done as a day case.

Section III: Fractures of the distal ulna

Gregoris Kambouroglou

3.5 OPEN REDUCTION AND INTERNAL FIXATION (ORIF) FOR DISTAL ULNAR FRACTURES

Indications

- Displaced isolated fractures of the distal ulna.
- Fractures of the distal ulna associated with distal radius fractures.

Pre-operative assessment

Clinical assessment

- High-energy fractures, often with an open wound over the ulnar fracture.
- Ensure the injury is in isolation and the arm remains neurovascularly intact.
- Specifically test for ulnar nerve impairment.

Radiological assessment

- Ensure adequate views are available.
- In complex fractures of the distal radius (Fig. 3.20) a CT scan may be helpful to delineate the injury and assist in reconstruction.
- Displaced fractures must be reduced with simple means to avoid complications but also to facilitate further imaging.
- Problems are often encountered related to the amount of fragmentation and the quality of the bone in the head of the ulna.

Operative treatment

Anaesthesia

- General anaesthetic is preferred. In acute injuries the use of regional blocks is discouraged as it may mask

underlying pressure phenomena or compartment syndrome.

Operative equipment

- Use the mini-fragment set with 2.7 mm screws for fractures proximal to the distal radio-ulnar joint. Use a tension band for the most distal fractures.
- In associated fractures of the distal radius with shortening, the small **external fixator** is also used as a reduction aid.

Set up and positioning

- Hand table at 45°.
- Imager intensifier.
- Rolled up towel.
- Surgeon on the head side of the table (Fig. 3.21).
- Prescrub the limb.
- Antibiotic prophylaxis and tourniquet if there are no contraindications.
- Prepare the arm to the elbow as occasionally it may be necessary to obtain a graft from the olecranon.

Draping and approach

- Upper limb drapes.
- Mark the incision almost parallel to the superficial branches of the ulnar nerve alongside the ulnar border (Fig. 3.22).
- Ensure that the branches of the ulnar nerve are identified and protected at the distal part of the incision (Fig. 3.23).

Fracture reduction

- The aim of reduction is to restore length alignment and rotation.

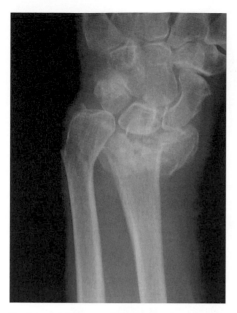

Fig. 3.20 High-energy distal forearm fracture.

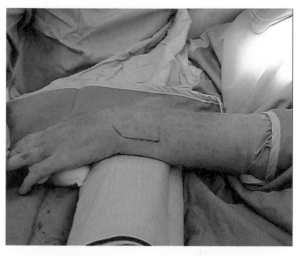

Fig. 3.22 Incision.

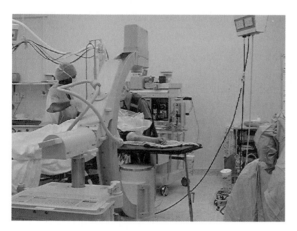

Fig. 3.21 Set up for distal forearm fracture surgery.

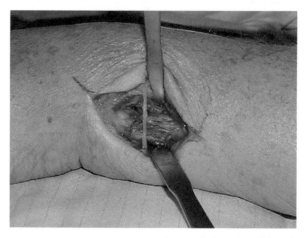

Fig. 3.23 Approach.

- In principle, avoid pointed reduction forceps as they may easily cut through the distal ulna and create more problems with bone stock and fixation.
- Reduction is often facilitated with traction with correction of the rotational deformity. An external fixator may be of use (see above).
- Use the indirect reduction technique whenever the fracture is stabilized with a plate.

Implant positioning

Plate fixation

- The 2.7 mm DCP is fashioned to a custom-made plate using the plate benders.

- The appropriate length of screw is estimated prior to the insertion of the plate (Fig. 3.24).
- The lateral cortex of the distal ulna is drilled twice with a 2 mm bit at the appropriate level using an image intensifier.
- Using small bone nibblers the entry point is widened and the 'blade' part of the plate is inserted. Thumb pressure is all that is needed in most cases.
- The proximal part of the plate is secured to the ulna using standard technique. It is worth attaching the plate to the shaft gently with a bone clamp to check that the fracture reduces or remains reduced and then secure the position with a screw.
- The predetermined-size screw is inserted via the plate through the distal hole of the 'blade'. The interlocking of the screw threads to the plate gives a surprisingly good fixation (Figs. 3.25, 3.26).

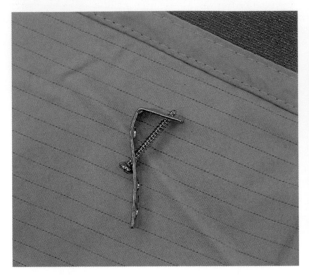

Fig. 3.24 Custom-made plate and strut screw measurement.

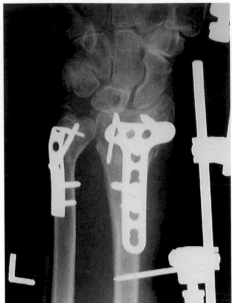

Fig. 3.26 Post-operative radiograph of the final construct using custom-made plating of the distal ulna.

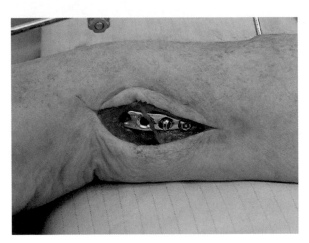

Fig. 3.25 Final construct. Custom-made plate of the distal ulna. Note the dorsal branch of the ulnar nerve.

Tension band fixation

- The fixation of the most distal ulnar fractures distal to the inferior margin of the DRUJ and fractures of the base of the styloid require more distal exposure and retinacular release.
- Depending on the fragment size 0.8 or 1.25 mm Kirschner wires are used.
- The wires are inserted in the distal fragment and are used as 'joysticks' to reduce and then transfix the fracture.
- A stainless steel suture or a thin wire is passed with the aid of an IV cannula under the triangular fibrocartilage complex (TFCC) complex and via a drill hole in the distal ulna.
- This is a fragile construct so the wire is tightened with care.
- The wires are cut and buried in a similar fashion to the TBW of the olecranon.

Closure

- It is imperative that the position of the fracture and the implants are checked with good-quality radiographs to ensure there is no penetration in the DRUJ or wrist joint.
- It is advisable to let the tourniquet down and achieve haemostasis.
- The wound is closed in layers with absorbable material for skin closure. Thick steri-strips are used longitudinally as dressings.
- In isolated fractures of the distal ulna, an above-elbow supination slab is applied.

Post-operative rehabilitation

- Depends on the fracture pattern and the stability of the final construct and associated injuries (fracture of the distal radius).

- For isolated distal ulnar fractures the wound is inspected in 48–72 h. A splint is fashioned with the forearm in supination but allowing flexion and extension of the wrist and elbow. The splint is maintained for 3 weeks.
- Radiographs are obtained on week 6 and if needed on week 12.
- Patients are discharged when there is evidence of clinical and radiological union and no ongoing problems with the hardware.

Implant removal

- Routing removal of the hardware is not routinely recommended although the subcutaneous position may cause discomfort and removal may be necessary.

Section I: Fractures of the proximal radius

Reinhard Meier

4.1 OPEN REDUCTION AND INTERNAL FIXATION OF RADIAL HEAD FRACTURES

Indications

- Open reduction and internal fixation (ORIF) for radial head fractures is used to stabilize displaced radial head fractures (Mason Type II) (Table 4.1).
- Non-displaced fractures (Mason Type I) are managed with early motion. To facilitate immediate motion aspiration of the joint fluid (haematoma) is recommended. Comminuted and displaced fractures (Mason Type III and IV) are best treated with complete early excision.

Pre-operative planning

Clinical assessment

- Pain localized in the affected elbow.
- Obliterated contour of the skin in the intracondylar recess ('soft spot').
- Assess and document neurovascular status of the arm.
- Careful examination of ligament stability is mandatory.

Radiological assessment

- Anteroposterior (AP) radiograph, a lateral view and a radial head view of the affected elbow (Fig. 4.1). A CT scan is helpful to demonstrate the exact fracture geometry. In children or in unclear situations (e.g. previous injury) the contralateral side should be evaluated.

Operative treatment

Anaesthesia

- Regional and/or general anaesthesia.
- At induction, administer prophylactic antibiotics according to local hospital protocol (e.g. 3rd generation cephalosporin).

Table and equipment

- Small-fragment instrumentation set or Herbert screw set – ensure the availability of the complete set of small compression screws.
- Radiolucent arm table.
- Image intensifier. Check for adequate visualization in 2 planes prior to draping.

Table set up

- The instrumentation is set up on the side of the operation.
- Image intensifier is from the front side of the arm table.

Patient positioning

- Supine, supinated arm extended on arm table.

Surgical approach

- Prepare the skin over elbow, forearm and hand with usual antiseptic solutions (aqueous/alcoholic povidone–iodine).

Practical Procedures in Orthopaedic Trauma Surgery: A Trainee's Companion, ed. Peter V. Giannoudis and Hans-Christoph Pape.
Published by Cambridge University Press. © Cambridge University Press 2006.

Table 4.1. **Mason–Johnson classification of radial head and neck fractures**

I	Non-displaced
II	Minimally displaced with depression, angulation and impaction
III	Comminuted and displaced
IV	Radial head fractures associated with dislocation of the elbow

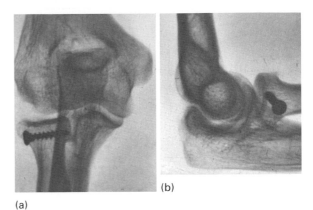

(a)

(b)

Fig. 4.3 a,b Screw fixation of radial head fracture.

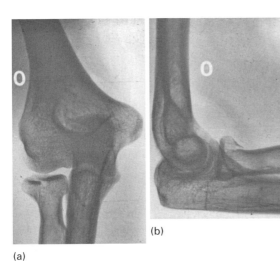

(a)

(b)

Fig. 4.1 (a) Anteroposterior and (b) lateral view.

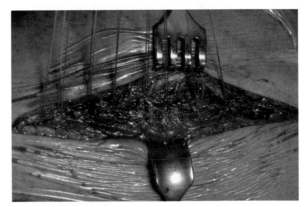

Fig. 4.4 Capsule repair with Vicryl.

- Evacuate haematoma.
- Rotate the forearm to expose the fragment.

Implant positioning

- Temporary fragment fixation can be made with a 0.45 K-wire if necessary.
- Ream, determine the screw length and reaming distance using the measuring device and tap the bone if no self-tapping screws are used.
- One or two small fragment screws (2.0) are inserted perpendicular to the fracture (Fig. 4.3 a,b).
- Take care that the head of the screw is countersunk and that the screw tip does not violate the opposite cortex. Correct positioning can be verified by rotation of the forearm.
- Obtain final radiographs in both AP and lateral planes (Fig.4.3 a,b).
- Check for stability of the joint.

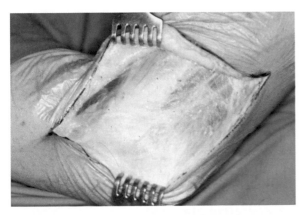

Fig. 4.2 Radial approach to the elbow joint.

- Make a longitudinal or s-shape incision proximally on the lateral humeral epicondyle (Fig. 4.2).
- Find the interval between the anconeus and the extensor carpi ulnaris distally.
- The capsule and anular ligament is incised proximal of the ulna and lateral of the ulno-humeral ligament.

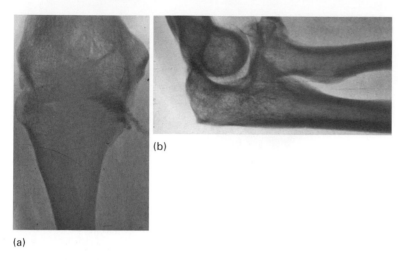

(b)

(a)

Fig. 4.5 (a) Anteroposterior and (b) lateral view.

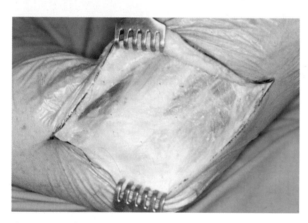

Fig. 4.6 Lateral approach to the elbow.

Closure

- Irrigate the wound thoroughly and achieve haemostasis.
- Repair the annular ligament and capsule (No. 3 PDS/Vicryl) (Fig. 4.4).
- Skin closure – monofilament non-absorbable suture or absorbable suture placed in the subcutis.

Post-operative rehabilitation

- Elevation of the operated arm and active movement of the finger.
- Routine radiographs within 24 hours.
- Immobilization in 90° of flexion and neutral rotation.
- Motion is begun as soon as possible and as determined by associated injuries.

Outpatient follow up

- Review at 6 weeks and 3 months with radiographs of the elbow.
- Discontinue as soon as clinical and radiological signs show evidence of fracture healing.

4.2 EXCISION OF RADIAL HEAD

Indications

Excision of radial head is indicated in the following situations:

(a) Comminuted radial head fracture (Mason Type III) (Table 4.1).
(b) Mason Type II fractures if open reduction and internal fixation is unachievable.
(c) Consider prosthetic replacement in complicated radial head fractures (Essex–Lopresti, fracture of coronoid, Monteggia, lateral ulnar collateral ligament disruption, Mason Type IV).

Pre-operative planning

Clinical assessment

- Localized pain in the affected elbow.
- Obliterated contour of the skin in the intracondylar recessus ('soft spot').
- Assess and document neurovascular status of the arm.
- Careful examination of ligament stability must be made.

Radiological assessment

- Anteroposterior (AP) radiograph, a lateral view and a radial head view of the affected elbow to demonstrate the fracture geometry (Fig. 4.5). In children or in unclear situations (e.g. previous injury), the contralateral side should be evaluated as well. In multifragmental fractures CT scan is helpful.

Operative treatment

Anaesthesia

- Regional and/or general anaesthesia.
- At induction, administer prophylactic antibiotics according to local hospital protocol (e.g. 3rd generation cephalosporin).

Table and equipment

- Small-fragment instrumentation set and oscillating saw.
- Radiolucent arm table.
- Image intensifier.

Table set up

- The instrumentation is set up on the side of the operation.
- Image intensifier is from the front side of the arm table. Check for adequate visualization in 2 planes prior to draping.

Patient positioning

- Supine, supinated arm extended on arm table.

Surgical approach

- Prepare the skin of the arm using usual antiseptic solutions (aqueous/alcoholic povidone–iodine).
- Make a longitudinal or s-shape incision proximally on the lateral humeral epicondyle (Fig. 4.6).
- Find the interval between the anconeus and the extensor carpi ulnaris distally.
- Incise the capsule and the anular ligament proximal to the ulna and lateral to the ulno-humeral ligament.
- Evacuate haematoma.
- Rotate the forearm and expose the radial head (Fig. 4.7).

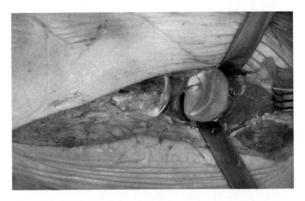
Fig. 4.7 Exposition of the radial head.

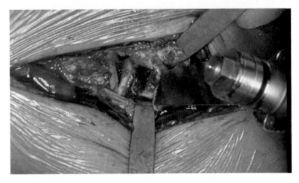
Fig. 4.8 Oblique osteotomy at the radial head.

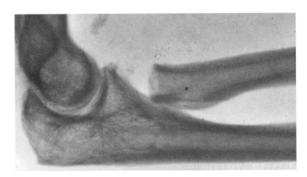
Fig. 4.9 Lateral view of radial head excision.

- Perform an oblique osteotomy at the radial head with the oscillating saw at the level of the anular ligament (Fig. 4.8).
- Remove all fragments carefully.
- Obtain final radiographs in both the AP and lateral planes (Fig. 4.9).

Closure

- Irrigate the wound thoroughly and achieve haemostasis.

- Repair the lateral ligament complex and capsule (No. 3 PDS/Vicryl).
- Skin closure – monofilament non-absorbable suture or absorbable suture placed in the subcuticular layer.
- Check for stability especially at the distal radio-ulnar joint by exerting an axial load on the radius at the wrist.

Post-operative rehabilitation

- Elevation of the operated arm and active movement of the finger.
- Routine radiographs within 24 hours.

- Immobilization in 90° of flexion and neutral rotation in a cast splint for 2 weeks.
- Motion is begun as soon as possible out of the splint and as determined by associated injuries.

Outpatient follow up

- Review at 6 weeks and 3 months with radiographs of the elbow.
- Discontinue follow up as soon as clinical and radiological evidence show stability and full range of movements.

Section II: Fractures of the radial shaft

Christopher C. Tzioupis, Peter V. Giannoudis (4.3)
and Brian W. Scott (4.4)

4.3 OPEN REDUCTION AND INTERNAL FIXATION (ORIF): ANTERIOR APPROACH

Indications

- Displaced isolated fracture of the radius (rotational deformity).
- Open fractures.
- Combined fractures of radius and ulna.
- According to AO/Muller Classification 22-A3.2, 22-B2.2, 22-C2.2.

Pre-operative planning

Clinical assessment

- Obtain a careful history, including the mechanism of injury.
- Determine concurrent ipsilateral injuries to the upper arm, wrist and hand.
- Assess and document neurovascular status of the arm: medial, radial, ulnar, and posterior interosseous nerves; and axillary, brachial, radial, ulnar pulses.
- Evaluate the soft tissue compartments of the forearm.
- Look for signs indicative of ischaemia.

Radiological assessment

- High-quality AP and lateral views of the forearm (Fig. 4.10 a,b).
- The radiographs should include the elbow and wrist joints.
- Exclude associated articular fractures or specific fracture types such as Monteggia or Galeazzi.

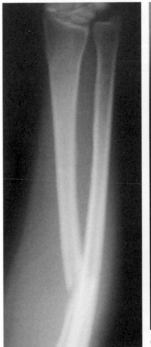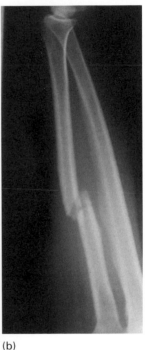

(a)   (b)

Fig. 4.10 (a) Anteroposterior and (b) lateral pre-operative radiographs of radius shaft fracture.

Timing of surgery

- Early operative treatment permits decompression of the fracture haematoma and reduction of fracture fragments, minimizing soft tissue trauma.
- Surgery can be delayed to allow either systemic or local conditions to improve.

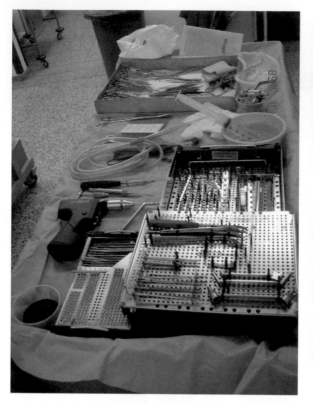

Fig. 4.11 Table instrumentation.

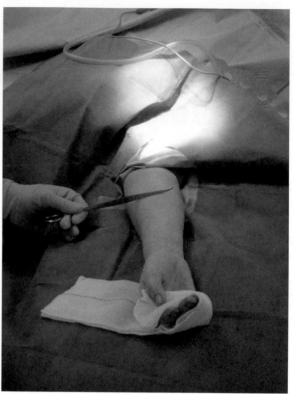

Fig. 4.13 The forearm is draped free with single use U-drapes over the side of the table.

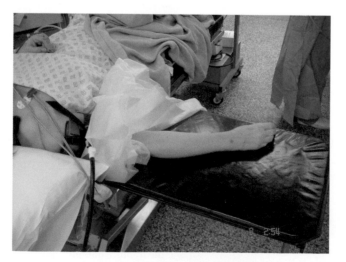

Fig. 4.12 The patient is supine with the arm over a radiolucent hand table.

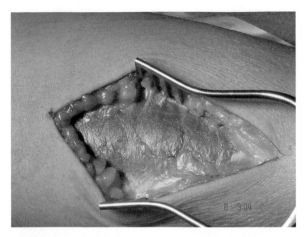

Fig. 4.14 Make a straight skin incision and reflect the skin edges. Take care not to damage intact superficial veins.

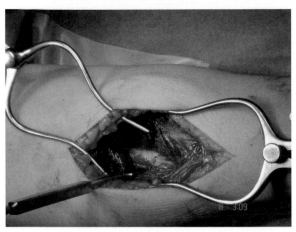

Fig. 4.17 After deep-dissection exposure of the fracture plane.

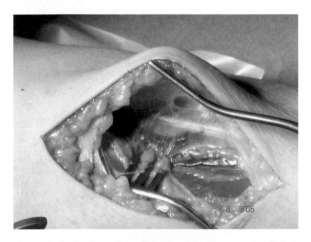

Fig. 4.15 The fascia on the radial side of the flexor carpi radialis is released, exposing the deep tissue.

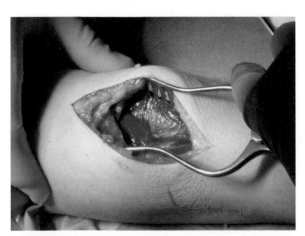

Fig. 4.16 Exposure of the pronator quadratus, the flexor digitorum sublimes (FDS) and flexor policis longus (FPL).

Operative treatment

Anaesthesia

- At induction administration of prophylactic antibiotics as per local hospital protocol.
- General anaesthesia is preferable. Avoid regional anaesthetic/block in acute injuries as they mask symptoms indicating compartment syndrome in the immediate post-operative period.
- Apply a tourniquet to the upper arm if not contraindicated (situations in which the soft tissue envelope is extremely traumatized).

Table and equipment

- AO small-fragment set 3.5 mm.
- Standard osteosynthesis set as per local hospital protocol (Fig. 4.11).
- Ensure availability of the preplanned plate length.
- Fluoroscopy is necessary for intraoperative imaging.

Table set up

- The instrumentation is set up on the side of the operation.
- Image intensifier is from the ipsilateral side.

Patient positioning

- The patient is supine with the arm abducted and supinated over a radiolucent hand table (Fig. 4.12).

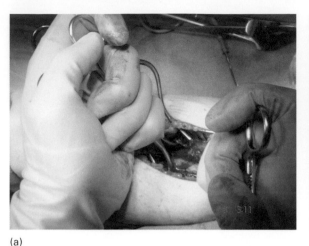

(a)

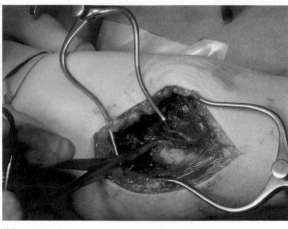

(b)

Fig. 4.18 a,b Reduction of the fracture with the use of two clamps restoring length and alignment.

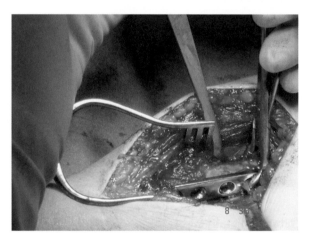

Fig. 4.19 Placing of the appropriate dynamic compression plate and holding it in place with clamps.

Draping and surgical approach

- Prepare the whole upper extremity with usual antiseptic solutions (aqueous/alcoholic povidone–iodine).
- The forearm is draped free with single use U-drapes over the side of the table (Fig. 4.13).
- If bone grafting is anticipated prepare the ipsilateral iliac crest as well.
- Draw the skin incision over the volar aspect of the forearm with a skin marker.
- Landmarks: groove between brachioradialis and distal biceps tendon proximally and styloid process of radius distally.

- Make a straight skin incision and reflect the skin edges.
- Take care not to damage intact superficial veins (Fig. 4.14).
- Identify the flexor carpi radialis (FCR) tendon ulna ward.
- Incise the subcutaneous fascia between the FCR and the brachioradialis.
- Identify and protect the anterior cutaneous nerve of the forearm and the superficial radial nerve that run along the brachioradialis muscle.
- Retract FCR to the ulnar side and the brachioradialis radial ward (Fig. 4.15).
- Now the pronator quadratus, the flexor digitorum sublimes (FDS) and flexor policis longus (FPL) are exposed (Fig. 4.16).
- Subperiosteally elevate the FPL and pronator quadratus and strip them towards the ulna.
- Proximally release FDS, FDP and pronator muscles from the volar radial aspect (Fig. 4.17).

Fracture reduction

- The aim is to restore length, alignment and rotation.
- Limit periosteal stripping to a minimum (1 mm around on each fragment).
- Expose the fracture ends using small Weber clamps and right angle retractors.
- If a butterfly fragment exists, fix it with a lag screw back to one of the fracture ends.
- Deliver the bones jointly, accentuate the deformity and rotate and fit the bones together.

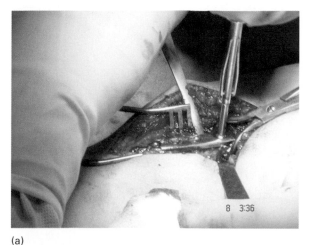
(a)

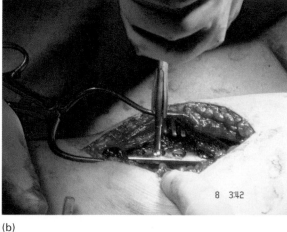
(b)

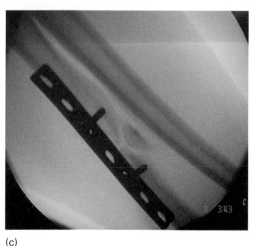
(c)

Fig. 4.20 a,b,c Using the offset drill guide, place the first cortical screw in a neutral position without inserting it completely into the plate. On the opposite side of the fracture place a second screw eccentrically in a similar fashion. By compressing these two screws against the plate the fracture is translated and compressed.

- Push them back into the wound obtaining alignment and rotation (Fig. 4.18 a,b).

Implant insertion

- The plate must be long enough to neutralize the torsional forces (at least 6 cortices in each main fragment).
- It is appropriate to prebend the plate to avoid developing a fracture gap in the contralateral side.
- Place the appropriate dynamic compression plate and hold it in place with clamps (Fig. 4.19).
- In fractures with extensive fragmentation an indirect reduction technique can be used with a long plate anchored distally and a push–pull technique.
- Use intraoperative fluoroscopic views to verify maintenance of reduction.

- Using the offset drill guide, place the first cortical screw in a neutral position without inserting it completely into the plate.
- On the opposite side of the fracture place a second screw eccentrically in a similar fashion.
- By compressing these two screws against the plate the fracture is translated and compressed (Fig. 4.20 a,b,c).
- Continue by placing the rest of the screws (Fig. 4.21 a,b,c,d,e).
- Use intraoperative fluoroscopic views of the whole forearm to assess location of the plate, length and positioning of the screws and reduction accuracy (Fig. 4.22).
- Clinically assess alignment and rotation, pronating and supinating the forearm. Confirm with fluoroscopic control images.
- Prior to closure, assessment and documentation of the radial pulse is mandatory (Fig. 4.23 a,b).

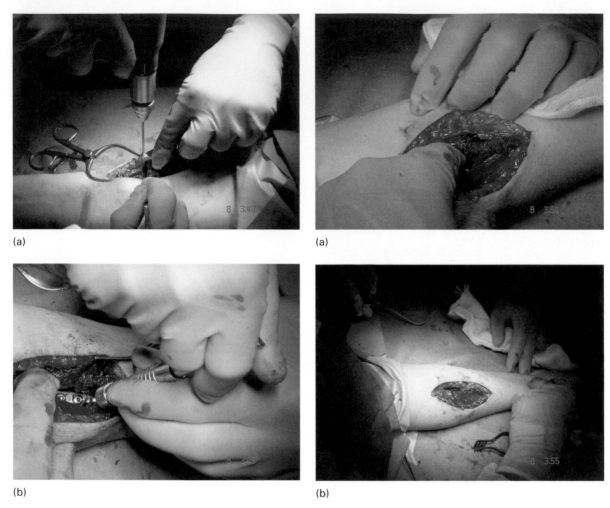

(a)

(a)

(b)

(b)

Fig. 4.21 a,b Insertion of the rest of the screws.

Fig. 4.23 a,b Prior to closure assessment and documentation of the radial pulse is mandatory.

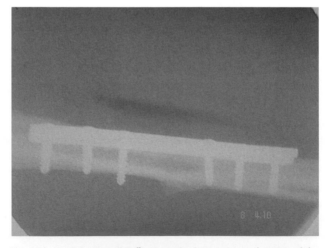

Fig. 4.22 Use intraoperative fluoroscopic views to assess location of the plate, length and positioning of the screws and reduction accuracy.

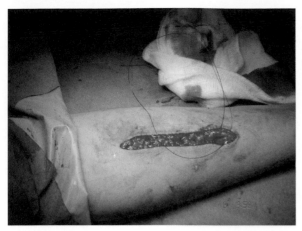

Fig. 4.24

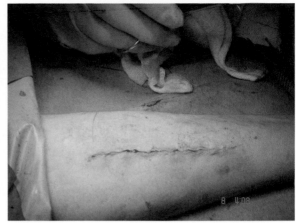

Fig. 4.25

Figs. 4.24 and 4.25 Closure in two layers with a subcuticular absorbable (3/0 PDS) material for the skin.

- If bone grafting is necessary, place it away from the interosseous border.

Closure

- Release the tourniquet and perform haemostasis.
- Reattach only the supinator proximally and the pronator distally.
- Do not reattach the deep fascia.
- Continue in 2 layers with a subcuticular absorbable (3/0 PDS) material for the skin. (Fig. 4.24, Fig. 4.25)
- Thick steri-strips can be used as dressings with dry gauze and cotton wool.
- Apply an above-elbow back slab.

Post-operative treatment

- The arm is elevated using a Bradford sling.
- Assess neurovascular status of the forearm in the immediate post-operative period.
- Finger motion is encouraged on the day after surgery.
- Inspect the wound at 48 hours.
- Remove the plaster splint in 3–5 days and encourage shoulder, elbow, forearm and wrist motion.

Outpatient follow up

- Review in clinic with routine X-ray evaluation at 6 and 12 weeks and after 1 year.

- Advise the patient to perform most daily activities 6 weeks after surgery, avoiding sports and heavy lifting.
- Removal of the implant is not mandatory.

4.4 ELASTIC INTRAMEDULLARY NAILING FOR DIAPHYSEAL FOREARM FRACTURES IN CHILDREN

Introduction

Angulated and displaced diaphyseal fractures are unforgiving injuries in both children and adults. Whilst bayonet apposition may be accepted and will remodel in children, angular deformities are poorly tolerated in both children and adults and tend not to remodel irrespective of age. As a guideline it has been suggested that a 15° angulation is acceptable under 9 years and 1° if older. For this reason control of alignment of forearm fractures is important and this is particularly difficult in this type of fracture which is inherently unstable.

In children younger than 6–7 years, with experience and skill with plaster, a satisfactory reduction can be achieved and maintained in most cases. Older children should be treated along the same lines as adults.

Open reduction and fixation with metal plates is an established and popular treatment for this type of injury but it has the disadvantage of a wide exposure and a very visible surgical wound(s).

Over the last decade intramedullary stabilization using thin steel or titanium nails has become increasingly

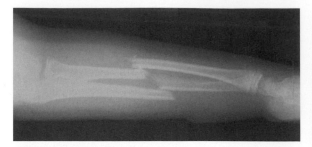

Fig. 4.26 Diaphyseal fractures.

popular. It has the advantage of limited exposure to insert the wire, and usually the fracture does not need to be exposed. With experience it is also a fairly quick procedure, sometimes taking as little as 20 minutes.

Indications/contradictions

- Suitable for children between 7–15 years. In younger children the medullary cavity tends to be narrow and the insertion technique is technically more difficult. In adults, where bone healing is slower than in children, the rigidity of open reduction and plating is a significant advantage in the early rehabilitation. With time the indications for intramedullary nailing will probably extend.
- Diaphyseal fractures (Fig. 4.26). Metaphyseal fractures of the radius and ulna can both be treated satisfactorily with other techniques such as plastering or wiring.
- Radial neck fractures. There is a well-described technique for this particular injury which is an extension of the technique for radial wiring. The reader is referred to other texts for further information.
- Isolated diaphyseal fractures. This technique is appropriate for Monteggia and Galeazzi-type injuries.
- Malunion/non-union. Where an open precision osteotomy is required the likelihood is that the exposure would permit plating also. The medullary cavity is likely to be at least partially obliterated and passage of the wire is likely to be very difficult.

Patient positioning

- Supine on operating table (Fig. 4.27).
- Hand table.
- Tourniquet.

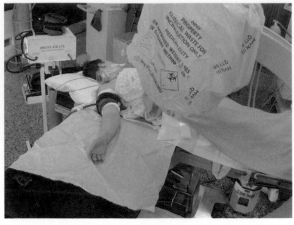

Fig. 4.27 Patient positioned supine.

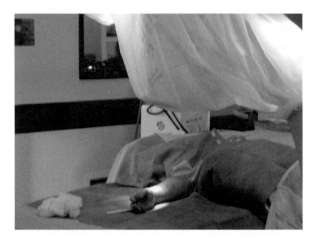

Fig. 4.28 Application of exclusion drapes to upper arm, exposing the whole of the upper limb.

- Exclusion drapes to upper arm, exposing the whole of the upper limb (Fig. 4.28).
- Pre-operative broad spectrum antibiotics.

Surgical technique

- Use a nail diameter of approximately 40% of the narrowest diameter of medullary cavity. Usual nail diameters in children aged 7–11 years: 2 mm; 11–16 years: 2.5 mm.
- Select length based on full length of bone segment from growth plate to growth plate (Fig. 4.29).
- Use the image intensifier to mark growth plates and skin incisions.

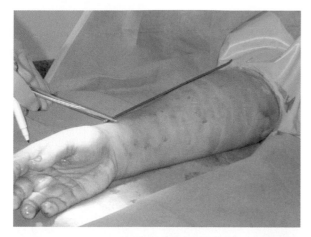

Fig. 4.29 Select length based on full length of bone segment from growth plate to growth plate.

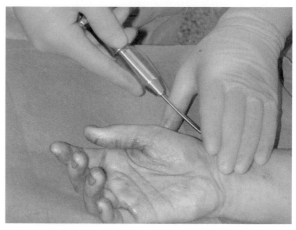

Fig. 4.31 Hold the nail in a Jacobs chuck and advance, introducing a progressive bend concave laterally, i.e. against the normal bow in the radius.

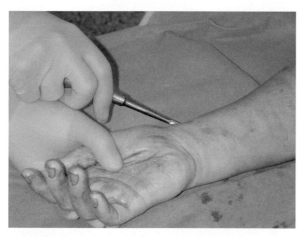

Fig. 4.30 Use an awl or drill to perforate the cortex approximately 2 cm proximal to the growth plate.

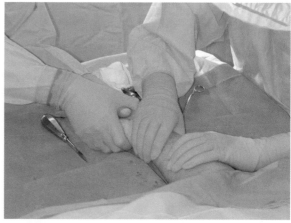

Fig. 4.32 Progress the tip of the wire to the level of the fracture site. The assistant attempts to reduce the fracture by gripping the forearm firmly with both hands.

- Make a 1–2 cm incision over the lateral distal radius. Take care with incision and dissect bluntly to avoid superficial radial nerve damage.
- Use an awl or drill to perforate the cortex approximately 2 cm proximal to the growth plate (Fig. 4.30). If a drill is used, use one that is 1 mm wider than the nail size.
- Bend the tip of the wire slightly to facilitate entry into the medullary cavity. Too much of a bend will make it difficult to pass across the fracture site.
- Hold the nail in a Jacobs chuck and advance, introducing a progressive bend concave laterally, i.e. against the normal bow in the radius (Fig. 4.31).

- Progress the tip of the wire to the level of the fracture site. The assistant attempts to reduce the fracture by gripping the forearm firmly with both hands (Fig. 4.32).
- Manipulate the nail across the fracture through a combination of feel and periodic image intensification, using a hammer as necessary.
- Advance the wire to the proximal metaphysis under image intensifier control.
- For the ulna, two entry sites are possible. The first approach is distal to the growth plate through the radial border of the proximal ulna. The second approach is

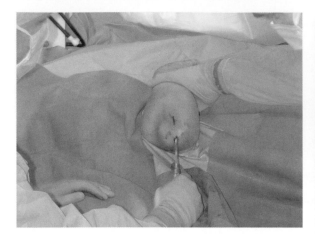

Fig. 4.33 For the ulna, two entry sites are possible. The first approach is distal to the growth plate through the radial border of the proximal ulna. The second approach is directly through the tip of the elbow and across the growth plate.

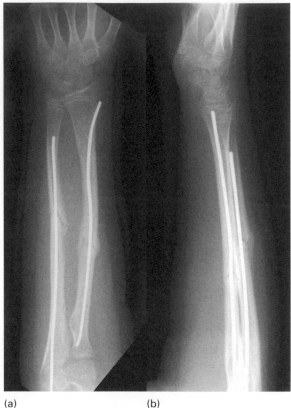

(a)   (b)

Fig. 4.35 a,b X ray at 6 weeks.

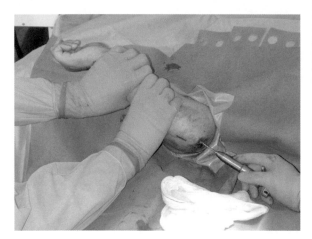

Fig. 4.34 Advance nail to the level of the fracture. Reduce fracture closed as for the radius.

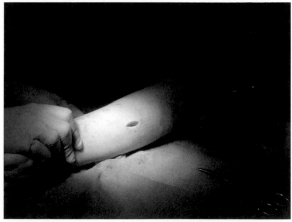

directly through the tip of the elbow and across the growth plate (Fig. 4.33). It is probably better to avoid transgressing the growth plate in younger children.

- Incision and perforation of the cortex as for the radius.
- Slightly bend the tip of the wire unless a direct trans-olecranon approach is adopted.
- Advance the nail to the level of the fracture. Reduce fracture closed as for the radius (Fig. 4.34).
- Manipulate the wire across the fracture and advance under image intensifier guidance to the distal meta-physic.
- Returning to the radius, firmly clamp the nail in the chuck and rotate the wire through 180° to restore the

Fig. 4.36 If the nail cannot be advanced across the fracture site despite repeated attempts then open reduction will be needed. This is usually possible through a 2–3 cm incision following the planes of a Henry incision for the radius and the direct approach for the ulna.

normal bow. If the end of the wire requires trimming do so to leave 1 cm of wire protruding and leave lying adjacent to the bone. Avoid wire tenting the skin. Close the skin over the wire.

- Although the ulna is a straight bone there will be a tendency to some slight radial bowing of the ulna unless a counter bow is introduced convex towards the ulnar side.
- Trim and bury the tip of the nail. Care is needed to avoid tenting of the skin using a direct trans-olecranon approach.
- Apply a below-elbow back slab.

Post-operative care

- Little post-operative splintage is required. It is reasonable to use a below-elbow back slab for 2 weeks and a sling for possibly a little longer.
- X-ray showing full length of forearm bones, wrist and elbow.

- X-ray at 6 weeks (Fig. 4.35 a,b). Assuming healing to be well advanced, permit an increase in normal activities and arrange a 6-month review to plan removal of wires shortly thereafter, if X-rays demonstrate sound union.

Tips and pitfalls

- If the nail cannot be advanced across the fracture site despite repeated attempts then open reduction will be needed. This is usually possible through a 2–3 cm incision following the planes of a Henry incision for the radius and the direct approach for the ulna (Fig. 4.36).
- Single bone fixation is sometimes advocated.
- It is generally recommended that the more displaced fracture be nailed first.

Implant Removal

- Nail should be removed between 6 and 9 months after insertion.

Section III: Fractures of the distal radius

Peter V. Giannoudis (4.5), Doug Campbell (4.6) and Reinhard Meier (4.7, 4.8)

4.5 OPEN REDUCTION AND INTERNAL FIXATION (ORIF) FOR DISTAL RADIUS FRACTURES: VOLAR APPROACH

Indications

- Displaced, irreducible extra-articular fractures (A3).
- Unstable, partial intra-articular fractures (B1, B2, B3), or complete (C2, C3).
- Fractures requiring bone grafting.
- Palmarly displaced short oblique fractures.
- Volar Barton's.
- Fractures with primary instability.

Pre-operative planning

Clinical assessment

- Mechanism of injury: grading from low- to high-velocity trauma.
- Typical deformity, swelling, tenderness.
- Evaluate neurovascular status of the hand.
- Assess soft tissue damage.
- Evaluate patient for age, hand dominance, occupation, and level of activity.
- Check for associated ligamentous lesions of fractures of carpal bones.

Radiological assessment

- High-quality anteroposterior and lateral radiographs (Fig. 4.37a,b).
- Oblique films (45° pronated and supinated).
- Assess degree of fragment displacement, quality of bone, whether the fracture is intra-articular or extra-articular, direction of displacement, metaphyseal comminution.
- CT scan if the diagnosis is not clear in plain radiographs.

Timing of surgery

- Immediately when the fracture is open or primary compression of the median nerve is present.
- After 5–6 days if there is important soft tissue swelling (after reduction of the initial displacement and immobilization in a plaster splint).

Operative treatment

Anaesthesia

- At induction, administration of prophylactic antibiotics as per local hospital protocol.
- General anaesthesia is preferable. Avoid a regional anaesthetic/block in acute injuries as it masks symptoms indicating compartment syndrome in the immediate post-operative period.
- Apply a tourniquet to the upper arm if not contraindicated (situations in which the soft tissue envelope is extremely traumatized).

Table and equipment

- AO small-fragment set 3.5 mm or Jupiter plating system (Fig. 4.38).
- Standard osteosynthesis set as per local hospital protocol.
- Fluoroscopy is necessary for intraoperative imaging.

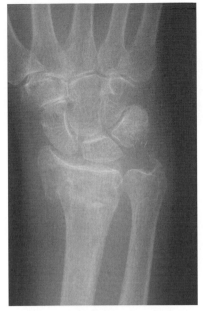

(a)

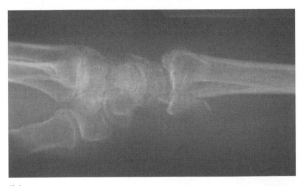

(b)

Fig. 4.37 Anteroposterior and lateral views of a distal radius fracture.

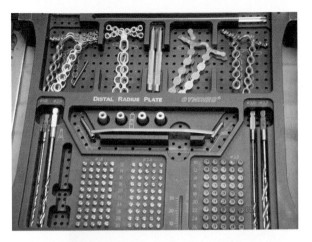

Fig. 4.38 Jupiter plating system.

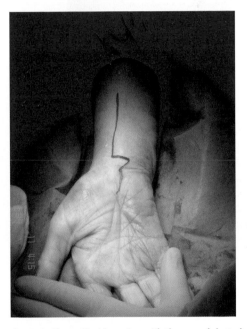

Fig. 4.39 The patient is supine with the arm abducted and supinated over a radiolucent hand table.

Table set up

- The instrumentation is set up on the side of the operation.
- Image intensifier is from the ipsilateral side.

Patient positioning

- The patient is supine with the arm abducted and supinated over a radiolucent hand table (Fig. 4.39).
- Apply a rolled towel under the wrist.

Draping and surgical approach

- Prepare the whole upper extremity with the usual antiseptic solutions (aqueous/alcoholic povidone–iodine).
- The hand is draped free with single use U-drapes over the side of the table.
- Make an incision over the distal portion of flexor carpi radialis (FCR).

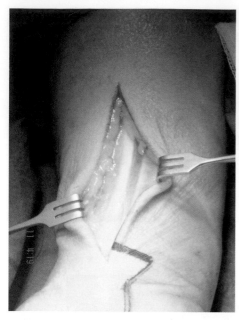

Fig. 4.40 An incision is made over the distal portion of flexor carpi radialis (FCR) going through the subcutaneous tissue to the palmar sheath of FCR.

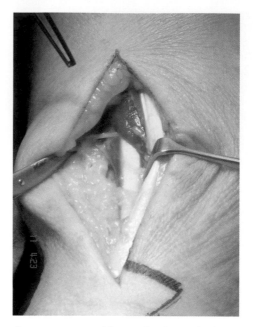

Fig. 4.41 Exposure of flexor policis longus (FPL) by incising the posterior sheath of FCR.

- Incise the subcutaneous tissue and the palmar sheath of FCR (Fig. 4.40).
- Expose flexor policis longus (FPL) by incising the posterior sheath of FCR (Fig. 4.41).
- Retract FPL and the radial artery radial ward.
- Expose pronator quadratus by retracting the median nerve and the extrinsic flexor tendons ulna ward (Fig. 4.42).
- Incise along its radial insertion.
- Elevate pronator quadratus from the periosteum of the distal radius and expose the fracture (Fig. 4.43).

Fracture reduction

- Identify any interposed intra-articular fragments before reduction.
- Apply a rolled towel under the wrist.
- Hyperextend the wrist over the towel and achieve reduction.
- Evaluate reduction with fluoroscopic control images.

Implant positioning

- Place a prebent Jupiter volar plate in a buttress position (Fig. 4.44).

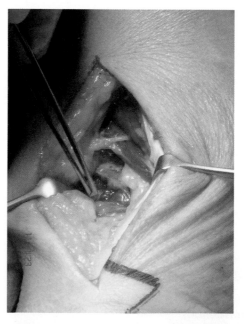

Fig. 4.42 Exposure of the pronator quadratus by retracting the median nerve and the extrinsic flexor tendons ulna ward.

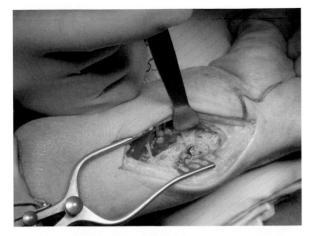

Fig. 4.43 Elevate pronator quadratus from the periosteum of the distal radius and expose the fracture.

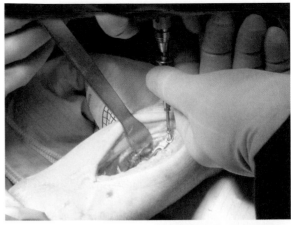

(a)

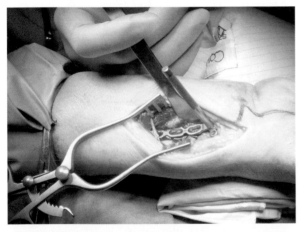

Fig. 4.44 After achieving reduction with hyperextension over an under-wrist towel place a prebent Jupiter volar plate in a buttress position.

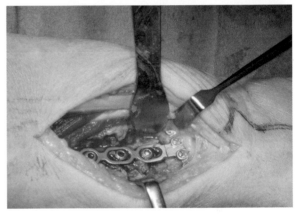

(b)

Fig. 4.46 a,b Securing the plate by placing the rest of the screws.

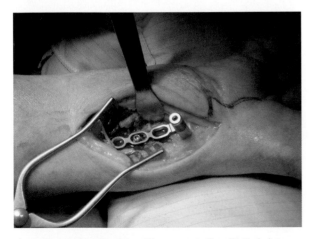

Fig. 4.45 Securing the plate with a screw in the elliptical plate hole.

- Confirm that the plate is adjacent to the distal fracture rim.
- Using the offset drill guide first drill a hole in the oval plate hole of the plate stem.
- Identify the screw length with the depth gauge.
- Prepare the screw hole with a 3.5 mm tap.
- Secure the plate with a screw in the elliptical plate hole (Fig. 4.45).
- Ensure reduction maintenance with fluoroscopic control.
- Secure the plate by placing the rest of the screws in the same manner (Fig. 4.46 a,b).
- Prior to closure clinically assess flexion and extension of the wrist joint.

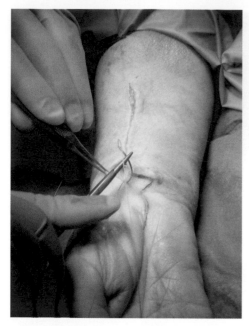

Fig. 4.47 Continue in 2 layers with a subcuticular absorbable (3/0 PDS) material for the skin.

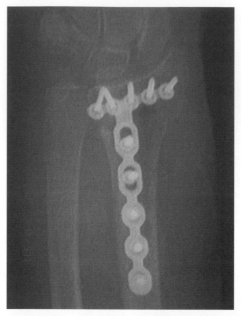

(a)

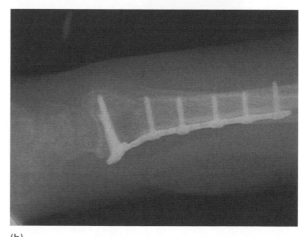

(b)

Fig. 4.48 a,b Post-operative AP and lateral radiographs.

Closure

- Release the tourniquet and perform haemostasis.
- Irrigate the wound.
- Avoid reapproximating pronator quadratus in case of existing tension.
- Do not repair the fascia.
- Continue in 2 layers with a subcuticular absorbable (3/0 PDS) material for the skin (Fig. 4.47 a,b).
- Thick steri-strips can be used as dressings with dry gauze and cotton wool.
- Apply a posterior sling with the forearm in neutral rotation.

Post-operative treatment

- The arm is elevated using a Bradford sling.
- Assess and document neurovascular status of the hand.
- Obtain AP and lateral post-operative radiographs (Fig. 4.48 a,b).
- Finger motion is encouraged on the day after surgery.
- Inspect the wound at 48 hours.
- Remove the plaster splint in 3–5 days and encourage shoulder, elbow, forearm and wrist motion.

Outpatient follow up

- Review at the clinic in 2, 6, and 12 weeks, with radiographs on arrival.
- Retain the splint for 3 weeks after surgery.
- After that encourage the patient to perform finger motion exercises, wrist flexion–extension and circumduction, as well as strengthening exercises using a sponge.

Complications

- Infection.
- Malunion.
- Non-union.
- Median neuropathy.
- Post-traumatic arthritis.

Implant removal

- Rarely required.

4.6 OPEN REDUCTION AND INTERNAL FIXATION (ORIF) FOR DISTAL RADIUS FRACTURES: DORSAL APPROACH

Indications

Dorsal plating of distal radial fractures is performed for:

(a) Comminuted, dorsally displaced intra-articular fractures.
(b) Unstable dorsally displaced extra-articular fractures untreatable by less invasive methods.
(c) Early malunion.

Pre-operative assessment

Clinical assessment

- Assess vascularity of the hand.
- Assess for evidence of neural compromise – particularly in the median nerve distribution.
- Assessment of the condition of the skin in the area of proposed incision.
- Assessment of oedema and compartment syndrome.

Radiological assessment

- Anteroposterior and lateral radiographs of the wrist and elbow (if indicated).
- Assess radial length, radial inclination, palmar inclination and intercarpal areas.
- Pay particular attention to *both* joints in the wrist: the radiocarpal and distal radioulnar joints (DRUJ) (Figs. 4.49, 4.50).

Operative treatment

Anaesthesia

- General or regional (axillary, supra- or infraclavicular block).

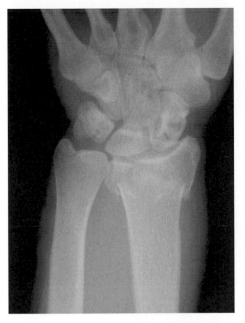

Fig. 4.49 Anteroposterior radiograph of fracture.

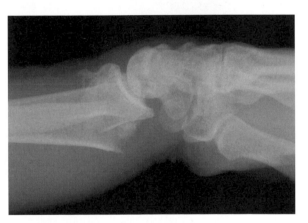

Fig. 4.50 Lateral radiograph of fracture.

- Intravenous dose of antibiotic as prophylaxis prior to inflation of tourniquet.

Tourniquet

- Well-padded upper arm cuff inflated to 250 mmHg.
- Plastic exclusion drape to prevent any soaking of padding by skin preparation.

Equipment

- Distal radial plating system of choice with full selection of implants and screws.

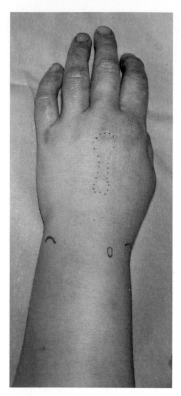

Fig. 4.51 Surface marking of radiocarpal joint level
and Lister's tubercle.

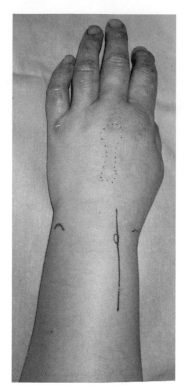

Fig. 4.52 Surface marking for incision.

- Radiolucent hand table securely fastened to operating table.
- Image intensifier or mini C-arm fluoroscan.

Operating room set up

- The arm must lie centrally on the hand table.
- Surgeon is best seated cephalad, assistant seated at patient's axilla, scrub nurse seated at the distal end of the affected limb.
- Image intensifier or mini C-arm is brought in from the assistant's side at the appropriate time.

Draping and surgical approach

- Skin is prepared from fingertips to tourniquet with aqueous antiseptic solution.
- Entire limb from tourniquet distally visible and mobile during the procedure.
- A single use drape with expandable aperture for limb recommended.
- Dorsal longitudinal incision based on Lister's tubercle (Figs. 4.51, 4.52).

- Raising of thick skin flaps to level of extensor retinaculum.
- Identification of 3rd extensor compartment containing tendon of extensor pollicis longus (EPL) – immediately ulnar to Lister's tubercle (Fig. 4.53).
- Opening of 3rd extensor compartment along its entire length.
- Tendon of EPL is lifted out of its compartment and protected to the side.
- The floor of the 3rd compartment is cut directly onto bone, and sub periosteal flaps are raised from the 2nd to the 4th extensor compartments (Fig. 4.54).
- If necessary, the radiocarpal joint is opened for direct visualization of the intrinsic ligaments of the proximal carpal row.

Fracture reduction

- The radial length is restored and held with a temporary 1.2 mm Kirschner wire placed through the tip of the radial styloid (Fig. 4.55).
- The articular pieces of both wrist joints are elevated and reduced.

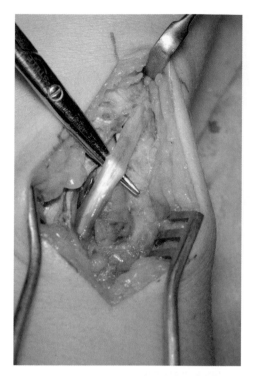

Fig. 4.53 Extensor pollicis longus lifted out of the 3rd compartment.

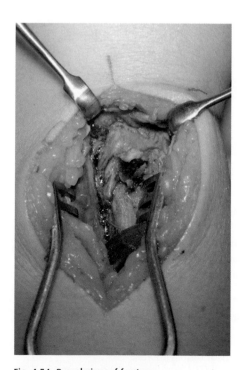

Fig. 4.54 Dorsal view of fracture.

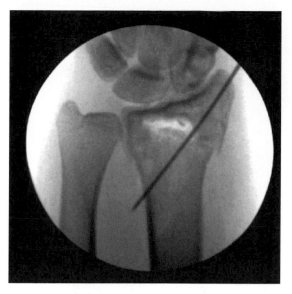

Fig. 4.55 Radial length restored and temporarily stabilized by Kirschner wire.

Implant positioning

- The transverse limb of the plate is applied to ensure an anatomical reduction of the articular surfaces.
- The longitudinal limb(s) of the plate are applied to stabilize radial length (Fig. 4.56).
- The Kirschner wire is removed and passive range of motion is assessed.
- At this stage, the passive stability of the DRUJ is also assessed (Fig. 4.57).
- Intraoperative radiographic screening is used at each stage to ensure adequate reduction.

Closure

- The edges of the 3rd extensor compartment are closed over the plate (4/0 Vicryl).
- The tendon of the EPL is left superficial to the extensor retinaculum.
- Skin closure with interrupted fine monofilament (5/0 Novafil) or continuous subcuticular monofilament (3/0 Prolene).

Dressing

- Bulky, not tight, wool roll.
- Palmar plaster of Paris slab with the wrist in 20° of extension.
- External crepe bandage.
- High elevation in Bradford sling.

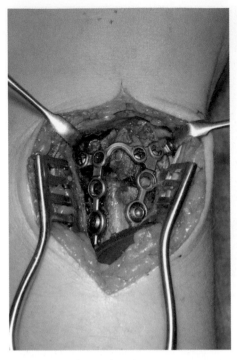

Fig. 4.56 Dorsal view after plating.

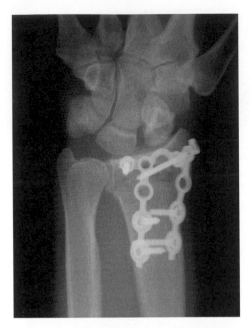

Fig. 4.58 Anteroposterior radiograph after surgery.

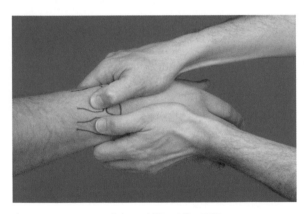

Fig. 4.57 Assessment of the stability of the DRUJ.

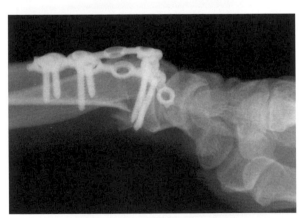

Fig. 4.59 Lateral radiograph after surgery.

Post-operative rehabilitation

- High elevation in Bradford sling and subsequently high arm sling for 72 hours.
- Routine check radiograph at first convenient opportunity (Figs. 4.58, 4.59).

Outpatient follow up

- Review at 2 weeks with check radiograph, removal of plaster splint and sutures, and referral for thermoplastic wrist gauntlet manufacture and out-patient physiotherapy.
- Further reviews at 6 weeks (to discard splint) and thereafter to monitor recovery of range of motion and grip strength, and radiological union.

Implant removal

- Often required after fracture healing in cases of secondary extensor tenosynovitis.
- May present with attrition rupture of extensor tendons if tenosynovitis is not recognised.

4.7 CLOSED REDUCTION AND K-WIRE FIXATION OF DISTAL RADIUS FRACTURES

Indications

- Extra-articular distal radial fractures with good bone stock, except flexion fractures.

Pre-operative planning

Clinical assessment

- Local pain and swelling.
- Assess and document neurovascular status.

Radiological assessment

- Standard anteroposterior (AP) and lateral radiographs of the wrist. Special projections like Stecher's view (AP view in ulnar adduction) can be helpful to find associated lesions of carpal bones or ligaments.
- High-resolution spiral computed tomography (1–2 mm, 120 kV, 80–100 mAs, axial and sagittal) helps define the degree of comminution within a fracture as well as suspected impaction of the articular surface. It should be considered in intra-articular fractures (Fig. 4.60).

Operative treatment

Anaesthesia

- Brachial plexus block, intravenous regional anaesthesia, intrafocal anaesthesia or general anaesthesia.
- At induction, administer prophylactic antibiotic according to local hospital protocol (e.g. 3rd generation cephalosporin).

Table and equipment

- Power drill.
- K-wires 1.2 to 1.8 mm.
- Extension device.
- Image intensifier.

Table set up

- The instrumentation is set up on the side of the operation.
- Image intensifier is from the side of the fracture. Check for adequate visualization in 2 planes prior to draping.

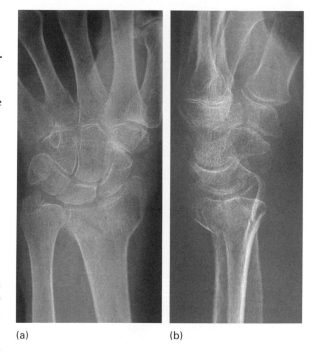

(a)   (b)

Fig. 4.60 (a) Anteriorposterior and (b) lateral view of distal radius fracture.

Patient positioning

- Supine arm extended in extension device in 90° flexion of the elbow, weight on upper arm of 2.5 to 5 kg (Fig. 4.61).

Draping, surgical approach and implant positioning

- Prepare the skin over elbow, forearm, wrist and hand with antiseptic solutions (aqueous/alcoholic povidone–iodine).
- Apply adherent drape above the elbow, to allow free elbow motion.
- To reduce the fracture, first increase the fracture deformity by extending the wrist, then manipulate the distal fragment in a palmar and ulnar direction whilst traction is maintained, and finally lock the fracture in place by rotating patient's hand and fragment carefully. Avoid repetitive and brusque manipulation.
- Dorsal skin incisions over the fracture, long enough to ensure that pins will neither be driven through the extensor tendons nor through the superficial branch of the radial nerve.
- In placing the pins 2 proceedings are preferable.

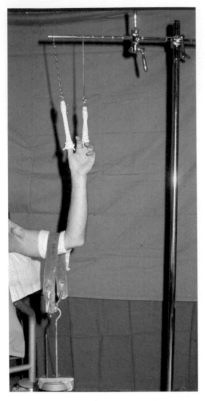

Fig. 4.61 Arm positioning in extension device.

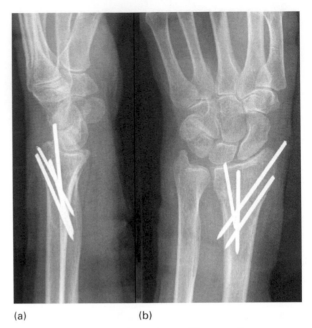

(a)   (b)

Fig. 4.62 Intrafocal pinning as advocated by Kapandji.

Intrafocal pinning as advocated by Kapandji (Fig. 4.62)

- Insert two to three 1.6 to 1.8 K-wires into the dorsal cortex of the fracture from proximal to distal by hand whilst protecting nerve and tendons.
- Correct persisting loss of dorsal angulation by levering the proximal end of the pins distally.
- Drive K-wire proximally into the palmar cortex of the proximal fragment.
- To correct radial inclination insert at least one K-wire into the radial cortex of the fracture and lever distally before driving the pin into the ulnar cortex of the proximal fragment.

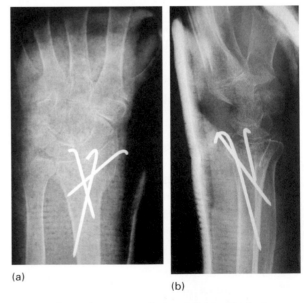

(a)

(b)

Fig. 4.63 a,b Interfragmentary pinning of distal radius fracture.

Interfragmentary pinning (Fig. 4.63 a,b)

- After manual reduction of the fracture and skin incision, drill one 1.6 to 1.8 K-wire from the tip of the radial styloid toward the fracture in an angle of approximately 45° to the dorso-ulnar cortex of the radius, proximal of the fragment.
- Depending on the size and count of fragments, drill at least two 1.6 to 1.8 K-wires from distal–dorsal to proximal–palmar.
- Control reposition and correct implant positioning with the image intensifier.

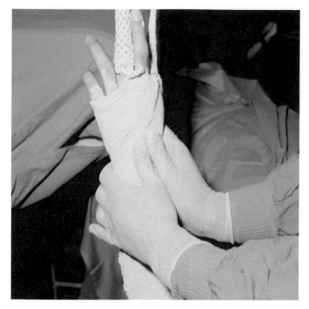

Fig. 4.64 Short-arm, cast splint.

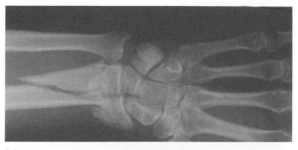

(a)

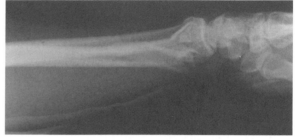

(b)

Fig. 4.65 a,b Comminuted fracture of the forearm and distal radius.

- In both procedures cut K-wires long enough not to interfere with tendons.
- Wound and skin closure (monofilament non-absorbable suture).
- Sterile and slightly compressing dressing from palm to forearm. Short-arm, cast splint with the wrist in 20° of extension (Fig. 4.64).

Post-operative rehabilitation

- Elevation of the operated arm. Active exercises of fingers, elbow and shoulder.
- Routine radiographs within 24 hours.
- Short-arm, cast for 4 to 6 weeks, depending on the stability obtained at surgery.

Outpatient follow up

- Review at day 1 and day 3 and control cast. Change cast at day 4 to 7 if correct fit is uncertain.
- Review at day 1, 4, 7 and day 28 with radiographs.
- Implant removal at day 28 if fracture healing is evident.
- Discharge from the follow up after clinical and radiological evidence of fracture healing.

4.8 CLOSED REDUCTION AND APPLICATION OF AN EXTERNAL FIXATOR IN DISTAL RADIUS FRACTURES

Indications

- Distal radial fractures, intra- and extra-articular, except flexion fractures.
- Comminuted fractures of the elderly.

Pre-operative planning

Clinical assessment

- Local pain and swelling.
- Assess and document neurovascular status.

Radiological assessment

- Standard anteroposterior (AP), and lateral radiographs of the wrist (Fig. 4.65 a,b). Special projections like Stecher's view (AP view in ulnar adduction) can be helpful to find associated lesions of carpal bones or ligaments.

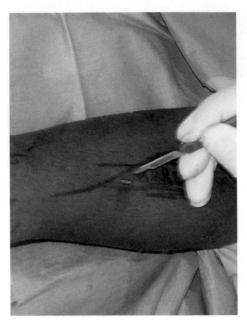

Fig. 4.66 Make a 5 mm incision over the bare area of the radius.

- High-resolution computed tomography (1–2 mm, 120 kV, 80–100 mAs, axial and sagittal) helps define the degree of comminution within a fracture as well as suspected impaction of the articular surface. It should be considered in intra-articular fractures.

Operative treatment

Anaesthesia

- Brachial plexus block, intravenous regional anaesthesia or general anaesthesia.
- At induction, administer prophylactic antibiotic according to the local hospital protocol (e.g. 3rd generation cephalosporin).

Table and equipment

- External fixation system
- Radiolucent arm table.
- Image intensifier.

Table set up

- The instrumentation is set up on the side of the operation.
- Image intensifier is from the front side of the arm table. Check for adequate visualization in 2 planes prior to draping.

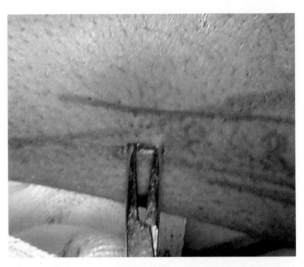

Fig. 4.67 Use a clamp to dissect gently down to bone to avoid damage to neurologic and vascular structures.

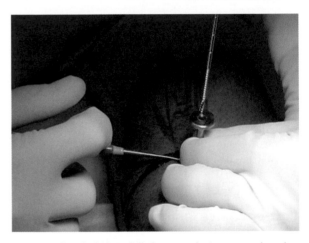

Fig. 4.68 After the hole is drilled remove the inner cannula and place the pin through the outer cannula.

Patient positioning

- Supine, pronated arm extended on arm table.

Draping, surgical approach and implant positioning

- Prepare the skin over elbow, forearm, wrist and hand with the usual antiseptic solutions (aqueous/alcoholic povidone–iodine).
- Apply adherent drape above the elbow, to allow free elbow motion.
- Make 2 small puncture skin incisions at a 45° angle to the plane of the radius and of metacarpal II.

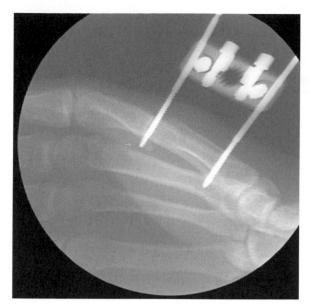

Fig. 4.69 At the metacarpal II place one pin in the base and one in the more distal aspect.

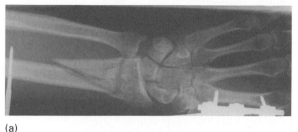

(a)

(b)

Fig. 4.70 Treatment with external fixation.

Place the 2 pins in the distal diaphysis of the radius, approximately 10 to 12 cm proximal to the radial styloid (Figs. 4.66, 4.67, 4.68). At metacarpal II place one pin in the base and one in the more distal aspect.

- Drill holes and insert the 4 fixator screws (2 mm at the metacarpal, 4 mm at the radius) by hand, creating an angle of 45 to 60° between the 2 pins at the metacarpal and between the 2 pins at the radius whilst protecting tendons and nerves by retracting them with forceps and drill guides (Fig. 4.69).
- Confirm position of the pins and their depths by image control.
- Attach joint bridging rods.
- Perform positioning after fracture reduction and fix the screws.

- Apply sterile, slightly compressing bandage from the palm to the forearm.

Post-operative rehabilitation

- Elevation of the operated arm. Active exercises of finger, elbow and shoulder.
- Routine radiographs, frontal and sagittal view, within 24 hours.

Outpatient follow up

- Review at 4 weeks with radiographs (Fig. 4.70).
- Implant removal after 4–6 weeks.
- Discharge from the follow up after clinical and radiological evidence of fracture healing.

Fractures of the wrist

Doug Campbell

5.1 PERCUTANEOUS FIXATION OF SCAPHOID FRACTURES

Indications

Percutaneous fixation of scaphoid fractures is performed for:

(a) Undisplaced scaphoid fractures in active individuals or multiple injuries.
(b) Do not use this technique if fractures are displaced >1 mm.

Pre-operative assessment

Clinical assessment

- Assess vascularity of the hand, particularly the radial artery.
- Assess for evidence of neural compromise – particularly in the median nerve distribution.
- Assess the condition of the skin in the area of proposed incision.
- Assess for tenderness in other areas around the wrist which may represent a second injury.

Radiological assessment

- Anteroposterior (AP), lateral, 45° oblique and long-axis radiographs of the scaphoid.
- Assess scaphoid length and look for evidence of fracture collapse (hump-back deformity, loss of carpal height).

Operative treatment

Anaesthesia

- General or regional (axillary, supra- or infraclavicular block).
- Intravenous dose of antibiotic as prophylaxis prior to inflation of tourniquet.

Tourniquet

- Well-padded upper arm cuff inflated to 250 mmHg.
- Plastic exclusion drape to prevent any soaking of padding by skin preparation.

Equipment

- Percutaneous screw system of choice with full selection of implants and screws.
- Radiolucent hand table securely fastened to operating table.
- Image intensifier or mini C-arm fluoroscan.

Operating room set up

- The arm must lie centrally on the hand table.
- Surgeon is best seated at the distal end of the affected limb.
- Image intensifier or mini C-arm is brought in from the head of the table throughout the procedure.

Practical Procedures in Orthopaedic Trauma Surgery: A Trainee's Companion, ed. Peter V. Giannoudis and Hans-Christoph Pape.
Published by Cambridge University Press. © Cambridge University Press 2006.

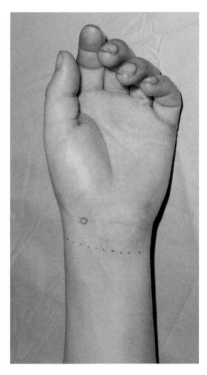

Fig. 5.1 Surface marking of the wrist joint and scaphoid tubercle.

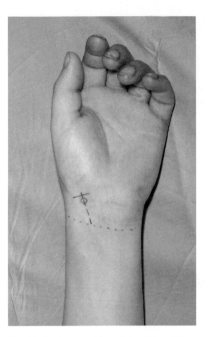

Fig. 5.2 Surface marking of the STJ and long axis of scaphoid.

Draping and surgical approach

- Skin is prepared from fingertips to tourniquet with aqueous antiseptic solution.
- Entire limb from tourniquet distally is to be visible and mobile during the procedure.
- Single-use drape with an expandable aperture for the limb is recommended.
- Mark the radiocarpal joint and scaphoid tubercle on the skin with a marker pen (Fig. 5.1).
- Using image intensifier, ascertain the level of the scaphotrapezial joint (STJ) and long axis of scaphoid with the wrist in extension. Mark these sites with a marker pen (Fig. 5.2).
- Make a 5 mm transverse incision just distal to the STJ.
- Blunt dissection through thenar musculature to reach STJ.
- Insert guide wire by hand into the STJ and confirm radiologically.

Fracture reduction

- Unnecessary.

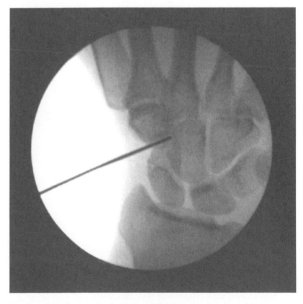

Fig. 5.3 Kirschner wire introduced by hand to localize the STJ.

Implant positioning

- Ensure the tip of the guide wire is deep in the STJ to guarantee correct entry point (Fig. 5.3).
- Introduce the guide wire under image intensifier control along the long axis of the scaphoid at 45° to the skin surface (Fig. 5.4).

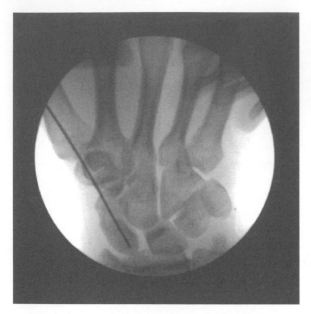

Fig. 5.4 Anteroposterior scan after guide wire insertion.

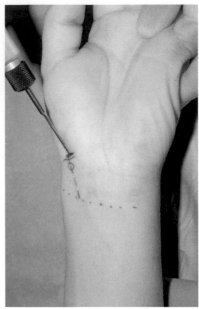

Fig. 5.6 Insertion of screw.

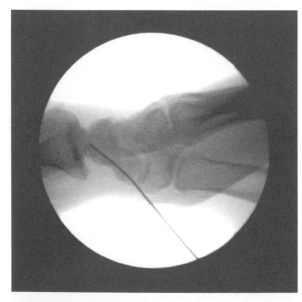

Fig. 5.5 Lateral scan after guide wire insertion.

into the STJ even though it is well buried in the articular surface.
- Measure the length of the guide wire.
- Choose and insert a screw of appropriate length (Fig. 5.6).
- Check position and length radiographically (Fig. 5.7a,b).

Closure

- Interrupted absorbable suture(s) (5/0 Vicryl Rapide).

Dressing

- Bulky, not tight, wool roll.
- Palmar plaster of Paris slab with thumb extension and wrist placed in 20° of extension.
- External crepe bandage.
- High elevation in Bradford sling.

- Check on AP, lateral and oblique views that the wire remains within the scaphoid throughout its course. Pay particular attention to ensure the tip does not penetrate the dorsal part of the proximal pole (Fig. 5.5).
- Countersink the cortex. The articular cartilage is very thick and the screw head will appear to be protruding

Post-operative rehabilitation

- High elevation in Bradford sling and subsequently high arm sling for 72 hours.
- Routine check radiograph at first convenient opportunity.

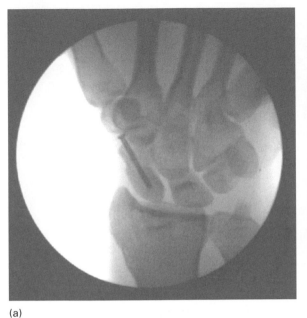

(a)

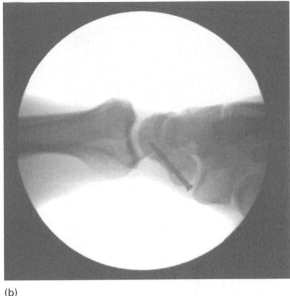

(b)

Fig. 5.7 a,b Anteroposterior and lateral radiograph after screw insertion.

Outpatient follow up

- Review at 1–2 weeks with check radiograph and removal of plaster splint.
- Referral for thermoplastic wrist gauntlet manufacture and outpatient physiotherapy.
- Further reviews at 6 weeks and 3 months to monitor recovery of range of motion and grip strength, and radiological union.

Implant removal

- Not required.

5.2 OPEN REDUCTION AND INTERNAL FIXATION (ORIF) OF ACUTE SCAPHO-LUNATE DISSOCIATION

Indications

Acute repair of a scapholunate ligament tear is performed:

(a) In the isolated case, within 2 months of injury; but preferably within the first 10 days.

(b) When the injury exists in combination with an intra-articular fracture of the distal radius or as part of a perilunate dislocation.

Pre-operative assessment

Clinical assessment

- Assess vascularity of the hand.
- Assess for evidence of neural compromise – particularly in the median nerve distribution.
- Assess the condition of the skin in the area of proposed incision.
- Assess for tenderness in other areas around the wrist which may represent a second injury.

Radiological assessment

- Anteroposterior (AP) and lateral radiographs of the wrist (Figs. 5.8, 5.9).
- Assess scapholunate gap (normally 2 mm distally, 3 mm proximally maximum).
- Assess scapholunate angle (>80° is suggestive of a complete tear of the scapholunate ligament).
- Look for the 'ring sign' of an excessively flexed scaphoid.
- Assess carpal height.

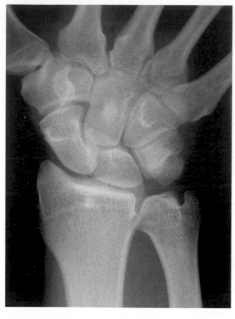

Fig. 5.8 Anteroposterior radiograph showing dissociation between the scaphoid and lunate.

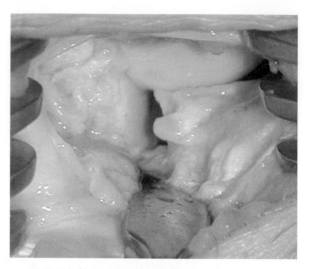

Fig. 5.10 Intraoperative view of scapho-lunate dissociation.

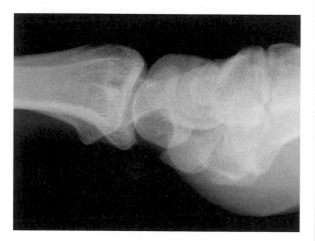

Fig. 5.9 Lateral radiograph showing increased scapho-lunate angle.

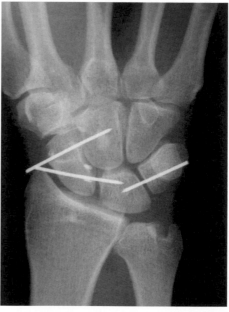

Fig. 5.11 Anteroposterior radiograph showing position of Kirschner wires.

Operative treatment

Anaesthesia

- General or regional (axillary, supra- or infraclavicular block).

Tourniquet

- Well-padded upper arm cuff inflated to 250 mmHg.

- Plastic exclusion drape to prevent any soaking of padding by skin preparation.

Equipment

- 1.0 mm and 1.2 mm Kirschner wires to act as 'joysticks' and to drill holes if required.
- Mini bone anchors with 4/0 non-absorbable suture.

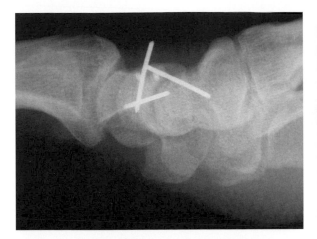

Fig. 5.12 Lateral radiograph showing correction of scapho-lunate angle.

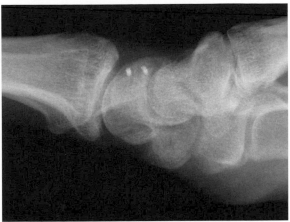

Fig. 5.14 Lateral radiograph at 3 months after surgery.

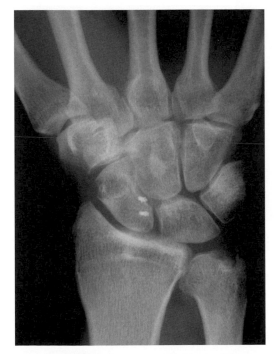

Fig. 5.13 Anteroposterior radiograph at 3 months after surgery. Note bone anchors.

- Radiolucent hand table securely fastened to operating table.
- Image intensifier, or mini C-arm fluoroscan.

Operating room set up

- The arm must lie centrally on the hand table.
- Surgeon best seated cephalad for a dorsal approach.

- Image intensifier or mini C-arm is brought in from the axilla of the patient.

Draping and surgical approach

- Skin prepared from fingertips to tourniquet with aqueous antiseptic solution.
- Entire limb from tourniquet distally to be visible and mobile during the procedure.
- Single-use drape with expandable aperture for the limb is recommended.
- Dorsal transverse skin incision just distal to the radiocarpal joint, centred over the scapho-lunate interval.
- Opening of the distal part of the 3rd and 4th extensor compartments and retraction of the extensor tendons therein.
- Transverse capsular incision from dorsal scaphoid to triquetrum, preserving the extrinsic ligaments.
- Identification of the scapho-lunate interval under direct vision (Fig. 5.10).

Surgical procedure

- Insert 1.0 or 1.2 mm Kirschner wire into the lunate and use it (like a joystick) to control rotation of the lunate and the width of the scapho-lunate gap.
- Assess for any small avulsion fractures attached to the ends of the torn ligament.
- Assess and document the condition of the articular cartilage on the surface of the distal radius.
- Reduce the rotated lunate and close the scapho-lunate gap using the joystick.
- Assess the reduction radiologically.

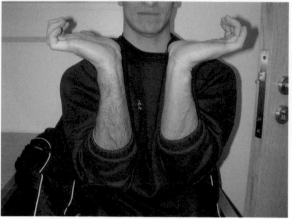

Fig. 5.15 Wrist extension 3 months after surgery.

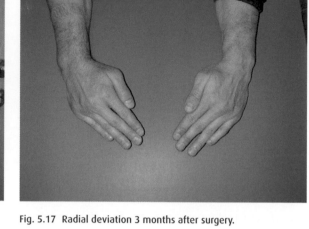

Fig. 5.17 Radial deviation 3 months after surgery.

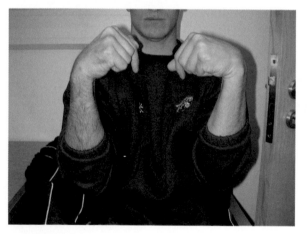

Fig. 5.16 Wrist flexion 3 months after surgery.

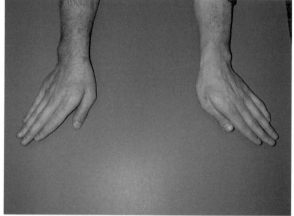

Fig. 5.18 Ulnar deviation 3 months after surgery.

- Insert percutaneous 1.2 mm Kirschner wires from scaphoid to lunate, lunate to triquetrum (to control lunate rotation) and scaphoid to capitate (to control carpal height) (Figs. 5.11, 5.12).
- Repair/reattach the torn edges of the scapho-lunate ligament using mini bone anchors or drill holes through scaphoid.
- Cut Kirschner wires deep to skin.
- Release the median nerve through the standard palmar approach if indicated.

Closure

- Interrupted absorbable sutures (4/0 Vicryl) to dorsal capsule/extrinsic ligaments.
- Reconstruction of extensor retinaculum (4/0 Vicryl).

- Continuous subcuticular non-absorbable suture (3/0 prolene).

Dressing

- Bulky, not tight, wool roll.
- Palmar plaster of Paris slab with thumb extension and wrist placed in 20° of extension.
- External crepe bandage.
- High elevation in Bradford sling.

Post-operative rehabilitation

- High elevation in Bradford sling and subsequently high arm sling for 72 hours.

- Routine check radiograph at the first convenient opportunity.

Outpatient follow up

- Review at 2 weeks with check radiograph, removal of suture and application of full scaphoid lightweight cast.

- Removal of plaster cast and Kirschner wires (under local anaesthesia) at 8 weeks (Figs 5.13, 5.14).
- Gentle exercise to regain range of movement with no heavy loading for a further month (Figs 5.15, 5.16, 5.17, 5.18).

Implant removal

- Not required.

Section I: Fractures of the first metacarpal

Reinhard Meier

6.1 KIRSCHNER WIRE FIXATION OF BASAL FRACTURES OF THE FIRST METACARPAL

Indications

Fractures of the base of the first metacarpal tend to dislocate owing to forces from the tendons (e.g. abductor pollicis longus (APL) tendon in Bennett's fracture). Therefore operative treatment is necessary if stable retention cannot be achieved by casting. Closed reduction and internal K-wire fixation can be performed for:

(a) Fractures with small fragments.
(b) Fractures with good alignment after closed reduction but no stable retention without fracture fixation, in the absence of large impression defects.

Pre-operative planning

Clinical assessment

- Pain and swelling localized to carpometacarpal joint I.
- Assess and document neurovascular status of thumb.

Radiological assessment

- Standard anteroposterior (AP) and lateral radiographs of the trapezium (Kapandji) obtained by placing the hand for a true lateral view, with abduction of the thumb and directing the imaging beam centred over the trapeziometacarpal joint.
- Computed tomography helps to define the degree of comminution within a fracture, as well as suspected impaction of the articular surface.

Operative treatment

Anaesthesia

- Brachial plexus block, intravenous regional anaesthesia or general anaesthesia.
- Prophylactic antibiotic according to the local hospital protocol (e.g. 2nd generation cephalosporin).

Table and equipment

- Hand surgery instrumentation set, K-wires: 1.2 mm.
- Radiolucent arm table.
- Upper arm tourniquet.
- Image intensifier.

Table set up

- The instrumentation is set up on the side of the operation.
- Image intensifier is from the front side of the arm table.

Patient positioning

- Supine, supinated arm extended on arm table.

Fracture reduction

- Gentle axial traction and pressure on the displaced fragment usually reduces displaced fractures.
- Open anatomical reduction is indicated if closed reduction fails and/or stable reduction cannot be achieved.

Practical Procedures in Orthopaedic Trauma Surgery: A Trainee's Companion, ed. Peter V. Giannoudis and Hans-Christoph Pape.
Published by Cambridge University Press. © Cambridge University Press 2006.

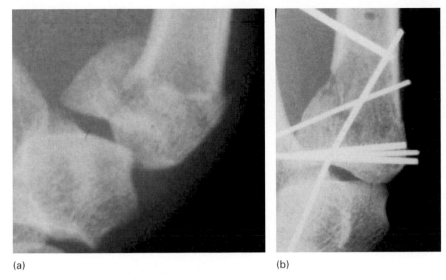

(a)   (b)

Fig. 6.1 a,b Fracture stabilized with K-wires.

Draping and surgical approach

- Place tourniquet at upper arm.
- Prepare the skin over elbow, forearm, wrist and hand using antiseptic solutions (aqueous/alcoholic povidone–iodine).
- Apply adherent drape above the elbow, to allow free elbow motion.
- If sufficient closed reduction is unachievable or large areas of impaction have to be filled with autologous bone grafting (e.g. for a Rolando fracture) a dorsoradial approach is made to the base of the first metacarpal bone after applying a tourniquet (required only for an open procedure).

Implant positioning

- Under fluoroscopic control insert a 1.2 mm K-wire from the dorsoradial-distal end of the first metacarpal bone to the trapezium for temporary transfixation of the thumb carpometacarpal joint.
- If stable retention cannot be achieved (e.g. fractures proximal to the APL tendon) the fragment is fixed by at least a second 1.2 mm pin monitoring its position on the image intensifier. If in doubt, a second K-wire appears to be the safer alternative (Fig. 6.1).
- Bending the ends of the pins, cut and sink them below the skin.

Post-operative rehabilitation

- Elevation of the operated arm. Active exercises of finger, elbow and shoulder are encouraged.
- Radiographic check within 24 hours.
- Short-arm, thumb spica cast splint, leaving the interphalangeal joint free for 4–6 weeks.

Outpatient follow up

- Follow up at 4 to 6 weeks (clinically and with X-ray check control).
- Normal use after 4 to 6 weeks when bone healing is secured.
- Remove the other pin when bone healing is secured.
- Discharge from the follow up after clinical and radiological evidence of fracture healing.

6.2 OPEN REDUCTION AND INTERNAL FIXATION (ORIF) OF BASAL FRACTURES OF THE FIRST METACARPAL

Indications

Fractures of the base of the first metacarpal tend to dislocate owing to forces of the tendons (e.g. abductor pollicis longus (APL) tendon in Bennett's fracture). Therefore open reduction and internal fixation is necessary if stable retention cannot be achieved by casting. Open reduction and internal fixation (ORIF) with screws and plates can be performed for:

(a) Fractures where the fragments are not too small.
(b) Fractures where closed reduction would be impractical.
(c) Combined fractures.
(d) Fractures with huge impression zones (e.g. a Rolando fracture).

Pre-operative planning

Clinical assessment

- Pain and swelling localized to carpometacarpal joint I.
- Assess and document neurovascular status of thumb.

Radiological assessment

- Standard anteroposterior and lateral radiographs of the trapezium (Kapandji) obtained by placing the hand for a true lateral view, with abduction of the thumb and directing the imaging beam centred over the trapeziometacarpal joint
- Computed tomography helps define the degree of comminution within a fracture, as well as suspected impaction of the articular surface.

Operative treatment

Anaesthesia

- Brachial plexus block, intravenous regional anaesthesia or general anaesthesia.
- At induction, administer prophylactic antibiotic as per local hospital protocol (e.g. 3rd generation cephalosporin).

Table and equipment

- Hand surgery instrumentation set.
- Hand small fragment implant system.
- A radiolucent arm table.
- An upper arm tourniquet.
- An image intensifier.

Table set up

- The instrumentation is set up on the side of the operation.
- Image intensifier is from the front side of the arm table.

Patient positioning

- Supine, supinated arm extended on arm table.

Draping, surgical approach and implant positioning

- Place tourniquet at upper arm.
- Prepare the skin over elbow, forearm, wrist and hand with usual antiseptic solutions (aqueous/alcoholic povidone–iodine).
- Apply adherent drape circularly above the elbow, so free motion of the elbow is possible.
- Tourniquet after exsanguination.
- Skin incision via a dorsoradial approach to the base of the first metacarpal bone.
- Longitudinal incision of the periosteal and subperiosteal reflection of the thenar musculature.
- Open carpometacarpal joint.
- Reduce fracture under direct vision.
- Huge zones of impression have to be filled with autologous bone grafting from the distal radius (e.g. for a Rolando fracture).
- In unstable situations temporary fixation with towel-clip forceps or K-wires.
- Drilling and interfragmentary lag screw fixation (self-tapping screws 1.5 to 2.3 mm) with fluoroscopic and direct visual control of correct repositioning, and stabilization with mini-plate (self-tapping screws 1.5–2.3 mm) (Fig. 6.2a, b).
- Suturing of the periosteum to cover the implants to minimize interferences with the tendons (No. 5 PDS/Vicryl).
- Wound and skin closure (monofilament non-absorbable suture).
- Sterile, slightly compressing dressing from thumb and palm to forearm. Short-arm, thumb spica cast splint leaving the interphalangeal joint free with the wrist in 20° of extension.
- Release of tourniquet.

Post-operative rehabilitation

- Elevation of the operated arm. Active exercises of finger, elbow and shoulder.
- Routine radiographs within 24 hours.
- Short-arm, thumb spica cast splint leaving the interphalangeal joint free for 1 to 6 weeks, depending on the stability obtained at surgery.

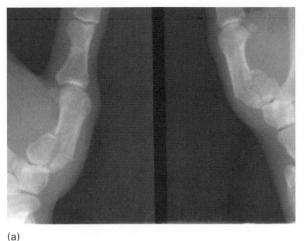

(a)

(b)

Fig. 6.2a, b Bennett's fracture: open reduction and internal fixation.

Outpatient follow up

- Review at 6 weeks with radiographs.
- If the implant gives rise to symptoms, removal after 12 weeks is possible.
- Discharge from the follow up after clinical and radiological evidence of fracture healing.

6.3 ULNAR COLLATERAL LIGAMENT REPAIR

Indications

- Ulnar collateral ligament rupture with a Stener lesion.

Pre-operative planning

Clinical assessment

- Pain and swelling localized over the ulnar aspect of metacarpophalangeal joint I.
- Assess and document neurovascular status of thumb.

Radiological assessment

- Standard anteroposterior and lateral radiographs of the trapezium (Kapandji) obtained by placing the hand for a true lateral view, with abduction of the thumb and directing the imaging beam centred over the trapeziometacarpal joint to verify lesions involving the bone.

- Ultrasound examination of the joint can verify a Stener lesion (Fig. 6.3).

Operative treatment

Anaesthesia

- Brachial plexus block, intravenous regional anaesthesia or general anaesthesia.
- At induction, administer prophylactic antibiotic as per local hospital protocol (e.g. 3rd generation cephalosporin).

Table and equipment

- Hand surgery instrumentation set.
- A radiolucent arm table.
- An upper arm tourniquet.
- An image intensifier.

Table set up

- The instrumentation is set up on the side of the operation.
- Image intensifier is from the front side of the arm table.

Patient positioning

- Supine, supinated arm extended on arm table.

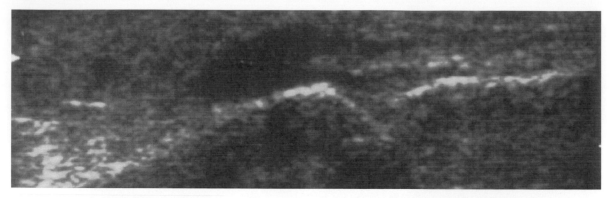

Fig. 6.3 Ultrasound view of metacarpal I and proximal phalanx I. Stener lesion: rupture of the ulnar collateral ligament.

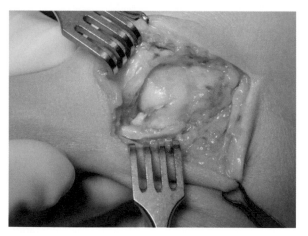

Fig. 6.4 Rupture of the ulnar collateral ligament.

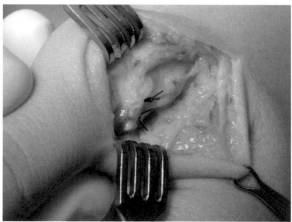

Fig. 6.5 Adaptation with PDS sutures.

Draping, surgical approach and implant positioning

- Place tourniquet at upper arm.
- Prepare the skin over elbow, forearm, wrist and hand with usual antiseptic solutions (aqueous/alcoholic povidone–iodine).
- Apply adherent drape circularly above the elbow, so free motion of the elbow is possible.
- Tourniquet after exsanguination.
- Skin incision from the mid-lateral aspect of the ulnar side of the thumb, curved over the metacarpophalyngeal (MP) joint and extended proximally ulnar to the extensor pollicis longus (EPL) tendon.
- Divide intertendinous lamina and joint capsule and expose the collateral ligament (Fig. 6.4).

- Verify a Stener lesion by identifying the extensor pollicis longus (EPL), its extensor hood, and the adductor aponeurosis.
- Depending on the type of rupture refixation can be performed as described below:
- If the ligament shows an intrasubstance rupture it should be sutured (No. 5 PDS) (Fig. 6.5). If there is an avulsion of the ligament it should be refixed with a screw (1.3–2.0 mm screws). If the fragment is too small, pins or bone sutures can be used.
- In unstable situations temporary fixation of the metacarpophalangeal joint is possible with a K-wire (1.2–1.4 mm).
- Drilling and interfragmentary lag screw fixation (self-tapping screws 1.5 to 2.3 mm) with fluoroscopic and direct visual control of correct repositioning, and

stabilization with mini-plate (self-tapping screws 1.5–2.3 mm).
- Suturing of the periosteum to cover the implants to minimize interferences with the tendons (No. 5 PDS/Vicryl).
- Wound and skin closure (monofilament non-absorbable suture).
- Sterile, slightly compressing dressing from thumb and palm to forearm. Short-arm, thumb spica cast splint leaving the interphalangeal joint free with the wrist in 20° of extension.
- Release of tourniquet.

Post-operative rehabilitation

- Elevation of the operated arm. Active exercises of fingers, elbow and shoulder.

Outpatient follow up

- Short-arm, thumb spica cast splint leaving the interphalangeal joint free for 4 weeks
- Full use is allowed after 6 weeks.

Section II: Fractures of the metacarpals II–V

Reinhard Meier

6.4 OPEN REDUCTION AND INTERNAL FIXATION (ORIF) OF MIDSHAFT FRACTURES OF THE METACARPALS

Indications

Screw and plate fixation is used to stabilize:

(a) Fractures of 2 or more metacarpal bones.
(b) Fractures irreducible by closed reduction.
(c) Open/comminuted fractures.
(d) Fractures with rotational mal-alignment.
(e) Angulation of more than 30°.
(f) Fractures if early mobilization is required.

Pre-operative planning

Clinical assessment

- Pain and swelling localized over the metacarpus.
- Assess and document neurovascular status of hand.
- Assess and document rotational alignment, axis and range of movement (ROM) of fingers.

Radiological assessment

- Anteroposterior, lateral, and oblique views (Fig. 6.6).
- A 30° pronated lateral view for 2nd and 3rd metacarpal fractures and 30° supinated lateral view for 4th and 5th metacarpal fractures are helpful.

Anaesthesia

- Brachial plexus block, intravenous regional anaesthesia or general anaesthesia.
- At induction, administer prophylactic antibiotic as per local hospital protocol (e.g. 2nd generation cephalosporin).

Table and equipment

- Hand surgery instrumentation set.
- Hand small-fragment implant system.
- A radiolucent arm table.
- An upper arm tourniquet.
- An image intensifier.

Table set up

- The instrumentation is set up on the side of the operation.
- Image intensifier is from the front side of the arm table. Check for adequate visualization in 2 planes prior to draping.

Patient positioning

- Supine, supinated arm extended on arm table.

Draping, surgical approach and implant positioning

- Place tourniquet at upper arm.
- Prepare the skin over elbow, forearm, wrist and hand with usual antiseptic solutions (aqueous/alcoholic povidone–iodine).
- Apply adherent drape above the elbow, to allow free elbow motion.
- Tourniquet after exsanguination.
- Skin incision via a longitudinal dorsal approach lateral to the metacarpal bone.
- Hold extension tendon laterally.
- Longitudinal incision of the periosteum and lateral moving of the periosteum and the insertion of the interosseous muscles (Fig. 6.7).
- Open reduction.

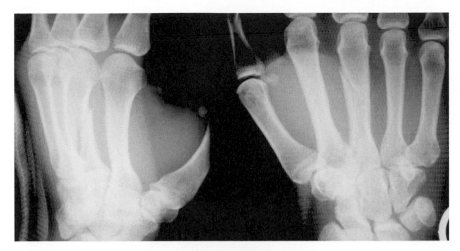

Fig. 6.6 Anteroposterior and oblique views of metacarpal III fracture.

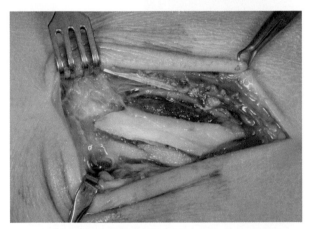

Fig. 6.7 Exposed fracture.

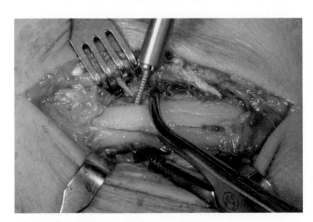

Fig. 6.8 Open reduction and lag screw fixation.

- Under fluoroscopic control of correct repositioning, drill and stabilize with mini-plate (self-tapping screws 1.5–2.3 mm) in lateral position and/or lag screws (self-tapping screws 1.5–2.3 mm) (Fig. 6.8).
- Suturing of the periosteum and the interosseous muscles (No. 5 PDS/Vicryl).
- Wound and skin closure (monofilament non-absorbable suture).
- Sterile, slightly compressing dressing from palm to forearm. Short-arm, cast splint leaving the interphalangeal joint free with the wrist in 20° extension.
- Release of tourniquet.

Post-operative rehabilitation

- Elevation of the operated arm. Active exercises of fingers, elbow and shoulder.
- Routine radiographs within 24 hours (Fig. 6.9).
- Short-arm, cast splint leaving the interphalangeal joint free for 1 week.

Outpatient follow up

- Review at 6 weeks with radiographs.
- If the implant gives rise to symptoms, removal is possible.
- Discharge from the follow up after clinical and radiological evidence of fracture healing.

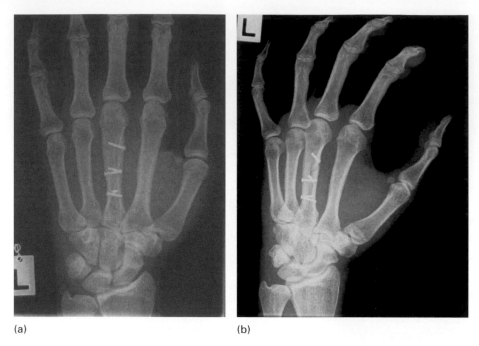

(a)   (b)

Fig. 6.9 (a) Anteroposterior and (b) oblique views of a metacarpal III fracture after internal fixation with lag screws.

6.5 CLOSED REDUCTION AND INTRAMEDULLARY FIXATION (CRIF) OF DISTAL THIRD FRACTURES OF METACARPALS II-V

Indications

Intramedullary fixation is used to stabilize:

(a) Subcapital fractures of metacarpal bones.
(b) Fractures with rotational malalignment.
(c) Angulation of more than 30°.

- Open reduction and screw and plate fixation can also be used for the above indications. However, interference with tendon sheaths is possible.
- Screw and plate fixation is preferable in fractures at the proximal or middle part of the metacarpal bone and, in cases were acceptable reposition and reduction cannot be achieved, with intramedullary fixation.

Pre-operative planning

Clinical assessment

- Pain and swelling localized over the metacarpals.
- Assess and document neurovascular status of the hand.

- Assess and document rotational alignment of the fingers.

Radiological assessment

- Anteroposterior, lateral and oblique views (Fig. 6.10a, b).
- A 30° pronated lateral view for 2nd and 3rd metacarpal fractures and a 30° supinated lateral view for 4th and 5th metacarpal fractures are helpful.

Operative treatment

Anaesthesia

- Brachial plexus block, intravenous regional anaesthesia or general anaesthesia.
- At induction, administer prophylactic antibiotic according to the local hospital protocol (e.g. 3rd generation cephalosporin).

Table and equipment

- Hand surgery instrumentation set.
- K-wires, at least 1.2 mm.
- Radiolucent arm table.

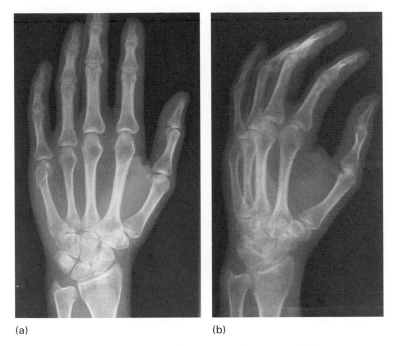

(a)   (b)

Fig. 6.10 (a) Anteroposterior and (b) oblique views of a metacarpal V fracture.

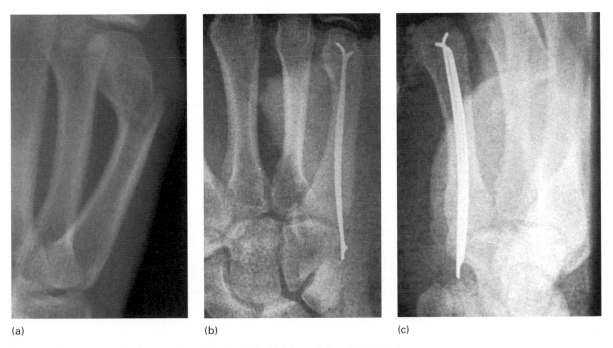

(a)   (b)   (c)

Fig. 6.11 a, b, c Metacarpal V fracture of a patient treated with intramedullary K-wire fixation.

- Upper arm tourniquet.
- Image intensifier.

Table set up

- The instrumentation is set up on the side of the operation.
- The image intensifier is from the front side of the arm table. Check for adequate visualization in 2 planes prior to draping.

Patient positioning

- Supine, supinated arm extended on arm table.

Draping, surgical approach and implant positioning

- Place tourniquet at upper arm.
- Prepare the skin over elbow, forearm, wrist and hand with antiseptic solutions (aqueous/alcoholic povidone–iodine).
- Apply adherent drape above the elbow, to allow free elbow motion.
- 1.2 mm-diameter Kirschner wires are prebent into shape.
- Tourniquet.
- Perform closed reduction of the fracture.
- Make a small stab incision in the proximal metaphysis on the dorsoulnar aspect of the metacarpal.
- Elevate the periosteum.
- Fenestrate the metacarpal bone with a 2 mm drill bit, that facilitates manual introduction of the Kirschner

wires into the diaphysis and across the fracture site.
- Place as many prebent K-wires (at least 1.2 mm diameter) as possible (3–4) under fluoroscopic control for correct repositioning and implant position before bending and cutting them (Fig. 6.11a, b, c).
- Suture of the periosteum to cover the implants and minimize interference with the tendons (No. 5 PDS/Vicryl).
- Wound and skin closure (monofilament non-absorbable suture).
- Sterile, slightly compressing dressing from palm to forearm.
- Release of tourniquet.

Post-operative rehabilitation

- Elevation of the operated arm. Active exercises of fingers, elbow and shoulder.
- Routine radiographs within 24 hours.

Outpatient follow up

- Clinical review weekly.
- Review if clinical evidence for dislocation occurs and before allowing full weight-bearing (at 6 weeks) with radiographs.
- Removal of the implants is usually not necessary; however, if the implant gives rise to symptoms, removal after secured bone healing is possible.
- Discharge from the follow up after clinical and radiological evidence of fracture healing.

Section III: Fractures of the phalanx

Reinhard Meier

6.6 OPEN REDUCTION AND INTERNAL FIXATION (ORIF) OF CONDYLAR FRACTURES

Indications

- Unstable dislocated intra-articular condylar fractures (Fig. 6.12).

Pre-operative planning

Clinical assessment

- Local pain and swelling.
- Assess and document neurovascular status of finger.
- Assess and document axial or rotational dislocation.

Radiological assessment

- Standard anteroposterior and lateral radiographs of the finger.

Operative treatment

Anaesthesia

- Brachial plexus block, intravenous regional anaesthesia or general anaesthesia.
- At induction, administer prophylactic antibiotic as per local hospital protocol (e.g. 3rd generation cephalosporin).

Table and equipment

- Hand surgery instrumentation set.
- Hand small-fragment implant system.
- K-wires 1.0–1.2 mm.
- A radiolucent arm table.
- An upper arm tourniquet.
- An image intensifier.

Table set up

- The instrumentation is set up on the side of the operation.
- Image intensifier is from the front side of the arm table. Check for adequate visualization in 2 planes prior to draping.

Patient positioning

- Supine, pronated arm on arm table.

Draping, surgical approach and implant positioning

- Place tourniquet at upper arm.
- Prepare the skin over elbow, forearm, wrist and hand with usual antiseptic solutions (aqueous/alcoholic povidone–iodine).
- Apply adherent drape circularly above the elbow, so free motion of the elbow is possible.
- Tourniquet after exsanguination.
- Skin incision via a dorsal 'S' or 'Z' approach to the metacarpophalangeal or interphalangeal joint. In combined fractures the skin incision is via the wound.
- Incision of the extensor tendons.
- Open joint.
- Reduce fracture under direct vision.

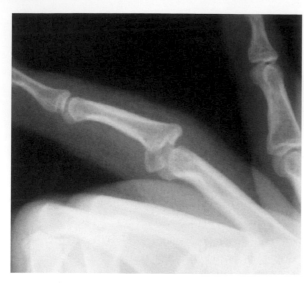

Fig. 6.12 Unstable fracture of the base of the proximal phalanx.

- Drilling and interfragmentary lag screw fixation (self-tapping screws 1.5 to 2.0 mm) with fluoroscopic and direct visual control of correct repositioning if fragments are big enough. Otherwise fix with K-wires (1.0–1.2 mm).
- Control reduction and implant position with image intensifier (Fig. 6.13a, b, c).
- Wound and skin closure (monofilament non-absorbable suture).
- Sterile, slightly compressing dressing. Short-arm, finger cast splint in intrinsic plus position.
- Release of tourniquet.

Post-operative rehabilitation

- Elevation of the operated arm. Active exercises of the elbow and shoulder.
- Routine radiographs within 24 hours.
- Short-arm, thumb finger intrinsic plus splint for 1 to 4 weeks, depending on the stability obtained at surgery.

Outpatient follow up

- Review before removing the splint with radiographs.
- If K-wires are implanted, remove after 4 weeks.

- Discharge from the follow up after clinical and radiological evidence of fracture healing.

6.7 OPEN REDUCTION AND INTERNAL FIXATION (ORIF) OF MIDSHAFT FRACTURES

Indications

- Unstable displaced midshaft fractures.
- Open fractures.

Pre-operative planning

Clinical assessment

- Local pain and swelling.
- Assess and document neurovascular status of the phalanx.
- Assess and document axial or rotational displacement (Fig. 6.14).

Radiological assessment

- Standard anteroposterior and lateral radiographs of the phalanx (Fig. 6.15a, b).

Operative treatment

Anaesthesia

- Brachial plexus block, intravenous regional anaesthesia or general anaesthesia.
- At induction, administer prophylactic antibiotic according to the local hospital protocol (e.g. 3rd generation cephalosporin).

Table and equipment

- Hand surgery instrumentation set.
- Hand small-fragment implant system.
- K-wires 1.0–1.4 mm.
- A radiolucent arm table.
- An upper arm tourniquet.
- An image intensifier.

Table set up

- The instrumentation is set up on the side of the operation.

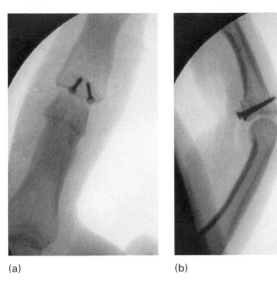

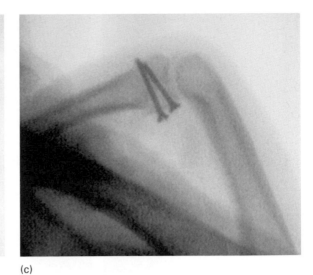

(a) (b) (c)

Fig. 6.13a, b, c After fixation with lag screws the joint is stable again.

- Image intensifier is from the front side of the arm table. Check for adequate visualization in 2 planes prior to draping.

Patient positioning

- Supine, pronated arm on arm table.

Draping, surgical approach and implant positioning

- Place tourniquet at upper arm.
- Prepare the skin over elbow, forearm, wrist and hand using antiseptic solutions (aqueous/alcoholic povidone–iodine).
- Apply adherent drape above the elbow, to allow free elbow motion.
- Tourniquet after exsanguination.
- Skin incision via a lateral approach to the phalangeal shaft.
- Prepare fracture at the proximal phalange via longitudinal incision between the extensor tendons and the tendons of the interosseous muscles.
- Remove debris from the fracture-line.
- Reduce fracture under direct vision.
- Drilling, interfragmentary lag screw fixation (self-tapping screws 1.5 to 2.0 mm) and/or mini-plate fixation in a lateral position with fluoroscopic and direct

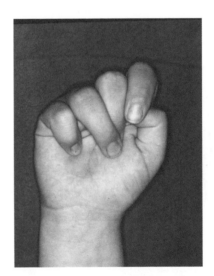

Fig. 6.14 Rotational displacement of the 4th phalanx.

visual control of correct repositioning if fragments are big enough (Fig. 6.16a, b). In case of very small fragments perform the fixation with K-wires (1.0–1.4 mm).
- Readaption of tendons and of the interosseous muscles if separated before.
- Wound and skin closure (monofilament non-absorbable suture).
- Sterile, slightly compressing dressing. Short-arm, phalanx cast splint in intrinsic plus position.
- Release of tourniquet.

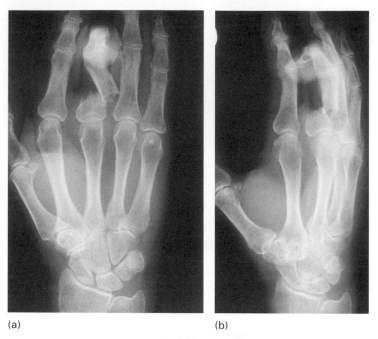

(a)   (b)

Fig. 6.15a, b Displaced fracture of the proximal phalanx II.

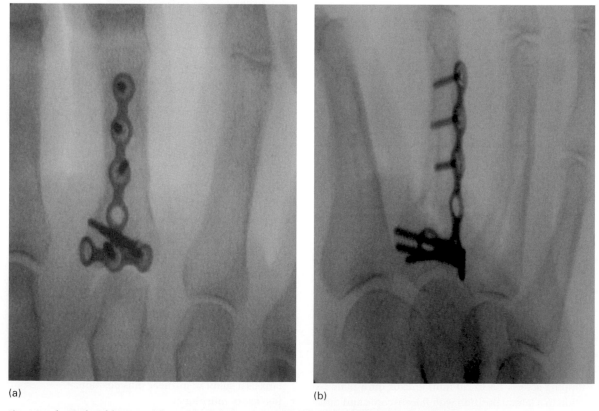

(a)   (b)

Fig. 6.16a, b Displaced fracture of the proximal phalanx II treated with open reduction and plate fixation.

Post-operative rehabilitation

- Elevation of the operated arm. Active exercises.
- Routine radiographs within 24 hours.
- Short-arm, phalanx intrinsic plus (40–45° extension of wrist, 70–80° flexion of metacarpophalangeal joint and extension in proximal and distal interphalangeal joints) splint for one to 4 weeks, depending on the stability obtained at surgery.

Outpatient follow up

- Review weekly.
- Review before removing the splint with radiographs.
- If K-wires are implanted, removal after 4 weeks.
- Discharge from the follow up after clinical and radiological evidence of fracture healing.

Part II

Pelvis and acetabulum

Fractures of the pelvic ring

Peter V. Giannoudis

7.1 APPLICATION OF ANTERIOR FRAME

Indications

Fixation of pelvic fractures associated with major bleeding including AP (anteroposterior) II, AP III, LC (lateral compression) II, LC III, vertical shear fractures and fractures with a combined mechanism of injury, according to Young's classification. Depending on the type of pelvic injury and when the physiological status of the patient has been normalized, the external fixator could be exchanged with an open reduction and internal fixation procedure of the pelvic ring. This usually takes place after the 4th or 5th day from the time of the injury.

Pre-operative planning

Clinical assessment

- Inspection of the anterior lateral and posterior aspect of the pelvic ring would allow evaluation about the extent of the soft tissue damage.
- Neurological examination of the lower limbs is of paramount importance.
- Careful inspection of the perineal region would allow identification of open fractures. Evaluation of the genitourinary system is of vital importance in order not to miss any injuries to the urethra, bladder and the vaginal walls.

Radiological assessment

- Standard anteroposterior radiographs demonstrate the type of fracture.

- Accurate evaluation of the injury to the posterior elements of the pelvic ring (sacrum and sacroiliac joint) require CT scan evaluation.
- Inlet and outlet views would allow accurate evaluation of the displacement of the hemi-pelvis, providing useful information to the surgeon regarding the manoeuvres necessary in theatre for accurate reduction of the fracture.

Timing of surgery

- The application of an external fixator on the pelvis in the presence of hypovolaemia is an emergency procedure. This can be performed either in a trauma room or in the operating theatre.

Operative technique

Anaesthesia

- General anaesthesia.
- Administration of prophylactic antibiotics as per local hospital protocol.

Table and equipment

- This includes the Hoffmann II external fixator pelvic tray.
- The instrumentation is set up on the site of the operation.
- An image intensifier is from the contralateral side.
- Position of the table diagonally across the operating room so that the operating area lies in the clean air field.

Practical Procedures in Orthopaedic Trauma Surgery: A Trainee's Companion, ed. Peter V. Giannoudis and Hans-Christoph Pape.
Published by Cambridge University Press. © Cambridge University Press 2006.

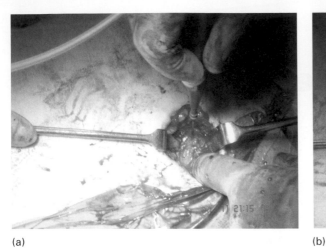

(a)

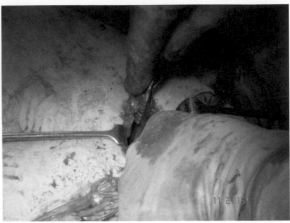

(b)

Fig. 7.1a, b The incision should cross the iliac crest at a right angle.

Draping and surgical approach

- Prepare the skin and drape the patient in the usual fashion from above the pubis symphysis to just below the umbilicus.

Operation details

- The tray is kept pre-assembled.
- The appropriate chucks and hand braces are included so that the tray can be used independently of other equipment including power tools.

Pin positioning: *two options of pin insertion are available*

(a) Either along the iliac crest.
(b) Or into the area of the anterior inferior iliac spine (this is just above the acetabulum where there is thick bone stock).

- However, in an acute trauma situation placement of the pins into the iliac crest is the only acceptable route.
- Landmarks for the pin insertion are easily identified even in the presence of quite extensive soft tissue swelling.
- The incision should cross the iliac crest at a right angle and be planned to take into consideration the final corrective position of the pelvis (Fig. 7.1a, b).
- It should be noted here that an incision above the crest will lead to extensive pressure on the skin from the pins as the pelvic position is reduced.

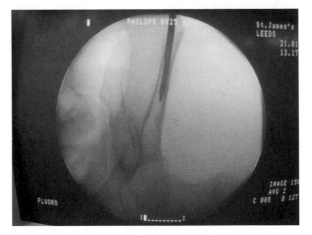

Fig. 7.2 Owing to the shape of the anterior iliac crest, the pins will converge interiorly and follow the plane of the iliac crest.

- The ideal site for pin placement extends posteriorly along the iliac crest from the anterior spine for 8–10 cm.
- Placement of 2 pins in each side of the crest is adequate to provide the necessary stability of the ring; however, if in any doubt, and if each one has been checked manually for security, then a third one could be inserted as well.
- Owing to the shape of the anterior iliac crest, the pins will converge interiorly and follow the plane of the iliac crest (Fig. 7.2).
- This requires that the fixator applied must accommodate free pin placement in all planes.
- After a bar is secured to the pins in each crest, a large alpha or quadro-lateral frame is constructed across the

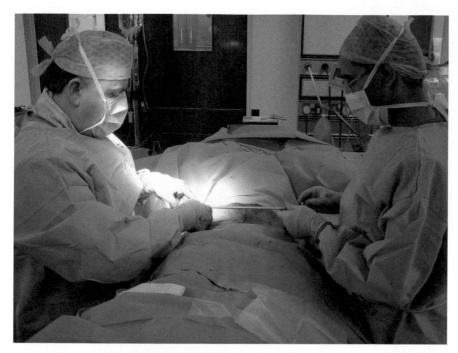

Fig. 7.3 After a bar is secured to the pins in each crest, a large alpha or quadro-lateral frame is constructed across the front of the patient, standing well up from the abdomen.

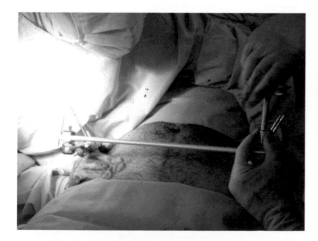

Fig. 7.4 The pelvic displacement is manually reduced and subsequently all the frame joints tightened.

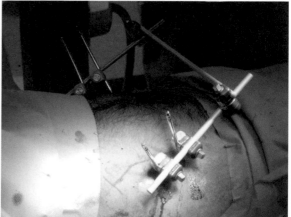

Fig. 7.5 It is of paramount importance that the emergency frame is well above the abdomen to accommodate the massive swelling that will develop.

front of the patient, standing well up from the abdomen (Fig. 7.3).

- Fracture reduction will create a loose application.
- The pelvic displacement is manually reduced and subsequently all the frame joints tightened (Fig. 7.4).
- It is of paramount importance that the emergency frame is well above the abdomen to accommodate the massive swelling that will develop (Fig. 7.5).

- After the insertion of the pins the wound should be checked and any pressure on the skin should be released.
- The wound is closed with 3.0 nylon and the pin sites can be covered with a prima pore dressing.

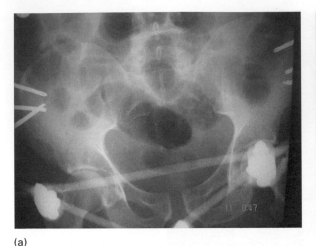

(a)

Fig. 7.6a Radiological examination.

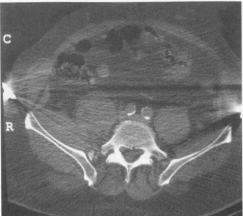

(b)

Fig. 7.6b CT examination.

Post-operative complications

(1) Be aware of contamination of the pin site.
(2) Loss of the initial reduction achieved.

- The pelvic frame is applied to aid the resuscitation process and nowadays it is very rarely used as a definitive method of treatment for pelvic ring injuries.

Implant removal

- The pins are usually removed in theatre during the ORIF procedure of the pelvic ring.
- If the surgeon has decided to keep the frame as a definitive method of treatment then the pins are usually removed after a period of approximately 6–8 weeks, from the time of the application.

7.2 PLATING OF THE PUBIC SYMPHYSIS

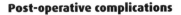

Indications

- When diastasis of the pubis symphysis exceeds 2.5 cm.
- According to Young's classification, use for such injury patterns as AP II, AP III, vertical shear injuries and injury patterns where there is a combined mechanism of injury.
- In cases where there is injury to the posterior elements of the ring, fixation of the ring alone (pubis symphysis) is insufficient and must be accompanied by reduction of the ligaments of the posterior pelvis.

- Contraindications for internal fixation of the symphysis pubis include unstable critically ill patients, open fractures with inadequate wound debridement and the crushing type of injuries where the extent of the injury to the skin could not tolerate a surgical incision.

Pre-operative planning

Clinical assessment

- These injuries require immediate evaluation and resuscitation of the patient and a multi-disciplinary team approach is necessary for their treatment including general surgeons, orthopaedic surgeons and urologists.
- In male patients it will be necessary to do a retrograde urethrogram to ensure that the urethra is intact before passing a Foley catheter. The presence of blood at the tip of the penile meatus is considered a sign of urethral trauma. When the urethra is intact a Foley catheter is passed and a cystogram obtained.
- In female patients because the urethra is only several centimetres in length a urethrogram is not required for the insertion of a Foley catheter.

Radiological assessment

- After the initial evaluation and resuscitation of the patient, radiographic studies are obtained. Radiological examination consists of an anteroposterior (AP) X-ray and inlet/outlet views (40° cephalad and 40° caudal) (Fig. 7.6a).

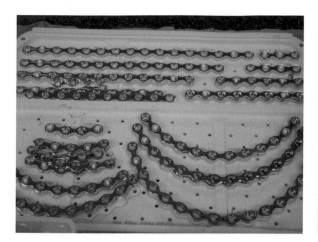

Fig. 7.7 The Matta plating system.

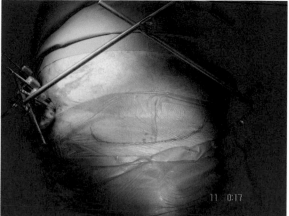

Fig. 7.8 The draping of the patient is in the usual fashion from 2 fingers below the pubis symphysis to 2 fingers superior to the umbilicus.

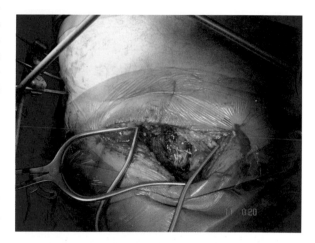

Fig. 7.9 A transverse Pfaennestiel incision is used for reduction and fixation of the symphysis.

- Computerised tomographic scans are recommended to assess the posterior pelvic anatomy and injury pattern (Fig. 7.6b). These views will allow the surgeon to determine the direction and magnitude of the symphysis pubis disruption and the relative position of the pubic bones. The most common injury pattern associated with disruption of the symphysis pubis is cephalad migration, posterior displacement and external rotation of one hemi-pelvis.

Timing of surgery

- It is usually 4 or 5 days after the injury.
- Initially as part of the resuscitation process, the pelvic injury may have been stabilized with an external fixator.

Operative treatment

Anaesthesia

- Prophylactic antibiotics are given as per local hospital protocol.
- General anaesthesia is administered with the patient in the supine position.

Table and equipment

- This includes the Matta plating system and several reduction tools (Fig. 7.7).
- An image intensifier is required from the beginning, and a radiolucent table (OSI table).
- The equipment tray is set up on the site of the operation.

- The image intensifier is on the opposite side of the surgeon.

Draping and surgical approach

- The skin is prepared with the usual antiseptics.
- The draping of the patient is in the usual fashion from 2 fingers below the pubis symphysis to 2 fingers superior to the umbilicus (Fig. 7.8).
- A transverse Pfaennestiel incision is used for reduction and fixation of the symphysis (Fig. 7.9).
- In cases where there has been marked disruption of the symphysis, detachment of one head of the rectus abdominis is a common finding.

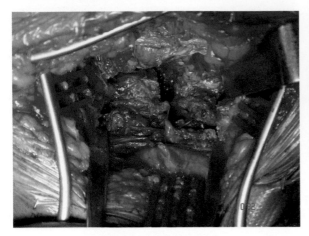

Fig. 7.10 Hofmann retractors are placed in the obturator foramen allowing enhancement of the exposure.

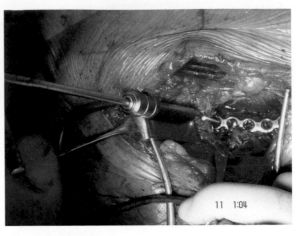

Fig. 7.12 Several different implants can be used for fixation of the disrupted symphysis and the most frequently used implants are pelvic reconstruction plates.

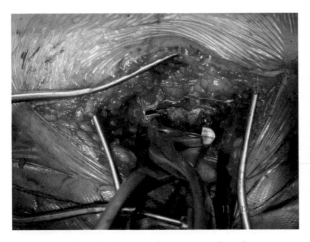

Fig. 7.11 For the reduction several manoeuvres have been described including the placement of large pointed reduction clamps on each side of the symphysis.

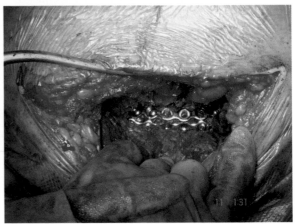

Fig. 7.13 The 3.5 mm plate could be applied superiorly, anteriorly or on the inner surface of the pelvic ring.

- The linea alba is divided longitudinally, with elevation of the insertion of the abdominis muscle laterally.
- Transverse sectioning of the rectus abdominis should be avoided as this will impair subsequent repair and healing of the abdominal wall.
- Hofmann retractors are placed in the obturator foramen allowing enhancement of the exposure (Fig. 7.10).
- For the reduction several manoeuvres have been described including the placement of large pointed reduction clamps on each side of the symphysis (Fig. 7.11).
- The pelvic reduction plate is secured to the pubis with 4.5 mm screws inserted into the pubic wall in an ante-rior to posterior direction (the screws are placed in such a way as to not interfere with the subsequent application of the symphysis plate).
- Several different implants can be used for fixation of the disrupted symphysis and the most frequently used implants are pelvic reconstruction plates (Fig. 7.12).
- Implants of 3.5 mm are considered the favoured option by many surgeons, with 3 screws inserted on each side of the symphysis.

Implant positioning

- The 3.5 mm plate could be applied superiorly, anteri-orly or on the inner surface of the pelvic ring (Fig. 7.13).

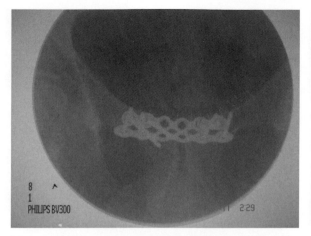

(a)

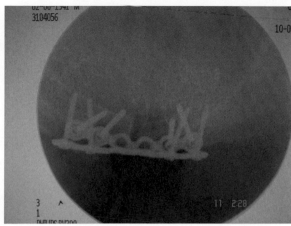

(b)

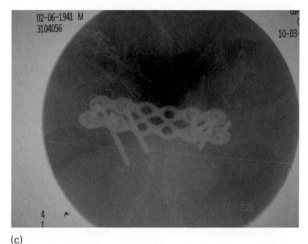

(c)

Fig. 7.14a, b, c Intra operatively, in addition to visualizing the reduction, screening with an image intensifier and obtaining AP, inlet and outlet views will confirm the adequacy of the reduction achieved.

- Intra operatively, in addition to visualizing the reduction, screening with an image intensifier and obtaining AP, inlet and outlet views will confirm the adequacy of the reduction achieved (Fig. 7.14a, b, c).

Closure

- Irrigate the wound thoroughly.
- A drain should be placed in the space of Retzius.
- Any detachment of the abdominis from the pubis symphysis should be re-attached with 1.0 Vicryl sutures Fig. 7.15a.
- The linea alba should be repaired with interrupted 1.0 Vicryl sutures (Fig. 7.15b).
- The fat layer should be approximated with 2.0 vicryl sutures.
- The skin should be closed with either surgical staplers or 3.0 nylon sutures in an interrupted manner.

Post-operative management

- Two further doses of prophylactic antibiotics.
- Anticoagulation therapy is prescribed in terms of low-molecular heparin until the patient is discharged home.
- Routine bloods and radiographs of the pelvis in 24 hours, including inlet/outlet views (Fig. 7.16a, b, c).
- Post-operatively watch for deep vein thrombosis (DVT) and infection.
- Partial weight-bearing on the injured side for 8 weeks for the isolated open book is advisable; however, in patients with combined internal fixation of the anterior and posterior pelvic ring, weight-bearing should be delayed for 8–12 weeks.
- When full weight-bearing is allowed, physiotherapy is indicated.
- Physiotherapy should be indicated at increasing hip abductor strength.

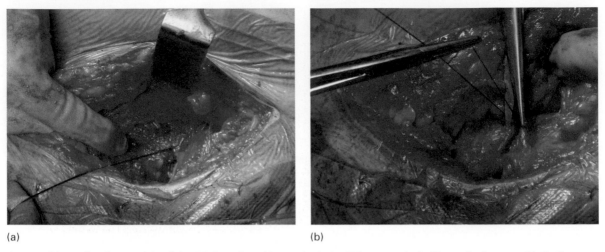

(a)   (b)

Fig. 7.15 (a) Any detachment of the abdominis from the pubis symphysis should be re-attached with 1.0 Vicryl sutures. (b) The linea alba should be repaired with interrupted 1.0 Vicryl sutures.

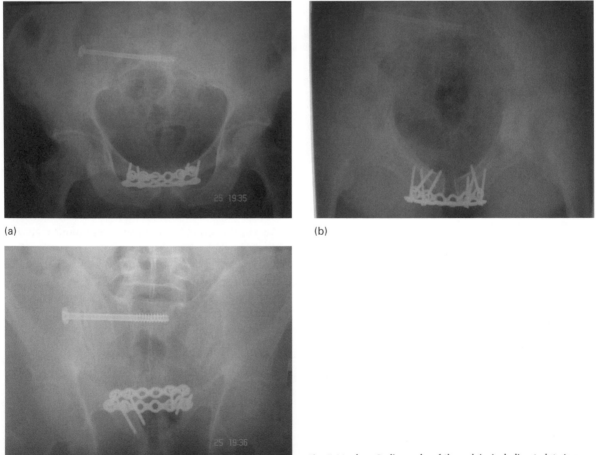

(a)   (b)

(c)

Fig. 7.16a, b, c Radiographs of the pelvis, including Judet views.

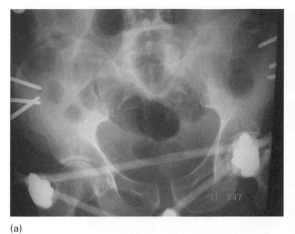

(a)

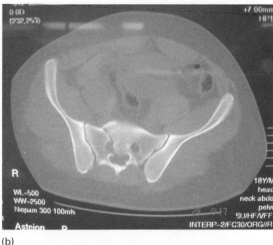

(b)

Fig. 7.17 (a) Radiograph of the pelvic ring demonstrating the degree and direction of displacement. (b) A CT scan is essential for accurate evaluation of the fracture pattern and for pre-operative planning for the insertion of the sacroiliac screws.

- For restoration of a normal gait, lower back strengthening exercises could be beneficial to the patient.

Post-operative complications

- Pneumonia, DVT, pulmonary embolism (PE) and dehiscence of the wound.
- Loss of fixation is usually associated with inadequate reduction and fixation of the posterior pelvic ring. If this occurs the entire fixation construct requires revision, reduction and fixation.
- Because of the physiological movement of the symphysis pubis, screw cut-out or plate failure are occasionally seen. However, it is unusual for these to become symptomatic and late hardware removal is infrequent.
- Other long term complications include impotence usually in the presence of an associated urethra injury or bladder injury.

Outpatient follow up

- Follow up at 2, 4, 8 and 12 weeks after surgery and then at 6 months and a year.
- The patient can be discharged and seen again at the request of their GP.

Implant removal

- Implant removal is not indicated unless there is good evidence to suggest that any ongoing symptoms are secondary to the presence of the implant.

7.3 SACROILIAC SCREW INSERTION

Indications

- Sacroiliac screw fixation is indicated in unstable fractures of the posterior pelvic ring, including sacroiliac joint dislocations, sacral fractures, certain iliac crescent fractures and a combination of the above injuries.

Pre-operative planning

Clinical assessment

- Evaluation of the soft tissue envelope both anteriorly and posteriorly of the pelvic ring. Assess and document the neurovascular status of the leg.
- Careful examination for other injuries must be made as quite frequently disruptions of the posterior pelvic ring are associated with other injuries and they are the result of high-energy trauma.
- Inspection of the perineal region is essential, as well as examination of the lumbar spine.

Radiological assessment

- Anteroposterior radiograph including inlet/outlet views of the pelvic ring (Fig. 7.17a). These would demonstrate the degree and direction of displacement.
- A CT scan is essential for accurate evaluation of the fracture pattern and for pre-operative planning for the insertion of the sacroiliac screws (Fig. 7.17b).

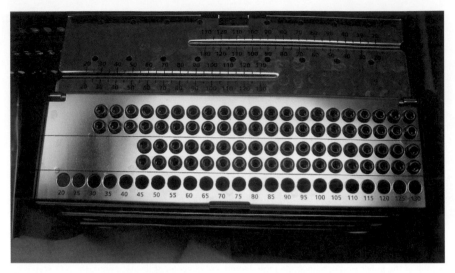

Fig. 7.18 A 7.3 mm cannulated screws set.

Anaesthesia

- General anaesthesia at induction.
- Administration of prophylactic antibiotics as per local hospital protocol.

Table and equipment

- A 7.3 mm cannulated screws set (Fig. 7.18).
- A radiolucent table with the appropriate traction devices is essential (OSI table).
- An image intensifier.

Table set up

- The instrumentation is set up on the site of the operation.
- Image intensifier is from the contralateral site.
- Position the table diagonally across the operating room.

Patient positioning

- Supine, with a well-padded radiolucent pudendal post.
- If there is a vertical shear disruption of the sacroiliac joint then a pin is inserted in the distal femur. This will facilitate the application of longitudinal traction for reduction of the joint dislocation.

Fracture reduction

- In cases of anteroposterior (AP) injury to the pelvic ring, internal rotation and immobilization of both lower limbs is adequate. In case of a vertical shear disruption, apply longitudinal traction for reduction of the ileum to the sacrum. Often anatomic reduction and stable fixation of the anterior pelvic injury improves the posterior pelvic displacement.

Draping and surgical approach

- Prepare the perineum, abdomen, part of the flanks and lower extremities with the usual antiseptic solutions (aqueous/alcoholic povidone–iodine).
- Using fluoroscopic control 3 views are taken: inlet, outlet and lateral, for the accurate verification of the entry point (Fig. 7.19).
- The skin is incised around the point selected for the insertion of the wire.
- Blunt deep dissection is accomplished with a narrow periosteal elevator.
- Following image intensifier control, the guide wire is progressed from the ilium across the sacroiliac (SI) articulation and into the lateral aspect of the sacral ala (using especially inlet and outlet pelvic images).
- The guide wire tip should be directed within the mid portion of the alar bone on the inlet view. It is then advanced up to the midline of the vertebral body of the sacrum (Fig. 7.20a, b, c).

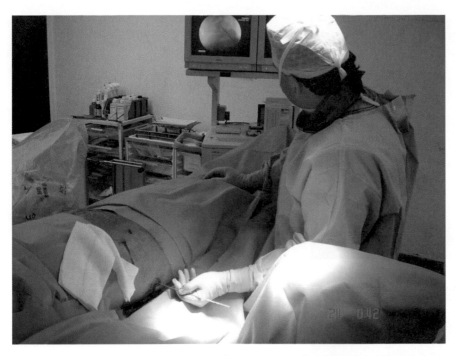

Fig. 7.19 Using fluoroscopic control 3 views are taken intraoperatively: inlet, outlet and lateral, for the accurate verification and marking of the entry point.

- Checking on the outlet view, the guide wire should be above the SI foramina and on the inlet view should be in the middle of the sacral ala.
- The guide wire depth is measured with the reverse ruler and the cannulated drill is advanced accordingly (Fig. 7.21a, b).
- The appropriate length 7.3 mm cannulated cancellous screw is inserted over the guide pin and tightened (Fig. 7.22).
- Partially threaded cancellous screws with 32 mm thread length or 16 mm thread length are chosen, when compression of fixation is indicated.
- Full threaded 7.3 mm cancellous screws are used when compression fixation is not desired such as after accurate reductions of transforaminal sacral fractures.
- During cannulated drilling and screw insertion, frequent fluoroscopic images should be obtained to assure no displacement of the guide wire.
- A washer should be used with the screw for better grip.
- The guide wire then is removed manually.
- Additional screws are used if residual instability is noted on the fluoroscopic stress examination.

Closure

- The percutaneous wound is then irrigated.
- The wound is closed with absorbable sutures 2.0 Vicryl for the subcutaneous fat layer.
- Skin closure could be performed either with stainless steel surgical staples or monofilament non-absorbable suture placed in a subcuticular layer.

Pitfalls to avoid and tips

- Screws inserted to treat sacral fractures are usually longer than those for SI joints.
- The initial iliosacral screw is positioned in such a way as to allow the insertion of a second screw if required.
- The SI joint screw is usually different from the sacral screw.
- Compression lag screws are routinely used to treat SI joint disruptions; however, sacral fractures may involve injury to the sacral neuroforamina and therefore, in this situation, compression with lag screws may produce nerve root injury.
- In the transforamina sacral fracture a fully threaded non-compression cancellous screw is indicated.

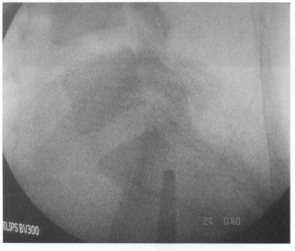

(a)

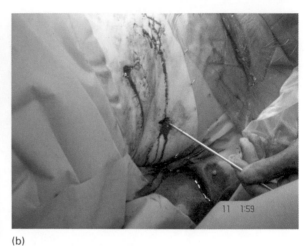

(b)

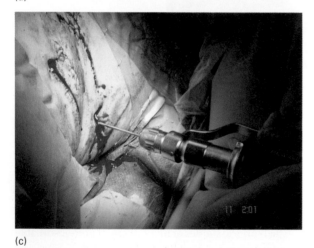

(c)

Fig. 7.20a, b, c Following image intensifier control, the K-wire is progressed from the ilium across the SI articulation and into the lateral aspect of the sacral ala (using especially inlet and outlet pelvic images).

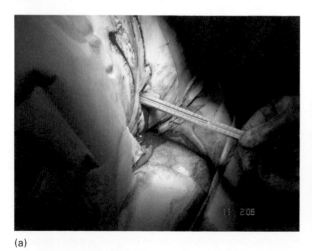

(a)

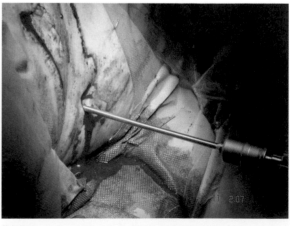

(b)

Fig. 7.21a, b The guide pin depth is measured with the reverse ruler and the cannulated drill is advanced over the K-wire.

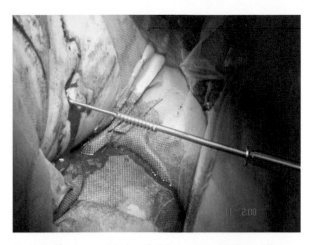

Fig. 7.22 The appropriate length 7.0 mm cannulated cancellous screw is inserted over the guide pin and tightened.

- The SI joint screws begin caudal/posteriorly on the ilium and are directed cephalad/anteriorly to be perpendicular to the oblique SI articulation. By obtaining such a direction a violation of the articular SI joint cartilaginous surfaces is usually avoided.

Post-operative rehabilitation

- Two further doses of prophylactic antibiotics, routine bloods and radiographs of the pelvis including AP inlet/outlet views (Fig. 7.23a, b, c).
- Chemical thromboprophylaxis or compression cuff pumps are indicated.
- The mobilization of the patient is dependent on the overall condition of the patient and other associated injuries.

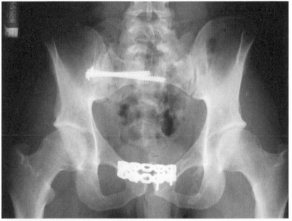

(a)

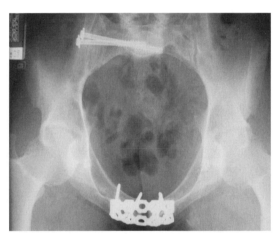

(b)

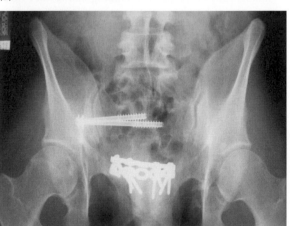

(c)

Fig. 7.23a, b, c Post-operative AP, inlet and outlet views demonstrating the SI screws position.

- Depending on the type of injuries sustained the sta-bilized hemi-pelvis is usually protected by means of partial weight-bearing with crutches for a period of 6–8 weeks.
- Progressive weight-bearing is subsequently allowed with a goal to progress to full weight bearing 3 months after the operation.
- It is essential post-operatively to accurately evaluate the neurological status of the patient. If there are any clinical signs of lumbar or sacral nerve root lesion, then a CT scan should be obtained to exclude perforation of the sacral foramina or insertion of the screw away from the safe anatomical zone. If this is the case then the screw should be removed immediately and should be re-inserted.

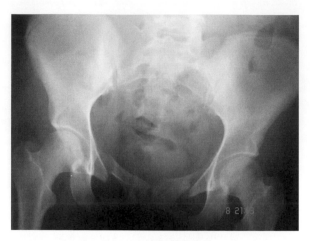

Fig. 7.24 Anteroposterior radiograph of the pelvis.

Outpatient follow up

- The patient is reviewed at 6 weeks initially and then at 3 months, 6 months and a year. Discharge from follow up after clinical and radiological evidence of fracture healing. Review again at the request of the GP, usually after a period of 18 months.

Implant removal

- No removal is indicated unless there is a good evidence of soft tissue irritation.

7.4 OPEN REDUCTION AND INTERNAL FIXATION (ORIF) OF THE SACROILIAC JOINT ANTERIORLY

Indications

- Disruptions of the sacroiliac joint posteriorly.
- AP III, LC III and vertical shear fracture patterns.

Pre-operative planning

Clinical assessment

- Pain localized at the affected hip site.
- Assessment and documentation of the neurovascular status of the leg is essential.
- In young patients careful examination must be made as this injury is usually the result of high-energy trauma and other associated injuries are usually present.

- Overall initial assessment should follow the Advanced Trauma Life Support (ATLS) protocol.
- After haemodynamic stability has been achieved following initial resuscitation with the administration of crystalloids and blood products, temporarily stabilization of the sacroiliac (SI) joint can be achieved with either an external fixator or a c-clamp posteriorly.

Timing of surgery

- The definitive procedure could be performed be 3–5 days after the day of injury.

Radiological assessment

- Radiological assessment includes anteroposterior (AP) radiographs of the pelvis including inlet/outlet views (Fig. 7.24).
- A CT scan will help to evaluate better the injury pattern and assist in the pre-operative planning.

Operative treatment

Anaesthesia

- General anaesthesia.
- Administration of prophylactic antibiotics as per local hospital protocol.

Table and equipment

- Radiolucent table (OSI) with the appropriate traction device.
- An image intensifier.

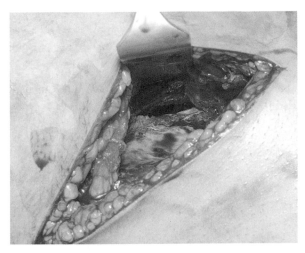

Fig. 7.25 The first window of the ilioinguinal approach is utilized where the abdominal muscles and the fascia of the iliacus are detached from the ilium following subperiosteal elevation. Access is made to the SI joint.

Table set up

- The instrumentation is set up at the site of the operation.
- Image intensifier is from the contralateral site.
- Position the table diagonally across the operating room so that the operating area lies in the clean air field.

Patient positioning

- Supine with a well-padded radiolucent pudendal post in cases where traction is indicated for the reduction of the fracture.

Reduction of the fracture

- Closed fracture reduction can be achieved with the application of axial traction through a distal femoral pin.

Draping and surgical approach

- Prepare the skin over the lower abdomen.
- Shaving of the pubic hair would allow simultaneous exposure of an anterior lesion (i.e. symphysis disruption).
- The first window of the ilioinguinal approach is utilized where the abdominal muscles and the fascia of the iliacus are detached from the ilium following subperiosteal elevation. Access is made to the SI joint (Fig. 7.25).

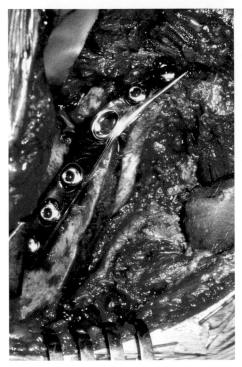

Fig. 7.26 A narrow 3-hole DCP 4.5 or 3.5 are the preferred implants. An angle of 6–9° between the two plates enables fixation in areas of dense bone and prevents shearing.

- Care has to be taken to avoid any injury to the lumbar sacral nerve root L5 which runs very close by, approximately 1.5 cm across the ala of the sacrum.
- Usually the reduction is achieved by manual lateral compression or the insertion of a lag screw into the iliac wing.
- Also a Farabeuf clamp can be applied by the insertion of two 3.5 screws on the sacral ala and the ilium for reduction of the dislocation.
- A narrow 3-hole DCP 4.5 or 3.5 are the preferred implants (Fig. 7.26).
- 2 plates enables fixation in areas of dense bone and prevents shearing.
- The holes of the sacral screws are drilled under direct vision and parallel to the joint.

Closure

- Irrigate the wound thoroughly and achieve haemostasis.

- The fascia is closed with No. 1 PDS or Vicryl over one drain.
- Subcutaneous fat is closed with absorbable sutures 2.0 PDS or Vicryl.
- Skin is closed with stainless steel surgical staples or monofilament nylon sutures in an interrupted manner.

Post-operative rehabilitation

- Two further doses of prophylactic antibiotics, routine bloods and radiographs of the pelvis at 24 hours including AP pelvis and inlet/outlet views.
- The drains are removed in 24 hours.
- The patient is mobilized toe touch, weight-bearing on the affected side.

- Post-operatively watch for DVT, PE, infection and loss of reduction.

Outpatient follow up

- Review at 3 weeks, 6 weeks, 6 months and 12 months with both clinical and radiographic assessment of the pelvis.
- Discharge from follow up after clinical and radiological evidence of fracture healing and full restoration of functional capacity, usually after 12–18 months from the time of the injury.
- Review again at the request of the GP.

Implant removal

- No removal is indicated.

Fractures of the acetabulum

Peter V. Giannoudis

8.1 OPEN REDUCTION AND INTERNAL FIXATION (ORIF) OF POSTERIOR WALL FRACTURES – KOCHER–LANGENBECK APPROACH

Indications

Fractures of:
- Posterior wall.
- Posterior column.
- Posterior column and wall.
- Transverse fractures.
- Transverse posterior wall and T-shaped fractures.

Pre-operative planning

Clinical assessment

- Examination of the injured limb is essential, including the soft tissue envelope.
- In cases of high-energy trauma examination for other potential associated injuries should be performed carefully.
- The Advanced Trauma Life Support (ATLS) evaluation protocol should be followed.

Radiological assessment

- Anteroposterior radiograph of the pelvis, as well as Judet views, can provide substantial diagnostic information in terms of fracture type and also indicate the need for emergency treatment (in cases of fracture dislocations of the femoral head) (Fig. 8.1a,b,c,).

- CT scan will supplement the plain radiographs and important additional information can be obtained for the pre-operative planning (Fig. 8.2a,b,c).

Timing of surgery

- Operative treatment is generally delayed for 3–5 days to allow stabilization of the patient's general status.
- Two to four units of blood should be made available, depending on the extent of the fracture pattern.

Indications for emergency acetabular fracture fixation

- Recurrent hip dislocation after reduction despite traction.
- Progressive sciatic nerve deficit after closed reduction
- Irreducible hip dislocation.
- Associated vascular injury requiring repair.
- Open fractures.

Anaesthesia

- General anaesthesia at induction.
- Administration of prophylactic antibiotics as per local hospital protocol.

Table and equipment

- Radiolucent fracture table which provides controlled traction and positioning, assisting the fracture reduction (OSI table).

Practical Procedures in Orthopaedic Trauma Surgery: A Trainee's Companion, ed. Peter V. Giannoudis and Hans-Christoph Pape.
Published by Cambridge University Press. © Cambridge University Press 2006.

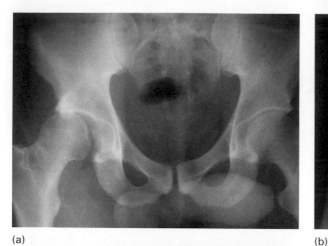

(a)

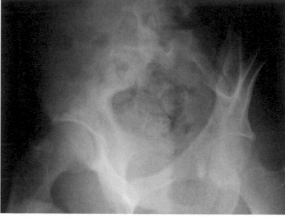

(b)

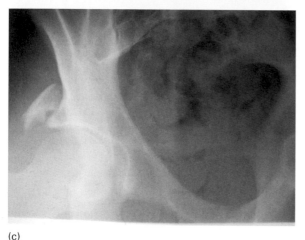

(c)

Fig. 8.1a,b,c, Anteroposterior, obturator oblique and iliac oblique views of a simple posterior wall fracture of the acetabulum.

- Traction is applied by using a distal femoral pin with the knee flexed approximately 90°.
- The angle of knee flexion places the sciatic nerve in a relaxed position minimizing the risk of intraoperative sciatic nerve injury.

Equipment

- Matta plating system.
- The instrumentation is set up on the site of the operation.
- Image intensifier is from the contralateral side.
- Position the table across the operating room so that the operating area lies in the clean air field.

Patient positioning

- Prone with a well-padded radiolucent pudendal post.
- A Foley catheter is inserted prior to the operation.

- For surgery, for instance on the right hip, the affected limb is placed in traction with the knee flexed to 90° and with the traction applied through the distal femoral pin (Fig. 8.3).

Draping and surgical approach (Kocher–Langenbeck)

- Prepare the skin of the buttock and the lateral aspects of the thigh (Fig. 8.4).
- The skin incision is centred over the greater trochanter.
- The proximal branch of the incision is directed towards the posterior superior iliac spine, ending approximately 6 cm short over this bony landmark.
- Distally the incision extends approximately 12 cm along the mid-lateral aspect of the thigh. The skin incision is carried through the subcutaneous tissue and

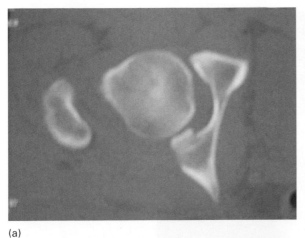

(a)

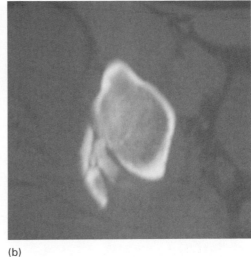

(b)

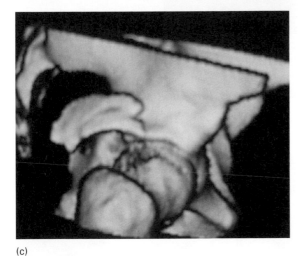

(c)

Fig. 8.2a,b,c CT scan of a posterior wall fracture of the acetabulum.

superficial fascia onto the fascia lata of the lateral thigh and the thin deep fascia overlying the gluteus maximus muscle.

- The fascia lata is then divided in line with the skin incision, beginning at the distal aspect of the wound, continuing approximately towards the greater tuberosity and ending at the first site of the gluteus maximus muscle fibres (Fig. 8.5a,b).
- Continue the proximal dissection by splitting the gluteus maximus muscle.
- The incision should be made between the upper 1/3 and lower 2/3 of the muscle as this is a relative avascular interval and in the desired plane of dissection. (Fig. 8.6a,b).
- There is no internervous plain.
- Release of the gluteus maximus insertion to the femur allows adequate posteromedial retraction of the large

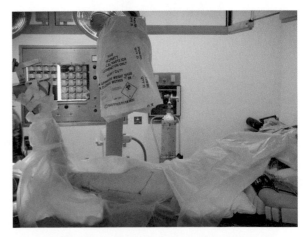

Fig. 8.3 The patient is prone with a well-padded radiolucent pudendal post. The affected limb is placed in traction with the knee flexed to 90° and with the traction applied through a distal femoral pin.

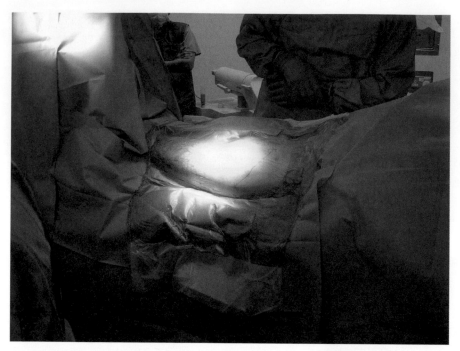

Fig. 8.4 Preparation of the skin and draping.

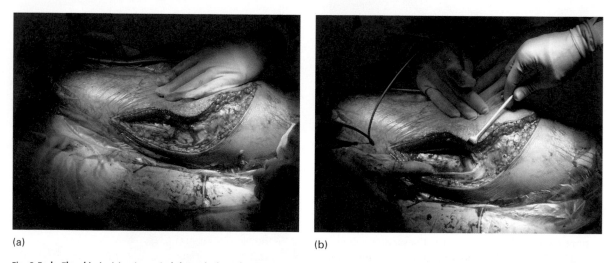

(a)

(b)

Fig. 8.5a,b The skin incision is carried through the subcutaneous tissue and superficial fascia onto the fascia lata of the lateral thigh and the thin deep fascia overlying the gluteus maximus muscle.

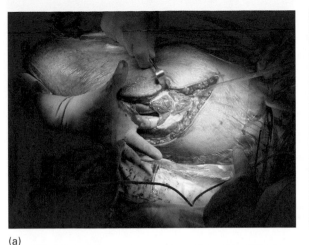

(a)

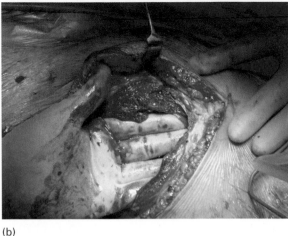

(b)

Fig. 8.6a,b The incision should be made between the upper 1/3 and lower 2/3 of the muscle as this is a relatively avascular interval and in the desired plane of dissection.

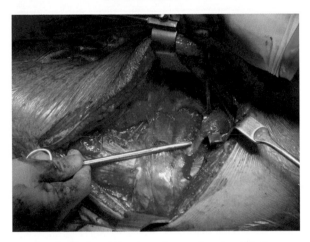

Fig. 8.7 Identify the piriformis tendon running alongside the gluteus minimus muscle.

mass of the gluteus maximus muscle without undue stretching on the inferior gluteal nerve.

• Whilst the tendon is released care should be taken to avoid damage of the first perforating branch of the profunda femoris artery, which runs in close proximity.

• Locate the sciatic nerve: the relationship between the sciatic nerve and quadratus femoris muscle should serve as a reference point.

• Identify the piriformis tendon running alongside the gluteus minimus muscle (Fig. 8.7).

• It must be noted here that variability exists in relation to the sciatic nerve and the piriformis muscle. One therefore should be aware of the anatomic variability in this

area and prior identification of the sciatic nerve on the posterior surface of the quadratus femoris muscle will prevent intraoperative confusion and decrease the risk of iatrogenic sciatic nerve injury.

• After the identification of the piriformis tendon it should be tagged with a suture and released from its insertion (Fig. 8.8a,b).

• Subsequently identify the obturator internus tendon with the superior and inferior gemeli muscles, which can be found just inferior and slightly deep to the piriformis.

• External rotation of the hip will relax the tendon allowing easier access to its deep surface. The obturator internus tendon is isolated, tagged with a suture and released from its insertion. Both the piriformis and obturator internus tendons should be incised approximately 1.5 cm from their insertion points into the greater trochanter to avoid injury to the blood supply of the femoral head (Fig. 8.9a,b).

• Elevate the obturator internus tendon away from the hip capsule along with the gemeli muscles.

• Access to the lesser sciatic notch is now possible and a specially designed sciatic nerve retractor can be placed with its tip anchoring to the lesser sciatic notch (Fig. 8.10a,b).

• With the appropriate position of the sciatic nerve retractor, access is now possible to the posterior hip capsule and retroacetabular surface of the posterior column, which can be explored and cleared of any debris (Fig. 8.11a,b).

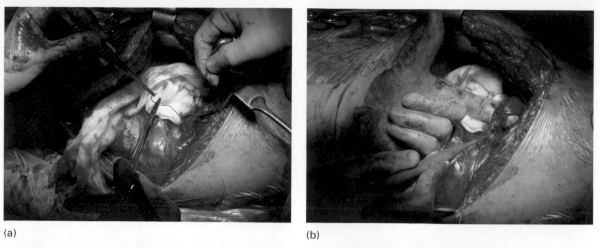

(a)   (b)

Fig. 8.8a,b After the identification of the piriformis tendon it should be tagged with a suture and released from its insertion.

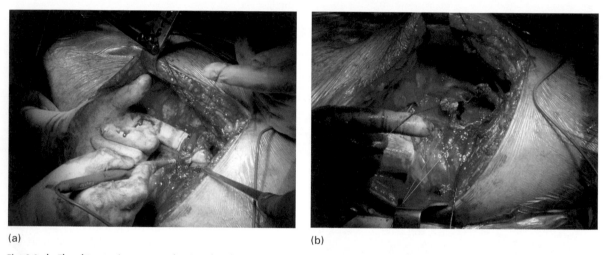

(a)   (b)

Fig. 8.9a,b The obturator internus tendon is isolated, tagged with a suture and released from its insertion. Both the piriformis and obturator internus tendons should be incised approximately 1.5 cm from their insertion points into the greater trochanter to avoid injury to the blood supply of the femoral head.

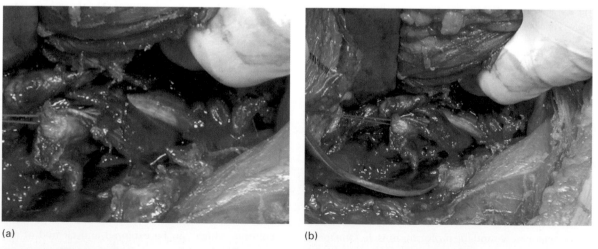

(a)   (b)

Fig. 8.10a,b With the piriformis being held back digitally, the sciatic nerve is visualized running posterior to the obturator internis tendon. A sciatic nerve retractor is placed anteriorly to the obturator internus tendon into the lesser sciatic notch.

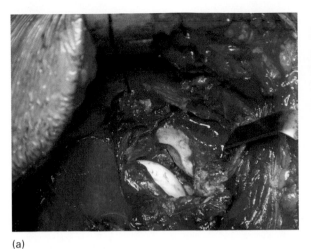

(a)

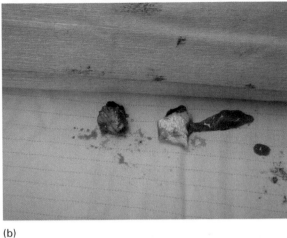

(b)

Fig. 8.11 (a) With the appropriate position of the sciatic nerve retractor access is now possible to the posterior hip capsule and retroacetabular surface of the posterior column, which can be explored and cleared of any debris (b).

- Superiorly the hip abductors are elevated from the external surface of the ilium with a curved retractor (Langenbeck).
- Care should be taken in the region of the greater sciatic notch not only to avoid injury to the sciatic nerve but also to the superior gluteal neurovascular bundle.
- The extent of the fracture pattern dictates the extent of the surgical approach; for instance, for isolated posterior wall fractures the dissection is completed at this stage.
- In cases where there is a transverse or a T-shape fracture, dissection must continue through the greater sciatic notch into the true pelvis and on to the quadrolateral surface of the acetabulum.
- Usually in cases where fracture dislocation has occurred visualization of the hip joint is possible without the need for any capsulotomy.
- The intra-articular surface of the hip joint could be better visualized by applying traction to the femur (Fig. 8.12).
- Osteotomy of the greater trochanter in an attempt to extend access of the Kocher–Langenbeck approach along the external surface of the anterior column is rarely required.
- In cases of an isolated posterior wall fracture, a posterior wall fracture fragment is reflected and reduced anatomically and held with the aid of K-wires.
- Lag screws can then be inserted from the wall to the posterior column (Fig. 8.13a,b,c).
- The screw length is usually determined by using the measuring gauge.

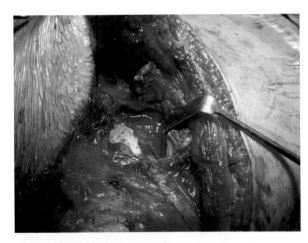

Fig. 8.12 The intra-articular surface of the hip joint could be better visualized by applying traction to the femur.

- Screws of 3.5 mm are used from the posterior wall to the posterior column.
- The overall fixation is then neutralized by the application of a 3.5 plate appropriately contoured to accommodate the shape of the posterior column (Fig. 8.14a,b).
- Intraoperative fluoroscopic images can assist in evaluating the accuracy of reduction and also the implant and screw positioning (Fig. 8.15a,b,c).

Closure

- The wound is irrigated thoroughly and haemostasis is achieved.

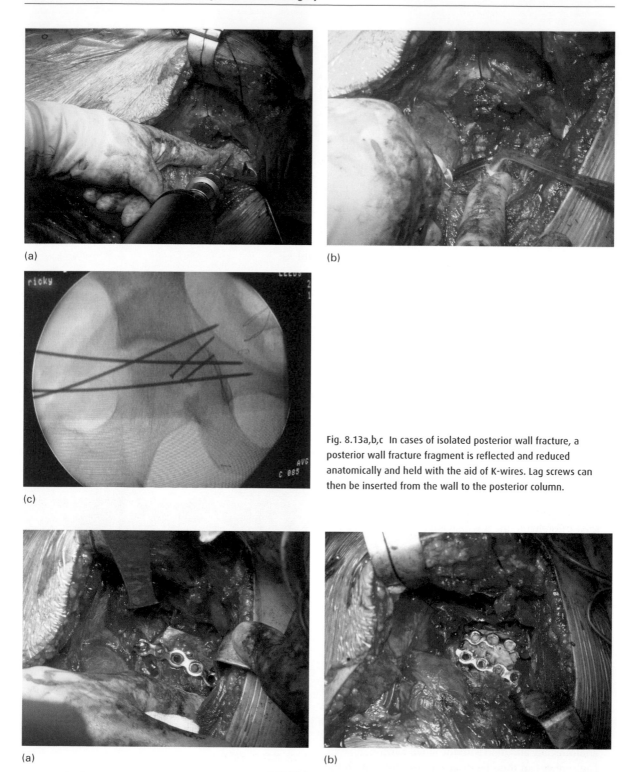

(a)

(b)

(c)

Fig. 8.13a,b,c In cases of isolated posterior wall fracture, a posterior wall fracture fragment is reflected and reduced anatomically and held with the aid of K-wires. Lag screws can then be inserted from the wall to the posterior column.

(a)

(b)

Fig. 8.14a,b The overall fixation is then neutralized by the application of a 3.5 plate appropriately contoured to accommodate the shape of the posterior column.

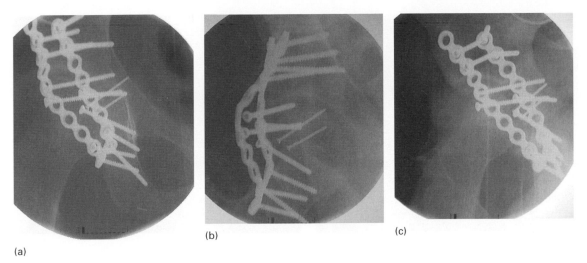

(a)

(b)

(c)

Fig. 8.15a,b,c Intraoperative fluoroscopic images can assist in evaluating the accuracy of reduction and also the implant and screw positioning.

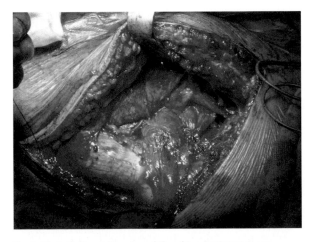

Fig. 8.16 Both the piriformis and the obturator internus are re-attached by using non-absorbable sutures.

- Both the piriformis and the obturator internus are re-attached by using non-absorbable sutures (Fig. 8.16).
- After the placement of a deep, closed suction drain, the fascia lata, gluteal fascia and subcutaneous tissues are closed in layers with 1.0 and 2.0 Vicryl absorbable sutures.
- The skin can be closed either with stainless steel surgical staples or monofilament nylon sutures in an interrupted manner.

Post-operative rehabilitation

- Two further doses of prophylactic antibiotics.

- Routine bloods and radiographs of the pelvis in 24 hours, including Judet views (Fig. 8.17a,b,c).
- The drain is removed in 24 hours.
- The patient is administered low-molecular weight heparin for thromboprophylaxis until discharged home.
- Subsequently the patient is prescribed 75 mg aspirin for a period of 6 weeks.
- Mobilize by toe touch weight-bearing for a period of 3 months.
- Subsequently progress to full weight-bearing and refer the patient to physiotherapy.

Outpatient follow up

- Review at 6 weeks and 3 months with radiographs of the hip.
- Follow the patient for a minimum of 2 years to evaluate the development of post-traumatic osteoarthritis with both clinical and radiological assessment.
- After a period of 3 years review again at the request of the GP.

Implant removal

- No removal is indicated unless there is evidence of low-grade infection or soft tissue irritation or development of heterotopic ossification.

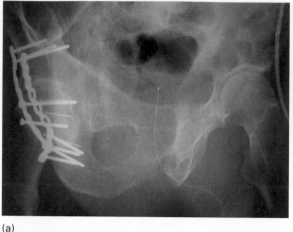

(a)

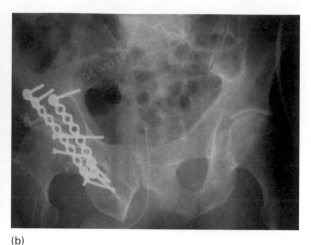

(b)

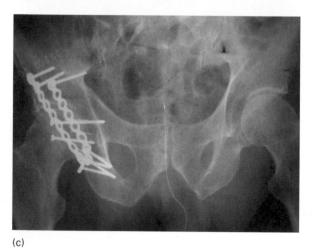

(c)

Fig. 8.17a,b,c Post-operative radiographs of the pelvis within 24 hours, including Judet views.

8.2 OPEN REDUCTION AND INTERNAL FIXATION (ORIF) VIA THE ILIOINGUINAL APPROACH

Indications

- Stabilization of the majority of both associated column fractures.
- Certain transverse fractures.
- Anterior column and anterior wall fractures.

Pre-operative planning

Clinical assessment

- Pain is usually localized in the affected hip site.
- Inspection of the soft tissue envelope of the pelvis anteriorly and posteriorly is of paramount importance.

- Accurate assessment and documentation of neurovascular status of the leg is imperative.
- In young patients careful examination or detection of other injuries must be made as they are frequently present as a result of the high-energy trauma sustained.

Radiological assessment

- Anteroposterior (AP) radiographs of the pelvis, including Judet views.
- CT scan adds important information regarding the fracture configuration and the presence of incarcerated or impacted fragments within the acetabulum (Fig. 8.18a,b,c).
- Drawing the fracture on a dry-bone, pelvic model helps ensure that the surgeon understands the fracture configuration.

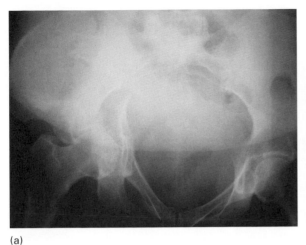

(a)

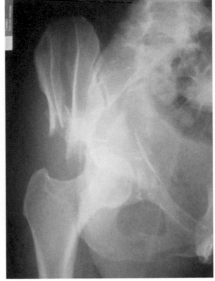

(b)

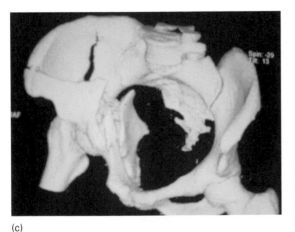

(c)

Fig. 8.18a,b,c Anteroposterior radiographs of the pelvis, including Judet views. CT scan adds important information regarding the fracture configuration and the presence of incarcerated or impacted fragments within the acetabulum.

Timing of surgery

- Surgery is usually performed 3–5 days after the date of injury.
- Chemoprophylaxis against development of deep vein thrombosis (DVT) and pulmonary embolism (PE) is administered when the patient's haemodynamic condition is stable (in cases where multiple injuries have been sustained).

Operative treatment

Anaesthesia

- General anaesthesia at induction.
- Administration of prophylactic antibiotics as per local hospital protocol.

Table and equipment

- The Matta plating system should be available with all the necessary reduction instruments.
- Radiolucent table (OSI) is used with the appropriate traction devices.
- An image intensifier.

Table set up

- The instrumentation is set up on the site of the operation.
- An image intensifier is from the contralateral site.
- Position of the table is diagonally across the operating room so that the operating area lies in the clean air field.

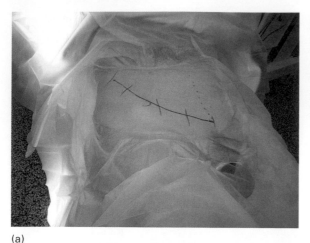

(a)

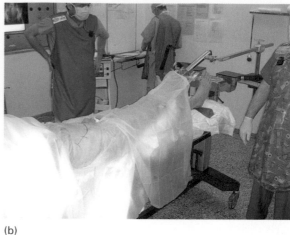

(b)

Fig. 8.19a,b During the operation the patient is placed supine with a well-padded radiolucent pudendal post to facilitate traction, which is exerted via the insertion of a distal femoral pin.

Patient positioning

- During the operation the patient is supine with a well-padded radiolucent pudendal post to facilitate traction, which is exerted via the insertion of a distal femoral pin (Fig. 8.19a,b).
- Traction can be applied intraoperatively and that can assist in the reduction of the fracture.

Draping and surgical approach

- The affected leg is positioned with the hip slightly flexed to relax the iliopsoas muscle, femoral nerve and external iliac vessels.
- Before surgery a Foley catheter is introduced into the bladder.
- Shaving of the pubic hair is indicated and the whole area of the lower abdomen is draped, as well as the gluteal region down to the middle of the thigh.
- The incision begins at the midline, 3–4 cm proximal to the symphysis pubis.
- It is directed laterally to the anterior superior iliac spine and then along the anterior two thirds of the iliac crest (Fig. 8.20).
- The periosteum is then incised along the iliac crest and the attachment of the abdominal muscles and the origin of the iliacus are released.
- By subperiosteal dissection the iliacus is elevated from the internal iliac fossa as far posterior as the sacroiliac joint and medially to the pelvic brim.
- The internal iliac fossa is then packed for haemostasis.

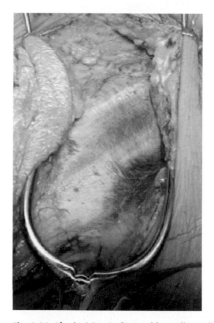

Fig. 8.20 The incision is directed laterally to the anterior superior iliac spine and then along the anterior two thirds of the iliac crest.

- Through the lower portion of the incision, the aponeurosis of the external oblique muscle and external rectus abdominis fascia are exposed.
- The incision is in line with the cutaneous incision at least 1 cm proximal to the external inguinal ring.
- The aponeurosis of the external oblique muscle is then reflected distally. This unroofs the inguinal canal and exposes the inguinal ligament.

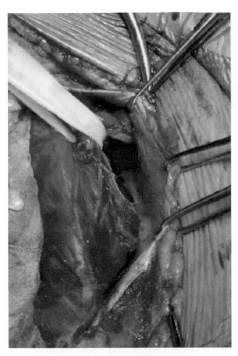

Fig. 8.21 A Penrose drain is placed around the spermatic cord or the round ligament and the adjacent ilioinguinal nerve.

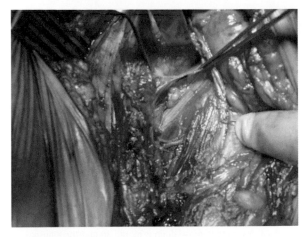

Fig. 8.23 The iliopectineal fascia separates vessels and lymphatics which are retracted from the medial aspect of the iliopectineal fascia, and the iliopsoas muscle and femoral nerve from the lateral aspect. Identify the iliopectineal fascia, lateral cutaneous femoral nerve, iliopsoas muscle and the external iliac vessels.

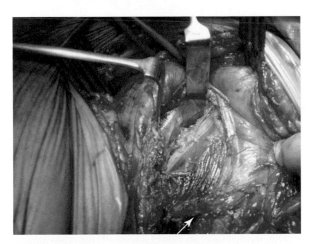

Fig. 8.22 Immediately beneath the inguinal ligament the lateral femoral cutaneous nerve exits into the thigh. Arrow indicates lateral femoral cutaneous nerve.

- The spermatic cord or the round ligament is visualized at the medial aspect of the incision.
- A Penrose drain is placed around the spermatic cord or the round ligament and the adjacent ilioinguinal nerve (Fig. 8.21).
- The inguinal ligament is sharply incised so that a 1–2 mm cuff of the ligament remains with the common

origin of the internal oblique and transversus abdominis muscles and the transversalis fascia.
- Immediately beneath the inguinal ligament the lateral femoral cutaneous nerve exits into the thigh (Fig. 8.22).
- Directly beneath the mid portion of the incision lie the external iliac vessels.
- Medial to these vessels the insertion of the conjoined tendon on to the pubis is incised.
- It may also be necessary to incise a portion of the rectus abdominis tendon just above its insertion on to the pubis.
- The retropubic space of Retzius is now accessible and is packed with swabs after evacuation of the fracture haematoma.
- The anterior aspects of the femoral vessels and the surrounding lymphatics are exposed in the mid portion of the incision within the lacuna vasorum.
- The iliopectineal fascia separates vessels and lymphatics which are retracted from the medial aspect of the iliopectineal fascia, and the iliopsoas muscle and femoral nerve from the lateral aspect (Fig. 8.23).
- The iliopectineal fascia is sharply incised to the pectineal eminence. Detaching the iliopectineal fascia allows access to the true pelvis and subsequently to the quadrilateral surface of the posterior column.
- A second Penrose drain is placed around the iliopsoas, femoral nerve and lateral femoral cutaneous nerve for retraction purposes.

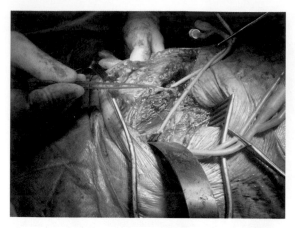

Fig. 8.24 A second Penrose drain is placed around the iliopsoas, femoral nerve and lateral femoral cutaneous nerve for retraction purposes. A third Penrose drain is placed around the femoral vessels and lymphatics.

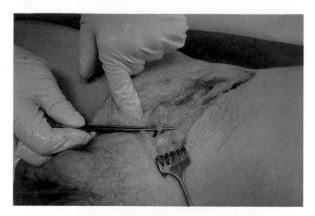

Fig. 8.25 A search is made for an anomalous origin of the obturator artery from the inferior epigastric artery or the presence of an anastomosis between the obturator and the external iliac vessels (Corona mortis).

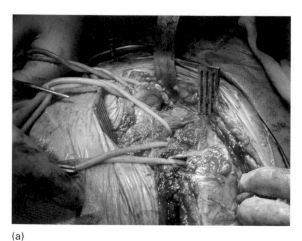

(a)

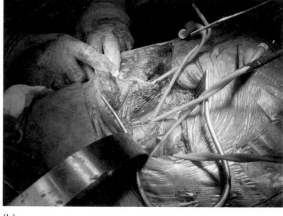

(b)

Fig. 8.26a,b The reduction and fixation of the fracture can now be completed by working back and forth in the three windows for vizualisation.

- A third Penrose drain is placed around the femoral vessels and lymphatics (Fig. 8.24).
- Care should be taken to leave undisturbed the fatty areolar tissues surrounding the vessels as this contains the lymphatic vessels.
- Before retraction of the external iliac vessels, the obturator nerve and artery should be identified posteromedial to the vessels.
- A search is made for an anomalous origin of the obturator artery from the inferior epigastric artery, or the presence of an anastomosis between the obturator and the external iliac vessels (Corona mortis) (Fig. 8.25).

- Subperiosteal dissection is used to expose the pelvic brim and superior pubic ramus.
- The periosteum can also be elevated from the quadrilateral surface.
- The reduction and fixation of the fracture can now be completed by working back and forth in the 3 windows for vizualisation (Fig. 8.26a,b).
- Medial retraction of the iliopsoas and femoral nerve allows vizualisation of the entire iliac fossa, the sacroiliac joint and the pelvic brim via the first window.
- Lateral retraction of the iliopsoas and the femoral nerve combined with medial retraction of the external iliac vessels opens the second window.

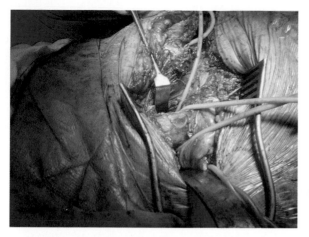

Fig. 8.27 Lateral retraction of the iliopsoas and femoral nerve combined with medial retraction of the external iliac vessels opens the second window as shown.

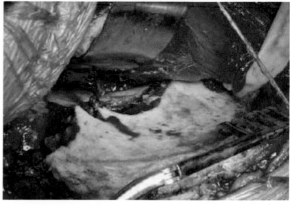

Fig. 8.28 Visualization of the fracture pattern through the lateral window.

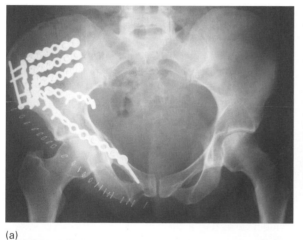

(a)

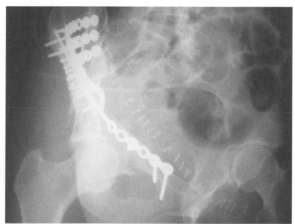

(b)

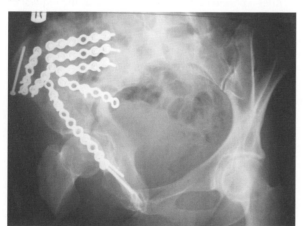

(c)

Fig. 8.29a,b,c Post-operative radiographs of the pelvis.

- This window gives access to the pelvic brim from the sacroiliac joint to the pectineal eminence as well as access to the quadrilateral surface for reduction of posterior column fractures. The pulse of the external iliac artery should be frequently checked when working within this window (Fig. 8.27).
- Medial retraction of the vessels gives access to the superior pubic ramus and the symphysis pubis if required.
- The spermatic cord or the round ligament is retracted medially or laterally as needed.

Technique of reduction and fixation

- Reduction usually starts from the back.
- The iliac crest and wing are reduced first.
- The reduction of fracture lines in the ilium must be perfect if the articular surface is to be reduced (Fig. 8.28).
- Traction could facilitate disimpaction of the iliac wing.
- Farabeuf and Weber clamps can be used for the reduction of iliac crest fracture fragments. Screws can be inserted between the tables of the ilium, parallel to the iliac crest.
- The anterior column fracture can then be reduced (the manoeuvre may be accomplished with the use of a Farabeuf clamp and ball spike).
- A screw placed from just lateral to the pelvic brim and directed towards the sciatic notch will hold the reduction.
- A long curved plate is then contoured to the superior aspect of the pelvic brim. This plate usually extends from the front of the sacroiliac joint to the body of the pubis. The plate must be twisted to match appropriately the contour of the ilium. It is important that the plate fits the bone as perfectly as possible to avoid loss of fracture reduction.
- The posterior column can be reduced with the use of an angled reduction clamp restoring the profile of the greater sciatic notch. The reduction clamp is usually placed entirely within the second window of the approach.
- Posterior column fixation is achieved by screws placed parallel to the quadrilateral surface. These screws can be placed either inside or separate from the pelvic brim plate to achieve fixation in the retroacetabular surface.

Closure

- Irrigate the wound thoroughly and achieve haemostasis.
- Closure of the ilioinguinal ligament is performed with non-absorbable sutures (2.0 Prolene). The closure extends up to the superior iliac spine.
- Drill holes can be made through the ilium to re-attach the iliacus fascia and external oblique abdominal muscles.
- A drain is inserted within the iliac fossa.
- The fat layer is closed with 2.0 Vicryl.
- The skin is closed with either stainless steel surgical staples or monofilament nylon interrupted sutures.

Post-operative treatment

- Two further doses of prophylactic antibiotics.
- Suction drains are generally removed after 24 hours or when drainage has ceased.
- Anticoagulation therapy is prescribed in terms of low-molecular heparin until the patient is discharged home.
- Subsequently a 6-week course of aspirin (75 mg) daily.
- A toe-touch, weight-bearing protocol is initiated for a period of 12 weeks.
- Subsequently the patient can progress to full weight-bearing.
- No heterotopic bone prophylaxis is necessary.

Outpatient follow up

- At 6 weeks, 3 months, 6 months, a year and yearly thereafter with radiographs of the pelvis, including Judet views (Fig. 8.29a,b,c).
- After a period of 2 years review again at the request of the GP.
- Patients are usually able to return to normal recreational activities after a period of 6 months and vigorous athletics after a period of a year.
- Be aware of post-operative complications of late infection, development of an inguinal hernia, deep vein thrombosis, pulmonary embolism and post-traumatic osteoarthritis.

Implant removal

- No removal is indicated.

Part III

Lower extremity

Section I: Extracapsular fractures of the hip

Raghu Raman and Peter V. Giannoudis

9.1 DYNAMIC COMPRESSION HIP SCREW

Indications

Sliding compression hip screw devices are used to stabilize

(a) Inter-trochanteric hip fractures (Fig. 9.1a,b).
(b) Intracapsular fractured neck of femur.

Pre-operative planning

Clinical assessment

- Pain localized in the affected hip site with radiation of pain to the knee.
- Limb is shortened and externally rotated.
- Assess and document neurovascular status of the leg.
- In young patients careful examination for other injuries must be made, as they are a result of high-energy trauma.
- A complete medical examination in elderly patients.

Radiological assessment

- Anteroposterior (AP) radiograph and a lateral view of the affected hip to demonstrate the fracture geometry.

Operative treatment

Anaesthesia

- Regional (spinal/epidural) and/or general anaesthesia.
- At induction, administer prophylactic antibiotic as per local hospital protocol (e.g. 3rd generation cephalosporin).

Table and equipment

- DHS instrumentation set – ensure the availability of the complete set of implants (Fig. 9.2).
- A radiolucent table or a fracture table with the appropriate traction devices.
- An image intensifier.

Table set up

- The instrumentation is set up on the side of the operation.
- Image intensifier is from the contralateral side.
- Position the table diagonally across the operating room so that the operating area lies in the clean air field.

Patient positioning

- Supine with a well-padded radiolucent pudendal post.
- Position the uninjured leg in a leg holder (i.e. Lloyd Davies with adequate padding over the peroneal nerve) or in wide abduction by a footplate attached to the leg extensions of the fracture table.
- A footplate attached to the other leg extension of the fracture table holds the injured leg (Fig. 9.3).

Fracture reduction

- Gentle traction and internal rotation reduces minimally displaced fractures.
- Apply longitudinal traction to restore the neck shaft angle (excessive traction may cause valgus over-reduction).

Practical Procedures in Orthopaedic Trauma Surgery: A Trainee's Companion, ed. Peter V. Giannoudis and Hans-Christoph Pape.
Published by Cambridge University Press. © Cambridge University Press 2006.

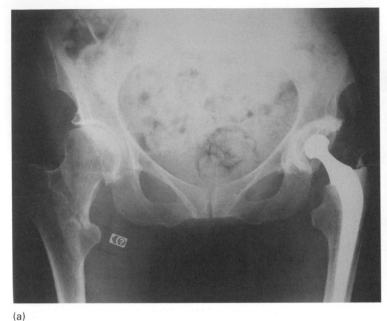

(a)

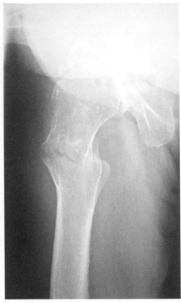

(b)

Fig. 9.1a,b Inter-trochanteric hip fracture.

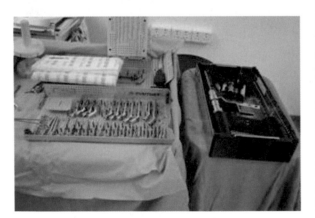

Fig. 9.2 DHS instrumentation set – ensure the availability of the complete set of implants.

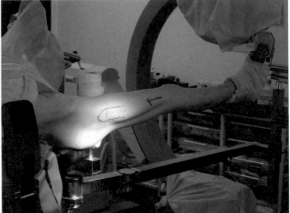

Fig. 9.3 A footplate attached to the other leg extension of the fracture table holds the injured leg.

- Open anatomical reduction is indicated if closed reduction fails to achieve a stable reduction.
- Non-anatomical methods such as a valgus osteotomy are reserved for failed reduction and unstable fractures.

Draping and surgical approach

- Prepare the skin over the proximal femur with the usual antiseptic solutions (aqueous/alcoholic povidone–iodine).

- Apply a transparent, plastic, adherent 'isolation' drape directly over the proposed incision site. This vertical drape is anchored above on a rail (Fig. 9.4).
- A direct lateral approach is made to the proximal femur from the greater trochanter, extending distally (Fig. 9.5).
- Divide the fascia lata in line with the skin incision (Fig. 9.6).
- Expose the proximal femur by splitting the vastus lateralis along its fibres or by elevating the vastus

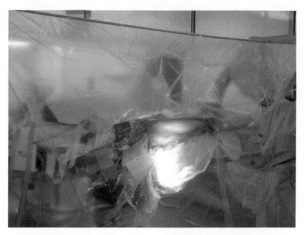

Fig. 9.4 Apply a transparent, plastic, adherent 'isolation' drape directly over the proposed incision site. This vertical drape is anchored above on a rail.

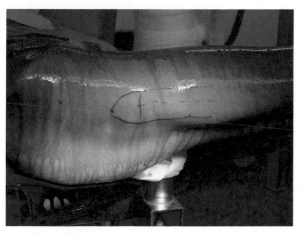

Fig. 9.5 A direct lateral approach is made to the proximal femur from the greater trochanter, extending distally.

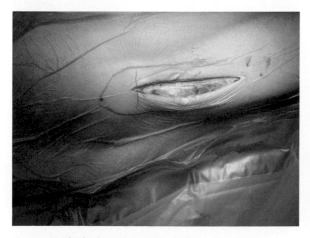

Fig. 9.6 Divide the fascia lata in line with the skin incision.

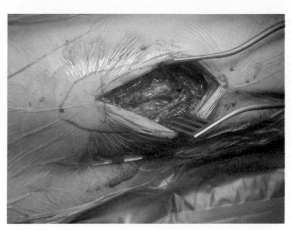

Fig. 9.7 Expose the proximal femur by splitting the vastus lateralis along its fibres or by elevating the vastus lateralis off the lateral intermuscular septum (beware of the perforators as they pierce the lateral intermuscular septum).

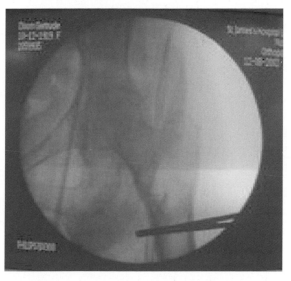

Fig. 9.8 The lesser trochanter marks the level of entry of a 135-degree angle plate.

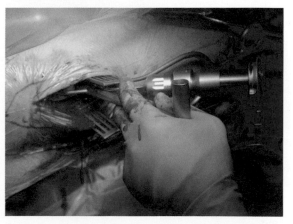

Fig. 9.9 Under fluoroscopic control insert a threaded 3.2 mm guide pin by power using the appropriate fixed angle guide.

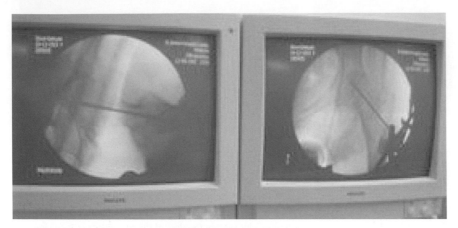

Fig. 9.10 Place the tip in the subchondral bone. The guide pin must lie in the centre of the femoral head in the anteroposterior and lateral views.

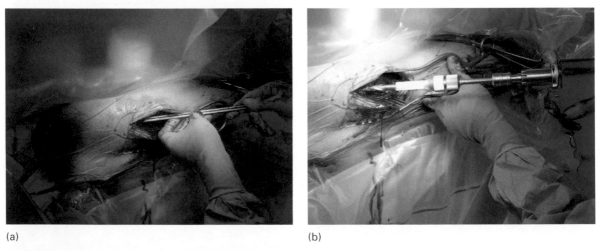

(a)   (b)

Fig. 9.11a,b Set the reamer 5 mm shorter than the length measured. Ream the femur by using the 'triple reamer'.

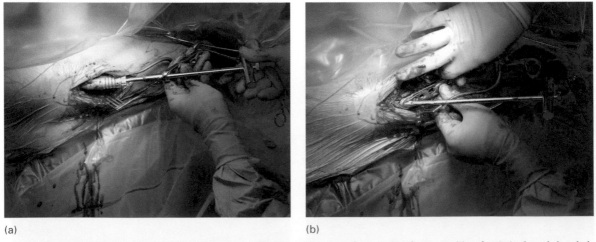

(a)   (b)

Fig. 9.12a,b Insert the lag screw over the centring sleeve after assembling it on the insertion device. Position the tip in the subchondral bone.

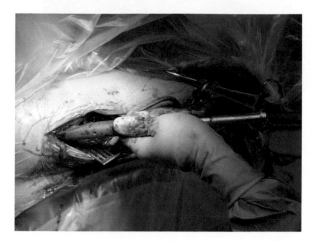

Fig. 9.13 Advance the side plate over the lag screw shaft and use the plate tamper to fully seat the plate.

lateralis off the lateral intermuscular septum (beware of the perforators as they pierce the lateral intermuscular septum) (Fig. 9.7).

Implant positioning

- The lesser trochanter marks the level of entry of a 135-degree angle plate (Fig. 9.8).
- Under fluoroscopic control insert a threaded 3.2 mm guide pin by power driver using the appropriate fixed angle guide (Fig. 9.9).
- The body of the guide must be flush and parallel with the lateral cortex.
- Advance the guide pin toward the apex of the femoral head, monitoring its position on the image intensifier.
- Place the tip in the subchondral bone. The guide pin must lie in the centre of the femoral head in the AP and lateral views (Fig. 9.10).
- Determine the lag screw length and reaming distance using the measuring device.
- Set the reamer 5 mm shorter than the length measured. Ream the femur by using the 'triple reamer' (Fig. 9.11a,b).
- Ream coaxially and use image intensification views to confirm that the guide pin is not advancing into the pelvis or being withdrawn at the conclusion of the reaming.
- Tap the bone in young patients and patients with hard sclerotic bones.

- Insert the lag screw over the centring sleeve after assembling it on the insertion device. Position the tip in the subchondral bone (Fig. 9.12a,b).
- The tip–apex distance (sum of the distances from the apex of the femoral head to the tip of the lag screw on both AP and lateral views, correcting for magnification) must ideally be less than 25 mm.
- On completion of the screw insertion, the handle of the insertion device must be parallel to the axis of the femoral shaft (perpendicular if a Richards compression screw is used) to allow the correct slotting of the lag screw to the plate barrel.
- Advance the side plate over the lag screw shaft and use the plate tamper to fully seat the plate (Fig. 9.13).
- Unscrew the lag screw retaining rod and remove the guide pin.
- Secure the plate to the femoral shaft using a plate clamp or a Haygroves clamp.
- Release traction (In unstable fractures, release traction after securing the plate). Using the 3.5 mm twist drill through the neutral drill guide, make screw holes corresponding to the holes in the plate.
- Determine the screw length using the measuring gauge. Use 4.5 mm screws after tapping to secure the plate (Fig. 9.14a,b,c).
- A compression screw through the lag screw to compress the fracture primarily (caution in osteoporotic bones) is optional and available for use.
- Obtain final radiographs in both the AP and lateral planes (Fig. 9.15a,b,c,d).

Closure

- Irrigate the wound thoroughly and achieve haemostasis.
- Close fascia lata (No.1 PDS/Vicryl) over a drain (12F) and the subcutaneous fat with absorbable sutures (2/0 PDS/Vicryl).
- Skin closure – stainless steel surgical staples, monofilament non-absorbable sutures or absorbable sutures placed in the subcuticular layer.

Post-operative rehabilitation

- Two further doses of prophylactic antibiotics.
- Routine bloods and radiographs of the pelvis in 24 hours.
- Remove drains in 24 hours.

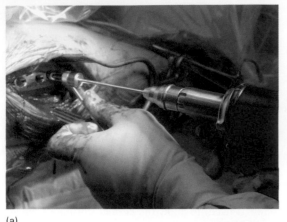

(a)

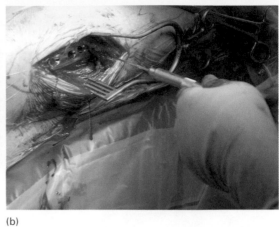

(b)

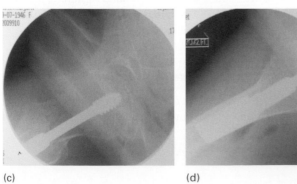

(c)

Fig. 9.14a,b,c Determine the screw length using the measuring gauge. Use 4.5 mm screws after tapping to secure the plate.

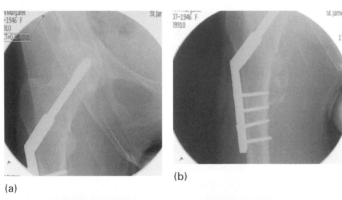

(a)

(b)

(c)

(d)

Fig. 9.15a,b,c,d Obtain final radiographs in both the AP and lateral planes.

- Mobilize full weight-bearing at the earliest opportunity and tailor physiotherapy to meet individual needs and demands.

Outpatient follow up

- Review at 3 months with radiographs of the hip.

- Discharge from the follow up after clinical and radiological evidence of fracture healing.
- Review again at the request of the GP.

Implant removal

- No removal is indicated unless there is good evidence of soft tissue irritation.

Section II: Intracapsular fractures of the hip

Christopher C. Tzioupis, Peter V. Giannoudis (9.2) and
David A. Macdonald (9.3)

9.2 CANNULATED SCREW FIXATION

Indications

- Undisplaced fractures of neck of femur (Garden Grade I, II).
- Displaced fractures in patients with adequate bone density and no severe chronic illness (rheumatoid arthritis, renal failure).
- Active individuals up to mid 70s.

Pre-operative planning

Clinical assessment

- Groin pain localized in the affected hip site – radiation of pain to the knee.
- Limb is shortened and externally rotated.
- Assess and document neurovascular status of the leg.
- In young patients careful examination for other injuries must be made, as they are a result of high-energy trauma.
- A complete medical examination in elderly patients.

Radiological assessment

- Anteroposterior radiograph and a lateral view of the affected hip (Fig. 9.16a,b).
- Evaluate head retroversion and posterior comminution.
- Assess primary and secondary compression and tension trabeculae on radiographs.
- CT or bone scans when physical signs are lacking.

Timing of surgery

- The outcome is improved if the surgery is performed within 8 hours.
- For young patients it is a true orthopaedic emergency.

Operative treatment

Anaesthesia

- Regional (spinal/epidural) and/or general anaesthesia.
- At induction, administer prophylactic antibiotic as per local hospital protocol.

Table and equipment

- Use a 7.0 or 7.3 cannulated screw set – ensure the availability of the complete set of implants.
- A radiolucent table or a fracture table with the appropriate traction devices.
- An image intensifier.

Table set up

- The instrumentation is set up on the side of the operation.
- Image intensifier is from the contralateral side.
- Position the table diagonally across the operating room so that the operating area lies in the clean air field.

Patient positioning

- Supine with a well-padded radiolucent pudendal post.
- Position uninjured leg in a leg holder (i.e. Lloyd Davies with adequate padding over the peroneal nerve) or in

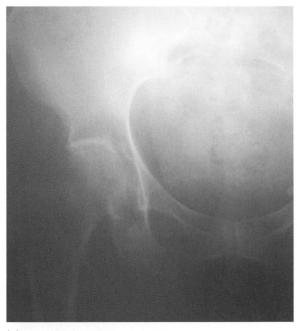

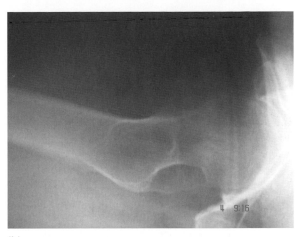

(b)

(a)

Fig. 9.16a,b Anteroposterior and lateral views of a right neck of femur undisplaced fracture.

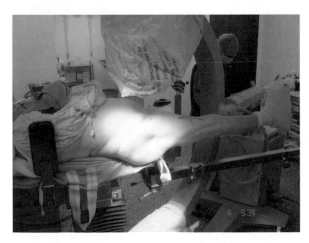

Fig. 9.17 The patient is positioned supine with a well-padded radiolucent pudendal post.

wide abduction by a footplate attached to the leg extensions of the fracture table.

- A footplate attached to the other leg extension of the fracture table holds the injured leg with up to 20° and up to 20° internal rotation (Fig. 9.17).

Fracture reduction

- Flex the affected limb at hip up to 90°.

- Internally rotate the thigh.
- Apply traction in line with the femur.
- Circumduct the limb into abduction maintaining the internal rotation.
- Bring it down to table level.
- Evaluate the reduction with the image intensifier using Garden alignment index.

Draping and surgical approach

- Prepare the skin over the proximal femur with usual antiseptic solutions (aqueous/alcoholic povidone–iodine).
- Apply transparent, plastic, adherent "isolation" drape directly over the proposed incision site. This vertical drape is anchored above on a rail (Fig. 9.18).
- A direct lateral approach is made to the proximal femur from the greater trochanter extending distally (Fig. 9.19).
- Divide the fascia lata in line with the skin incision (Fig. 9.20).
- Expose the proximal femur by splitting the vastus lateralis along its fibres or by elevating the vastus lateralis off the lateral intermuscular septum (beware of the perforators as they pierce the lateral intermuscular septum) (Fig. 9.21).

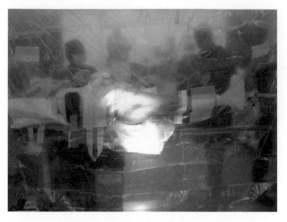

Fig. 9.18 A transparent, plastic, adherent 'isolation' drape is applied directly over the proposed incision site. This vertical drape is anchored above on a rail.

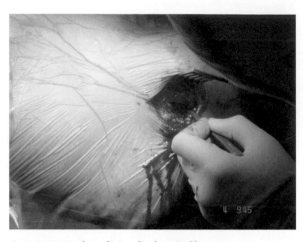

Fig. 9.21 Vastus lateralis is split along its fibres.

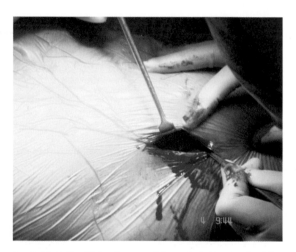

Fig. 9.19 A direct lateral approach is made to the proximal femur from the greater trochanter, extending distally.

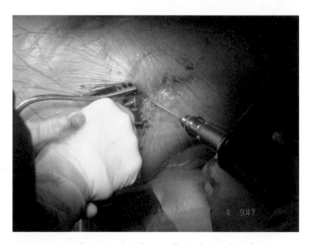

Fig. 9.22 A guide pin is placed centrally in the neck under fluoroscopic control in 2 planes.

Implant positioning

- A guide pin is placed centrally in the neck under fluoroscopic control in 2 planes (Fig. 9.22).
- Use image intensification to confirm the correct placement of the guide pin.
- Insert a guide pin into the subchondral bone of the femoral head through each of the outer triangle-patterned placement holes (Fig. 9.23a,b).
- Determine the insertion depth with the direct measuring device and calculate screw length (Fig. 9.24).
- Passing the cannulated tap over the guide pin tap the near cortex (Fig. 9.25).
- Insert the cannulated screw over the guide wire.

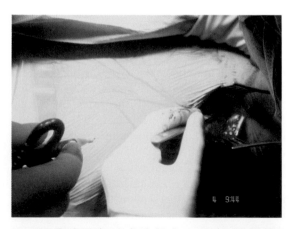

Fig. 9.20 The fascia lata is divided in line with the skin incision.

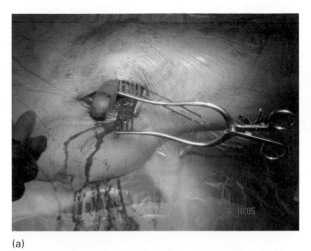

(a)

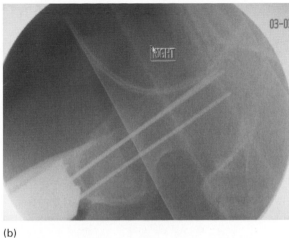

(b)

Fig. 9.23a,b Insertion of a guide pin into the subchondral bone of the femoral head through each of the outer triangle-patterned placement holes.

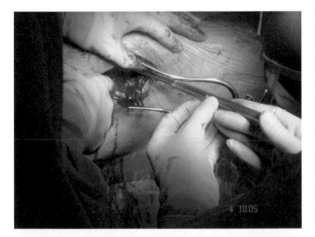

Fig. 9.24 Determination of the insertion depth with the direct measuring device and calculation of the screw length.

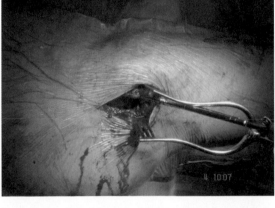

Fig. 9.26 Insertion of the cannulated screw over the guide wire using a washer to prevent the screw head from sinking into the cortex.

- Use a washer to prevent the screw head from sinking into the cortex (Fig. 9.26).
- Remove the guide pin and repeat the screw insertion technique for the remaining screws, inserting each screw before proceeding to the next.
- Obtain final radiographs in both the AP and lateral planes (Fig. 9.27a,b).

Closure

- Irrigate the wound thoroughly and achieve haemostasis.

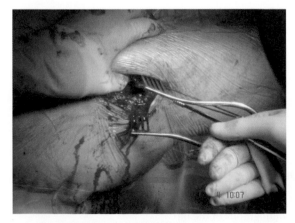

Fig. 9.25 Tapping of the near cortex.

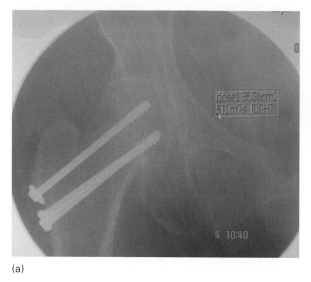

(a)

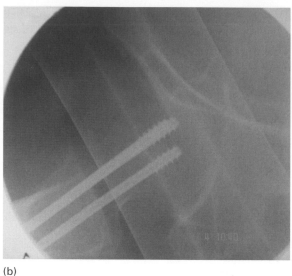

(b)

Fig. 9.27a,b Final radiographs in both the AP and lateral planes.

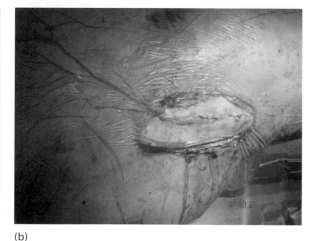

(a)   (b)

Fig. 9.28a,b Wound closure.

- Close fascia lata (No.1 PDS/Vicryl) and the subcutaneous fat with absorbable sutures (2/0 PDS/Vicryl).
- Skin closure with 3/0 monofilament absorbable sutures placed in the subcuticular layer (Fig. 9.28).

Post-operative rehabilitation

- Two further doses of prophylactic antibiotics.
- Routine bloods and radiographs of the hip in 24 hours.

- Remove drains in 24 hours.
- Mobilize by partial weight-bearing at the earliest and tailor physiotherapy to meet individual needs and demands.

Outpatient follow up

- Review at 2, 6, 12 weeks, 6 months, 1 and 2 years with radiographs of the hip.

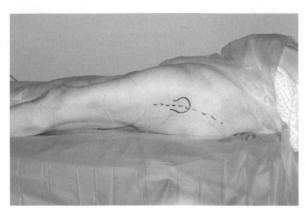

Fig. 9.29 Position in the anaesthetic room with a sand bag under the sacroiliac joint and U-drape to seal the perineum. The trochanter and proposed skin incision is highlighted.

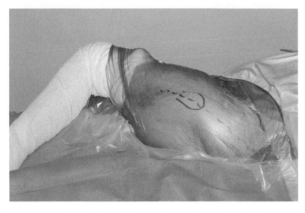

Fig. 9.30 'Prepped and draped', showing posterior and proximal access. Position of leg for initial skin incision.

- Discharge from the follow up after clinical and radiological evidence of fracture healing.
- Review again at the request of the GP.

9.3 HEMIARTHROPLASTY FOR INTRACAPASULAR HIP FRACTURES: AUSTIN MOORE UNCEMENTED HEMIARTHROPLASTY AND THOMPSON'S CEMENTED HEMIARTHROPLASTY

Indications and alternatives

- Displaced intracapsular (subcapital) hip fractures in the low-demand patient.

- In high demand/younger patients consider reduction (open or closed) and internal fixation or total hip replacement.
- Austin Moore requires an intact femoral neck and a 'normal' diameter proximal femur.
- Thompson's can be used when a fracture compromises the femoral neck.

Pre-operative planning

Clinical assessment

- Assess limb and patient.
- IVI.
- FBC, U&ES, Grp & Save.
- Social and mental assessment.
- Chest X-ray and ECG if indicated.
- Urinary catheter if indicated.
- Thromboembolic prophylaxis, 75 mg asprin once daily for 6 weeks post surgery. Mark the limb with an indelible marker on the thigh so that the mark can be viewed when the limb is draped.
- Consent, including a realistic assessment of the outcome.
- Start the discharge plan.

Radiological assessment

- X-rays of the pelvis, lateral hip, AP of the hip to show the proximal femur and the whole femur if a pathological fracture is suspected.

Anaesthesia

- Regional/general anaesthetic.
- Prophylactic antibiotics: 1.5 g intravenous cefuroxime.

Patient positioning

- Supine with a sandbag under the ipsilateral sacroiliac joint, plus perineal isolation drape (Fig. 9.29).
- Apply diathermy plate.
- Protect pressure areas.
- Check side.

Theatre

- Laminar flow.
- X-rays on viewing box.

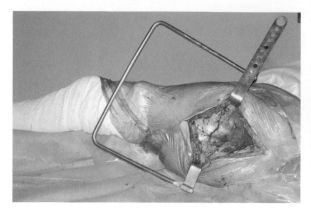

Fig. 9.31 Fascia lata incised in line with skin incision and initial incision retractor.

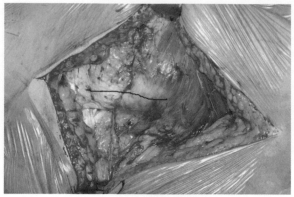

Fig. 9.32 The proposed line of incision is into the combined tendon of gluteus medius and vastus lateralis.

- Diathermy and suction on contralateral side – avoid where the leg will go when dislocated.

Draping and surgical approach

- Ensure 'prep and drapes' are far enough proximally and posteriorly to allow the skin incision to be centred on the greater trochanter (Fig. 9.30).
- Alcoholic betadine or chlorhexidene (if allergic to iodine).
- Waterproof drapes.
- Perineal seal.
- Adherent isolation drape, Ioband or similar.

Lateral approach

- The incision is centred on the greater trochanter with the leg flexed, adducted and internally rotated to create a posteriorly curved incision to aid delivery of the femur into the wound (Fig. 9.30).
- The fascia lata is divided in line with the skin incision – avoid curving anteriorly – and the initial incision retractor, such as the Charnley bow (Fig. 9.31).
- Incise from tip of the trochanter along the combined tendon of gluteus medius and vastus lateralis (Fig. 9.32).
- Elevate the anterior flap of the combined tendon to expose the anterior capsule of the hip (Fig. 9.33).
- NB: diathermy circumflex vessels below the trochanteric flare.
- Deliver the femur by external rotation and adduction to allow the tibia to be held parallel to the floor with the knee in 90° of flexion (Fig. 9.34).

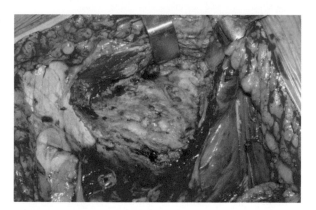

Fig. 9.33 Anterior femoral neck exposed to allow excision/incision of anterior capsule.

Neck resection

Austin Moore

- Resection is a finger's breadth above the lesser trochanter across to the piriformis fossa to ensure that the implant is supported by the femoral neck.
- Compare to a Thompson's in which resection is from the upper 1/3 of the lesser trochanter across to the piriformis fossa to ensure that the collar of the implant sits on the lesser trochanter (Fig. 9.35).
- Removal of the head with a 'corkscrew'. Keep twisting the corkscrew until the whole head rotates, indicating a disruption of the ligamentum teres (Fig. 9.36).
- Incise/excise the superior capsule to allow easy removal of the head and ease of relocation of the implant.

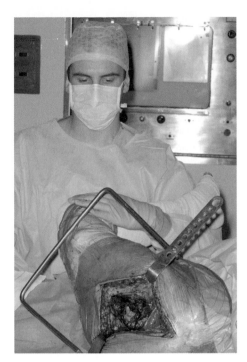

Fig. 9.34 The femur is delivered out of the wound by adduction and external rotation.

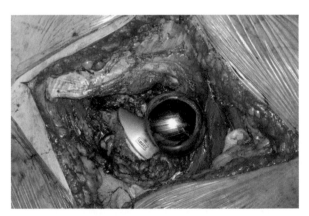

Fig. 9.35 Femoral neck cut for Thompson's down on to the lesser trochanter, so that the implant collar rests on the cut surface of the trochanter.

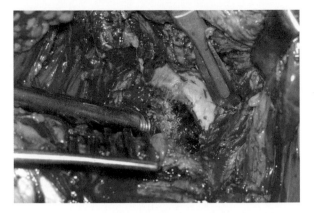

Fig. 9.36 Incise the superior capsule and labrum to allow easy removal of the head with a 'corkscrew', and relocation of the implant.

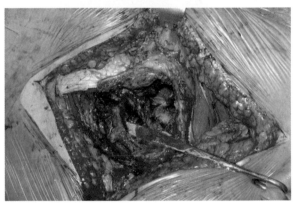

Fig. 9.37 Gently feel way down the shaft with the Trethowan to avoid perforation with broaches.

- Trial reduction or 'dummy' trial.
- Take care of performing a full reduction in porotic bone, as re-dislocation can cause a femoral fracture. Consider a 'dummy' trial with a swab in the acetabulum to prevent full relocation, but ensures that the hip is locatable, leg lengths are equal and the hip is stable.

Sizing of the head

- Canal entry with a blunt probe, such as a Trethowan spike (Fig. 9.37).
- Prepare canal with reamers (Fig. 9.38).
- Prepare a bone block from the femoral head to act as a cement restrictor for the Thompson's.

Cementation for a Thompson

- Bone block as a cement restrictor.
- Retrograde filling with a cement gun.
- Pressurize cement with thumb.
- Insert implant when the cement is 'doughy': approximately 4 minutes with Palacos R – the time varies with

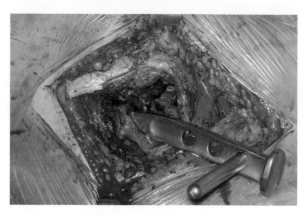

Fig. 9.38 Enlarge canal with the broach.

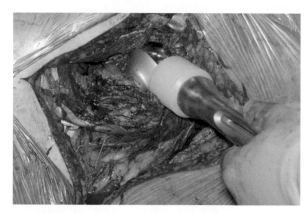

Fig. 9.39 Surgeon pushes implant into joint whilst assistant applies traction.

the type of cement and the theatre temperature and humidity.

Uncemented Austin Moore

- Ensure a firm fit and use light blows with a mallet. If not progressing down the canal, consider changing to a narrower implant or aborting to Thompson's.
- NB: 'It is the last blow that breaks the femur'!

Reduction

- Traction combined with internal rotation from an assistant, whilst the operator pushes the head into the joint (Fig. 9.39). Ensure the superior capsule and

labrum are not blocking the reduction. Divide/resect if this occurs.
- Check stability.

Closure

- Haemostasis.
- Drains: one in joint, one deep to fascia lata. In the obese patients, consider one drain in the fat layer.
- Abductor repair with 1 PDS or Vicryl.
- Fascia lata repair with 1 PDS or Vicryl.
- Fat layer – if anything, a few interrupted 2-0 PDS or Vicryl, but NOT continuous sutures.
- Skin closure: staples or subcuticular absorbable sutures.

Post-operative treatment

- Antibiotics: 750 mg cefuroxime, 8 hourly, 3 doses.
- Drains: remove the following morning.
- Mobilize.
- Check Hb and U&Es.
- Thromboembolic prophlaxis: early mobilization plus asprin 75 mg once daily for 6 weeks.

Discharge

- When safe.
- Follow up at GP's request.

Complications

Peri-operative

- Must ensure that the hemiarthroplasty is stable and the femur intact at the end of the operation. Do not adopt a 'hope for the best' attitude!
- Fractured femur or perforation. This must be identified and treated – don't 'hope for the best'.
- Unstable joint. May need revising.
- If unable to resolve instability, leave as an excisional arthroplasty.

Post-operative

- Wound leakage: if the wound is not dry by the 10th day or when sutures/clips are due for removal, return to theatre.

- Infection: culture, then treat aggressively with appropriate antibiotics. Early washout if infection is deep.
- Dislocation: maninupation and examination under anaesthetic. If recurrent or likely to be, then plan for either revison/excision.

- Pain: assess for infection.

Late failure

- Septic or aseptic.
- Conversion to a total hip replacement is not an 'easy' revision. Consider referral to a hip surgeon.

Section I: Subtrochanteric fractures of the femur

Peter V. Giannoudis

10.1 INTRAMEDULLARY FIXATION FOR SUBTROCHANTERIC FRACTURES USING A PROXIMAL FEMORAL NAIL (PFN)

Indications

- Low and extended subtrochanteric fractures.
- Ipsilateral femoral neck and shaft fractures.
- Unstable inter-trochanteric fractures.
- Failed plate fixation of subtrochanteric fractures.
- Pathological fractures.

Pre-operative planning

Clinical assessment

- Obtain a thorough patient's history (mechanism of injury, past medical records).
- Mechanism of injury: as a result of low-energy trauma in patients with osteoporotic bones (watch for underlying pathology).
- High-energy trauma: motor vehicle accidents, falls from a height, gunshot injuries.
- In polytrauma patients the Advanced Trauma Life support (ATLS) protocol must be followed.
- Look for associated injuries, especially in polytrauma patients.
- The extremity is shortened, the thigh is swollen and there is a prominence of the proximal fragment.
- Neurologic and vascular injuries are uncommon; however, neurovascular assessment is mandatory.
- Although rare, be alert for signs of compartment syndrome.

Radiological assessment

- High-quality anteroposterior (AP) and lateral radiographs of the femur including the knee, the femoral neck and head (Fig. 10.1a,b).
- Anteroposterior radiograph of the pelvis.
- Look for extension of the fracture into the greater trochanter and piriformis fossa.
- Contralateral radiographs of the unaffected femur are useful in assessing the width of the medullary canal, the shaft-neck angle and for the determination of the nail's length.

Operative treatment

Anaesthesia

- Spinal or general anaesthesia.
- Prophylactic antibiotic as per local hospital protocol.

Table and equipment

- PFN set (Fig. 10.2).
- Standard osteosynthesis set as per local hospital protocol.
- An image intensifier.

Table set up

- The instrumentation is set up on the side of the operation.
- Image intensifier is from the contralateral side.
- Position the table diagonally across the operating room so that the operating area lies in the clean air field.

Practical Procedures in Orthopaedic Trauma Surgery: A Trainee's Companion, ed. Peter V. Giannoudis and Hans-Christoph Pape.
Published by Cambridge University Press. © Cambridge University Press 2006.

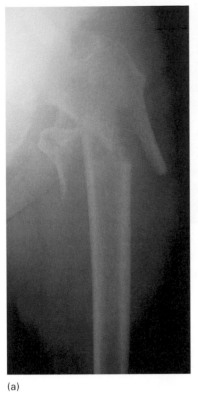

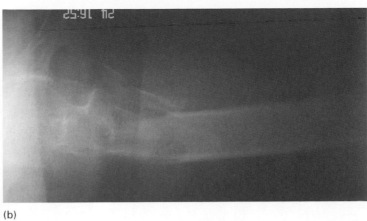

(b)

Fig. 10.1a,b Anteroposterior and lateral view of the hip and femur on the affected side.

(a)

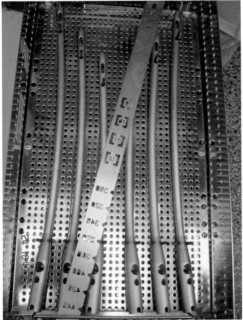

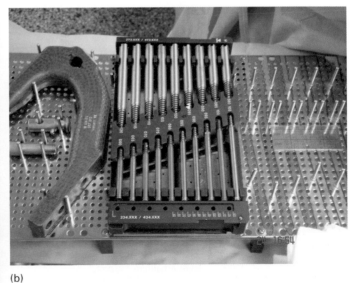

(b)

(a)

Fig. 10.2 PFN intramedullary osteosynthesis set.

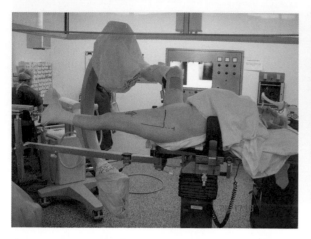

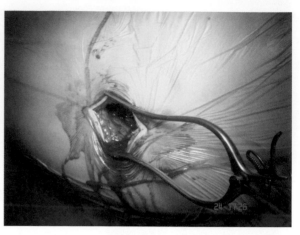

Fig. 10.3 Positioning for the PFN. The patient is supine on the fracture table, with the affected leg in a foot holder attached to the fracture table.

Fig. 10.5 Make a 5 cm incision, 5–8 cm proximal from the tip of the greater trochanter. Incise the gluteus maximus fascia and split the muscle in line with its fibres.

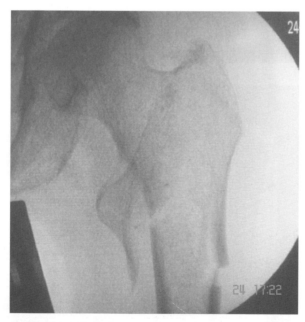

Fig. 10.4 Fluoroscopic image demonstrating the reduction of the subtrochanteric fracture.

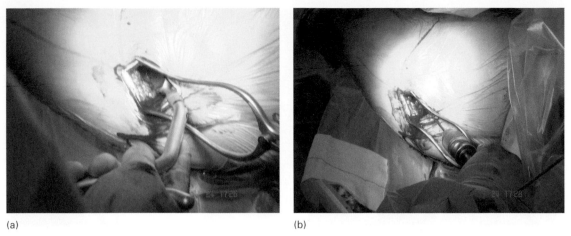

(a)   (b)

Fig. 10.6 (a) A curved awl is introduced to the tip of the greater trochanter and driven in gently in line with the femoral shaft of the proximal fragment. (b) An alternative technique is the use of a 2.8 mm guide wire inserted laterally at an angle of 60° to the shaft up to a depth of 15 cm.

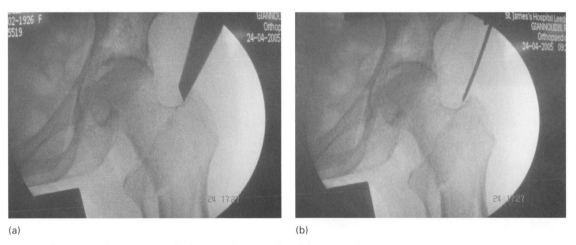

(a)   (b)

Fig. 10.7a,b Obtain radiographs to verify the exact determination of the entry point.

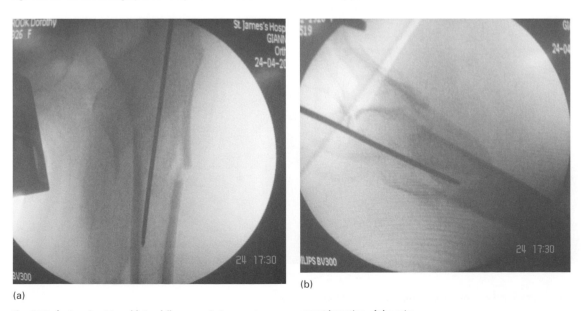

(a)

(b)

Fig. 10.8a,b Acquire AP and lateral fluoroscopic images to ensure correct insertion of the wire.

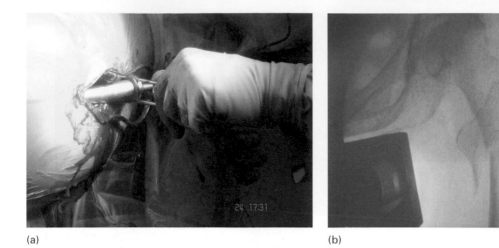

(a)   (b)

Fig. 10.9a,b Use the cannulated drill bit to ream as far as the stop on the protection sleeve.

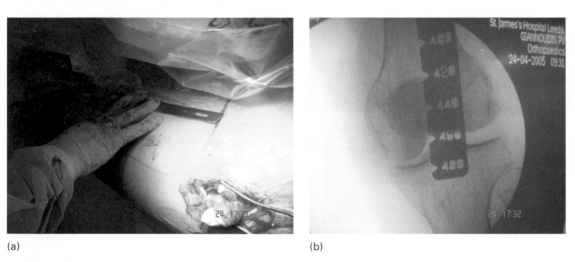

(a)   (b)

Fig. 10.10a,b Using a ruler, calculate the appropriate nail length.

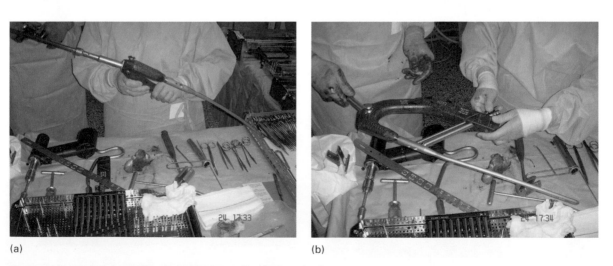

(a)   (b)

Fig. 10.11a,b Attach and assemble the appropriate nail to the insertion jig.

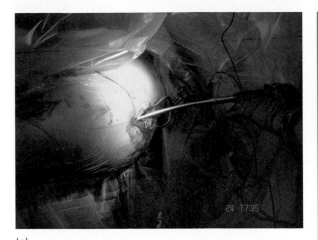

(a)

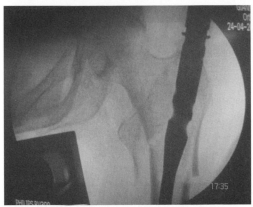

(b)

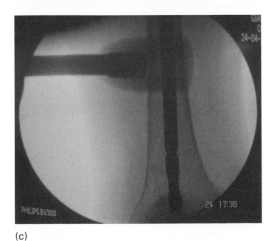

(c)

Fig. 10.12a,b,c Insert the nail over the guide wire into the medullary canal using manual force under fluoroscopic control.

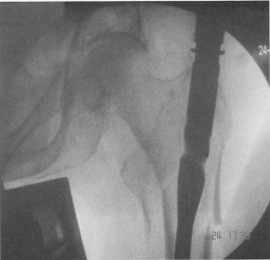

Fig. 10.13 The nail is passed until the proximal locking screw hole allows for placement of the screw in the inferior to central portion of the neck.

Patient positioning

- The patient is supine on the fracture table with traction applied to the affected leg through a skeletal pin in the proximal tibia or a foot holder attached to the fracture table.
- The affected leg is adducted about 10–15° to facilitate the nail's entrance.
- The unaffected leg is placed in a lithotomy position (Fig. 10.3).
- The arm of the affected side is draped over the body.
- Beware of maintenance of rotational mal-alignment.

Draping and surgical approach

- Prepare and drape the skin from the iliac crest together with the lateral thigh to the tibial tubercle with usual antiseptic solutions (aqueous/alcoholic povidone–iodine).
- Obtain fluoroscopic AP and lateral images of the fracture site (Fig. 10.4).
- Using a marker pen draw the fracture plane over the skin.
- Make a 5 cm incision, 5–8 cm proximal from the tip of the greater trochanter (Fig. 10.5).
- Incise the gluteus maximus fascia and split the muscle in line with its fibres
- Palpate the tip of the trochanter and the piriformis fossa.

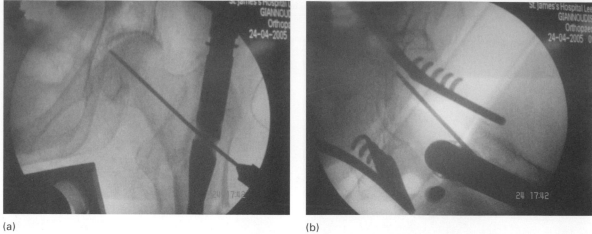

(a)

(b)

Fig. 10.14a,b The guide wire is advanced into subchondral bone.

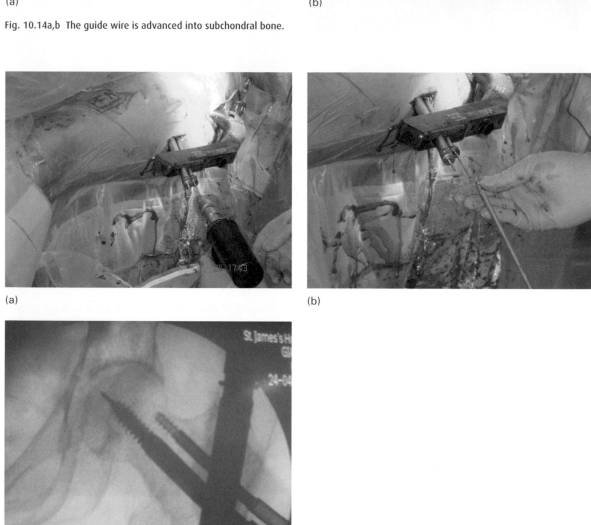

(a)

(b)

(c)

Fig. 10.15a,b,c Appropriate length reaming is performed and the appropriate femoral neck screws are placed.

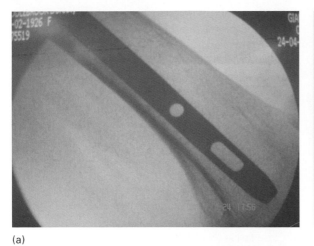

(a)

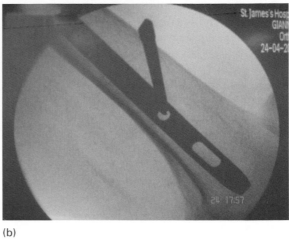

(b)

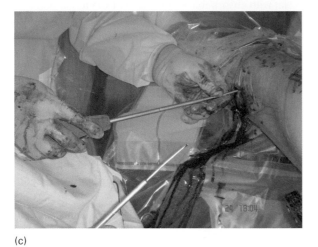

(c)

Fig. 10.16a,b,c For distal locking, a freehand perfect circle technique is used.

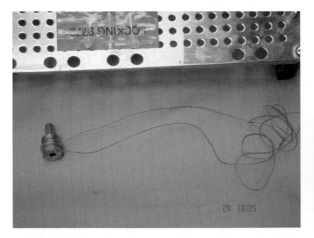

Fig. 10.17 Preparation of the end cap for insertion.

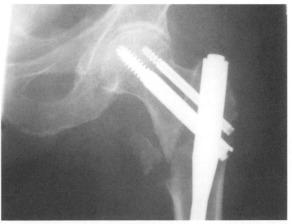

Fig. 10.18 Anteroposterior radiograph during follow up.

- Introduce a curved awl to the tip of the greater trochanter and drive it in gently in line with the femoral shaft of the proximal fragment.
- An alternative technique is the use of a 2.8 mm guide wire inserted laterally at an angle of 6° to the shaft, up to a depth of 15 cm (Fig. 10.6).
- Obtain radiographs to verify the exact determination of the entry point (Fig. 10.7a,b).
- Insert the guide wire in line with the proximal fragment and forward it down the medullary canal.
- Acquire AP and lateral fluoroscopic images to ensure correct insertion of the wire (Fig. 10.8a,b).
- Use the cannulated drill bit to ream as far as the stop on the protection sleeve. (Fig. 10.9a,b).
- Using a rule, calculate the appropriate nail length (Fig. 10.10a,b).
- Attach and assemble the appropriate nail to the insertion jig (Fig. 10.11a,b).
- Insert the nail over the guide wire into the medullary canal using manual force under fluoroscopic control (Fig. 10.12a,b,c).
- The nail is passed until the proximal locking screw hole allows for placement of the screw in the inferior to central portion of the neck (Fig. 10.13).
- Once the nail is inserted abduct the limb to correct any varus deformity.
- Once the nail is at its proper depth, a true lateral radiograph must be obtained.
- With the nail centred within the jig and both centred within the head and neck, the screw must be in the centre of the head when placed. This rotation must be maintained while the guide wire for the screw is advanced.
- Insert the stacked drill sleeves and push them to the bone.
- Advance the guide wire into the subchondral area of the bone.
- Confirm correct guide placement with image intensifier views (Fig. 10.14a,b).
- Perform appropriate length reaming and place the appropriate length femoral neck screw into the dense subchondral bone of the femoral head.

- Verify that the femoral neck screw threads are within the subchondral bone.
- Confirm correct screw placement with the image intensifier (Fig. 10.15a,b,c).
- For distal locking a freehand perfect circle technique is used (Fig. 10.16a,b,c).
- Insert the end cap (Fig. 10.17).
- Obtain AP and true lateral radiographs of the whole femur.

Closure

- Irrigate the wound thoroughly and achieve haemostasis.
- Close fascia (No.1 PDS/Vicryl) and the subcutaneous fat with absorbable sutures (2/0 PDS/Vicryl).
- Skin closure – stainless steel surgical staples, monofilament non-absorbable sutures or absorbable sutures placed in the subcuticular layer.

Post-operative rehabilitation

- Two further doses of prophylactic antibiotics and thromboembolic prophylaxis are administered.
- Partial weight-bearing is allowed from the 2nd postoperative day with the use of a walker or crutches.
- Routine bloods and radiographs of the whole femur in 24 hours.

Outpatient follow up

- Review in clinic with X rays every 3–4 weeks (Fig. 10.18).
- Allow progressive full weight-bearing after radiographic callus detection usually 4–8 weeks after the surgery.

Implant removal

- Rarely before one year after the operation.
- Ensure the radiographic existence of mature callus bridging the fracture ends in both AP and lateral radiographs.

Section II: Fractures of the femoral shaft

Hans-Christoph Pape, Stefan Hankemeier, Thomas Gosling (10.2, 10.3, 10.4, 10.6) and Brian W. Scott (10.5)

10.2 GENERAL ASPECTS

Pre-operative planning

Clinical assessment

- Pain, swelling, deformity, shortening, loss of function.
- Assess neurovascular status of the leg and evaluate soft tissue damage of closed fractures.
- Do not open dressings of open fractures placed on the scene in the emergency unit, but in the operating theatre.
- Assess compartment pressure (clinical signs of compartment syndrome: tense swollen compartment, severe ischaemic muscle pain, pain on palpation and passive stretching, nerve disturbances such as numbness, tingling and motor weakness). If in doubt, measure intracompartmental pressure: in case of compartment syndrome the difference in diastolic systemic pressure and compartment pressure is less than 30 mmHg.
- Femoral compartments:
  - Anterior (quadriceps femoris, sartorius, iliacus, psoas, pectineus muscles; femoral artery and vein; femoral nerve, lateral femoral cutaneous nerve).
  - Medial (gracilis, adductor longus, adductor brevis, adductor magnus, obturator externus muscles; profundus femoris artery, obturator artery and vein; obturator nerve).
  - Posterior (biceps femoris, semitendinosus, semimembranosus, portion of the adductor magnus muscle; branches of the profundus femoris artery; sciatic nerve, posterior femoral cutaneous nerve).
- Assess the local injury severity by the Abbreviated Injury Scale (AIS) and the total severity of injuries with the Injury Severity Score (ISS).

Closed fractures

Tscherne Classification:

Grade 0:
- No or minor soft tissue injury.
- Simple fracture types, indirect fracture mechanism (e.g. pathological fractures).

Grade I:
- Superficial abrasion or contusion by fragment pressure from the inside.
- Simple or medium to severe fracture types (e.g. spiral tibia fractures in a skiing injury).

Grade II:
- Deep contaminated abrasions and localized skin or muscle contusion through an indirect trauma (e.g. tibia fracture from a direct blow by a car bumper), blisters. Usually medium to severe fracture types.
- Also: imminent compartment syndrome.

Grade III:
- Extensive skin contusions.
- Destruction of musculature.
- Subcutaneous tissue avulsion.
- Also: manifest compartment syndrome and vascular injuries.
- Severe and mostly comminuted fracture types.
- Soft tissue treatment is often more difficult than a type III open fracture.
  The amount of soft tissue damage in closed fractures is often underestimated.

Open fractures

Gustilo Classification:

Type I:
- Skin wound less than 1 cm.
- 'Clean' wounds with little or no contamination.

- Skin wound results from a perforation from the inside by one of the fracture ends.
- No comminution.

Type II:

- Skin laceration larger than 1 cm; surrounding tissues have minor or no signs of contusion.
- No extensive soft tissue damage or dead musculature.
- No flaps or avulsions.

Type III:

- High-energy injury involving extensive soft tissue damage.
  - Type IIIa:
    - Adequate soft tissue coverage of bone despite extensive soft tissue damage.
  - Type IIIb:
    - Extensive soft tissue injury with periosteal stripping and bone exposure.
    - Major wound contamination.
  - Type IIIc:
    - Open fracture with arterial injury requiring reconstruction.

The main part of the tissue damage may be covered by intact skin. The severity of soft tissue damage does not always correlate with the size of the skin laceration. The correct amount of tissue damage is judged intraoperatively.

Radiological assessment

- Anteroposterior (AP) and lateral views including the adjacent joints.
- Assess the fracture geometry by the AO-classification:
  - 32-A: simple femoral shaft fractures (A1: spiral, A2: oblique, A3: transverse).
  - 32-B: wedge fractures (B1: spiral, B2: bending, B3: fragmented).
  - 32-C: complex fractures (C1: spiral, C2: segmental, C3: irregular).
- Assess fracture deformity and shortening:
  - Fractures of the proximal third are usually flexed and externally rotated owing to the pull of the iliopsoas muscle on the lesser trochanter. Gluteal muscles pulling on the greater trochanter cause abduction of the proximal fragment.
  - Adductor muscles exert strong axial and varus forces to the femoral shaft and can therefore cause adduction of the distal fragment and shortening.

- Pull of the gastrocnemius muscles in distal femoral shaft fractures usually causes recurvatum of the distal fragment.

Implant selection

- Closed intramedullary nailing offers the most biomechanical and biological advantages and is the preferred treatment for femoral shaft fractures.
- There is discussion about the advantages of reamed versus unreamed intramedullary nailing in open fractures. Reamed femoral nailing can be performed in Gustilo type I, II and IIIa open fractures. Unreamed femoral nailing can be performed in all closed femoral shaft fractures and open femoral shaft fractures, Gustilo type I to IIIb. After reamed nailing, interlocking screw breakage is observed less frequently owing to the larger locking screws.
- However, reaming of the medullary canal may cause systemic fat embolism. Unreamed nailing is associated with less damage to the endosteal and cortical blood supply, reduces heat necrosis, and therefore may also be beneficial in the treatment of open fractures, Gustilo type II, IIIa and IIIb. Solid nails seem to be less susceptible to infections than tubular nails.
- Damage control orthopaedic surgery: patients with femoral fractures, who are at high risk of developing post-traumatic systemic complications (e.g. multiple organ failure, Adult respiratory distress syndrome (ARDS)), or haemodynamically unstable patients, should be treated by minimally invasive, rapid fracture fixation with external fixation. Guidelines for primary external fixation are:
  - systolic blood pressure on arrival in the shock room <100 mmHg
  - necessity of catecholamines
  - anuria
  - signs of increased intracerebral pressure
  - hypothermia (rectal temperature <32°C)
  - thrombopaenia <80 000
  - severe thoracic trauma

Treatment of open fractures

- Do not open the dressing of open fractures in the emergency unit. Most commonly, infection follows contamination with bacteria from the hospital.
- In the anaesthesia room of the operating theatre, open the wound after adequate anaesthesia, take a smear from the wound, remove the hairs by shaving, and

scrub the skin with sterile gloves, sterile scrub, sterile soap and sterile, isotonic electrolyte solutions.

- Change sterile gloves, scrub and clean the wound and bone fragments mechanically. Rinse the wound with a sufficient amount of sterile, isotonic electrolyte solutions. Cover the wound with a sterile dressing.
- Intraoperatively, the wound is rinsed with high amounts of sterile, isotonic solutions. Debride necrotic and contaminated tissue. High-pressure irrigation ('Jet Lavage') increases decontamination from bacteria.

Intraoperative control of alignment, rotation and bone length

Techniques of closed, indirect fracture reduction do not rely on anatomical reduction of the fracture fragments. Exact intraoperative control of alignment, rotation and bone length is crucial. Tricks for intraoperative control are:

Axial alignment:

- 'Cable technique': The knee is fully extended and the patella faces anteriorly. With the image intensifier beam strictly vertical, the centre of the femoral head and the centre of the ankle are marked. Now the electrocauter cable can be spanned between these 2 points and the image intensifier centred on the knee joint. Varus/valgus mal-alignment can now be determined using the projection of the cable (Fig. 10.19.a,b).

Rotational alignment:

- 'Lesser trochanter shape sign' (most accurate method): Pre-operatively, the shape of the lesser trochanter of the uninjured limb with the patella facing anteriorly is stored on the fluoroscope screen. The X-ray contour of the lesser trochanter depends on the rotation of the bone. Before locking, with the patella facing anteriorly, the proximal fragment is rotated around the nail, until the shape of the lesser trochanter is symmetrical to the stored picture on the fluoroscope. External malrotation leads to a more prominent lesser trochanter, whereas the lesser trochanter decreases in internal malrotation.
- 'Cortical step sign': Especially in transverse or short oblique fractures, rotation of the main fragments may be judged roughly by the thickness of the cortices of the proximal and distal fragment.

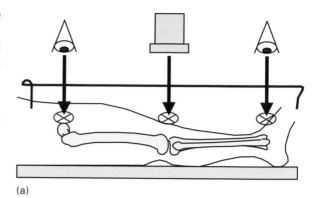

(a)

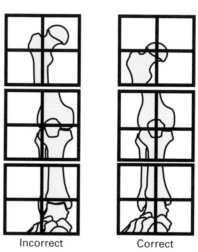

Incorrect   Correct

(b)

Fig. 10.19 (a) Intraoperative control of the alignment with the 'Cable Technique' after closed fracture reduction. The knee is fully extended and the patella faces anteriorly. With the image intensifier beam strictly vertical, the electrocauter cable is spanned between the centre of the femoral head and the centre of the ankle. Then the image intensifier is centred on the knee joint and the varus/valgus mal-alignment is determined using the projection of the cable. (b) Incorrect (left) and correct (right) position of the hip, knee and ankle joint centre on the image intensifier.

- 'Diameter difference sign': In case of malrotation, the transverse diameters of the proximal and distal fragment can be different.
- Clinical judgement of the rotational range of movement (ROM) in the hip joint in comparison to the contralateral side: depends on the position of the patient and of the leg during surgery.
- Pre-operative testing of radiologic imaging on the operating table is recommended to confirm sufficient intraoperative control options.

10.3 OPEN REDUCTION AND INTERNAL FIXATION (ORIF): PLATING

Indications

- Fractures involving the metaphyseal and diaphyseal area.
- Technical contraindications to intramedullary nailing (very small or sclerotic medullary canal).
- Complex shaft fractures in young patients with open growth plates.

Pre-operative planning

- Outlined earlier in this chapter (under 'General aspects', p. 179).
- Limited contact plates (e.g. LC-DCP) reduce the contact between implant and bone and improve bone–blood supply.
- To achieve compression in AO type A and B fractures, use interfragmentary lag screws in combination with a neutralization plate or compression plating.

Operative treatment

Anaesthesia

- General or regional anaesthesia.
- Pre-operative prophylactic single shot antibiotics (e.g. 2nd generation cephalosporin).

Table and equipment

- Instrumentation set and set of implants (e.g. broad LC-DCP 4.5 mm, 4.5 mm cortex screws/ 6.5 mm cancellous bone screws).
- Image intensifier.

Table set up

- Instrumentation is set up on the side of the operation.
- Image intensifier is set up on the contralateral side.

Patient positioning

- Supine position on a radiolucent table.
- Lift the buttocks to expose posterolateral aspect of the thigh and buttocks.

Draping and surgical approach

- Clean the skin from the hip to the foot with antiseptic solutions.
- Make a longitudinal lateral incision of the appropriate length in a line from the greater trochanter to the lateral femoral condyle.
- Incise the fascia lata longitudinally.
- Elevate the vastus lateralis off the lateral intermuscular septum, or incise the vastus lateralis muscle along its fibres.
- Ligate perforating branches of the profunda femoris artery perpendicular to the femur.
- For minimally invasive perentaneons plate osteosynthesis (MIPPO), make a small incision at the lateral femur over the lateral femoral condyle, tunnel the vastus lateralis muscle at the lateral femoral condyle and push the plate proximally, without opening of the fracture site.

Fracture reduction

- External manual traction.
- A distraction device (e.g. the AO distractor) can be helpful to restore length and resist major muscle forces.
- Pointed bone forceps for exact fracture reduction.
- Minimize soft tissue damage. Extensive deperiostation affects blood supply and bone healing.

Implant positioning

- Position the plate on the posterolateral aspect of the femur alongside the linea aspera.
- Use at least 3 bicortical screws on each side of the main fragments.
- Depending on the fracture localization, the plate needs contouring by a bending press or hand-held bending pliers to fit the individual anatomical shape of the bone.
- Predrill holes perpendicular to the bone. Minimize heat production by using sharp reamers and cool water irrigation.
- The screws are correctly positioned, when they penetrate the opposite cortex fully and protrude by at least one rotation of the screw.

Conventional plating

- Simple fractures, AO type A and B, can be reduced precisely and fixed rigidly by interfragmentary

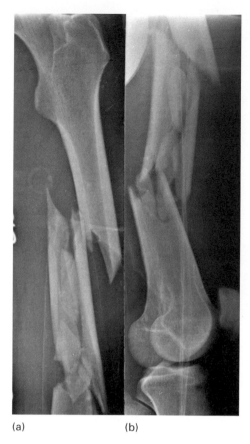

(a)   (b)

Fig. 10.20a, b Irregular complex femoral shaft fracture AO-type 32-C3.2 of a 38-year-old man.

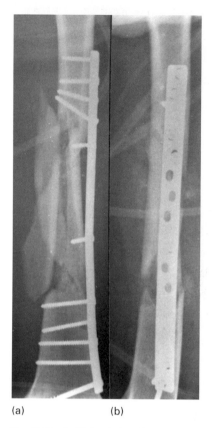

(a)   (b)

Fig. 10.21a, b Minimally invasive percutaneous plate osteosynthesis (MIPPO). No anatomical reduction of all fragments is performed, but indirect stabilization is achieved via stab incisions, in order to minimize soft tissue damage and preserve blood supply of the bone fragments.

compression. This can be achieved by lag screws, by overbending of the plate or by a combination of both.

- To fix simple oblique or spiral diaphyseal fractures, use lag screws combined with a plate (functions as a 'neutralization' plate). Lag screws generate high forces at the fracture gap and should be used whenever possible in conventional plating. The neutralization plate helps to neutralize bending forces at the fracture site. Lag screws generally produce their best efficiency when the screw is orientated perpendicularly to the fracture line.
- A fully threaded screw can be used as a lag screw: drill a gliding hole into the fragment close to the screw (larger hole diameter than the outer diameter of the screw thread).
- Wedge fragments can be reduced with the aid of a pointed reduction clamp and fixed by a lag screw.
- To compress transverse fractures, use a dynamic compression plate (DCP), and drill eccentrical holes with a DCP-drill guide. The design of the screw holes allows compression of 1.0 mm.
- For axial compression over a distance of more than 2.0 mm, an articulated tension device is helpful.
- Owing to the eccentric position of a plate on a tubular bone, compression forces are higher underneath the plate and less at the opposite site, where a small gap of the fracture is frequent. If a lag screw cannot be applied for technical reasons, i.e. in transverse fractures, bend the plate slightly at the height of the fracture. By inserting the screws, the bent plate is straightened, which leads to compression of the opposite cortex.
- Be careful not to disturb fracture healing by extensive deperiostation: conventional plating of femoral shaft fractures with open fracture reduction generally causes soft tissue damage at the fracture site, increases the risk to devitalize fracture fragments, and increases blood loss and the risk of infection.

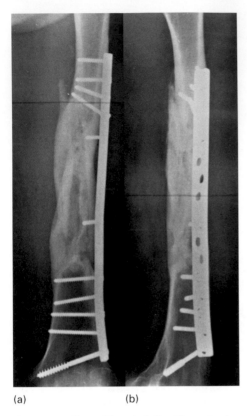

(a)   (b)

Fig. 10.22 Radiographic control after 12 months demonstrates solid consolidation with correct axial alignment.

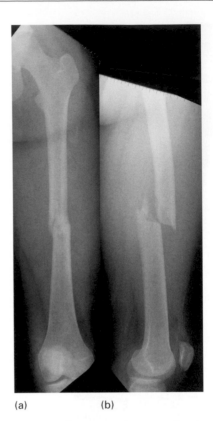

(a)   (b)

Fig. 10.23a, b Accuracy of pre-operative planning with templates depends upon the X-ray magnification. Selection of the nail can be based on intraoperative measurements.

Minimally invasive percutaneous plate osteosynthesis (MIPPO)

- In an effort to limit the amount of soft tissue dissection at the fracture site, indirect reduction and minimally invasive fixation techniques have been developed: via a small incision, usually at the lateral distal femur, the plate is pushed proximally below the vastus lateralis muscle along the femur without opening of the fracture site (Fig. 10.20a, b).
- The fracture is reduced in a closed manner and fixed by a minimum of 3 bicortical, percutaneous plate screws in each main fragment.
- Owing to indirect fracture reduction, precise control of alignment, rotation and bone length is mandatory (Fig. 10.21a, b).

Closure

- Irrigate the wound thoroughly and achieve haemostasis.
- Subfascial drainage in conventional plating.

- Close fascia lata over subfascial drainage and close subcutaneous fat with absorbable sutures.
- Close the skin with monofilament non-absorbable sutures.

Post-operative care

- Post-operative radiographs in 2 planes.
- Routine post-operative blood laboratory control.
- Physiotherapy on the 1st post-operative day with active range of motion exercise.
- Remove drains within 48 hours.
- Partial weight-bearing (15 kg).

Outpatient follow up

- Serial radiographs at 6 weeks, 3 months, 6 and 12 months post-operatively (Fig. 10.22a,b).
- Full weight-bearing usually after 6–12 weeks, depending on the fracture pattern and radiographic signs of fracture healing.

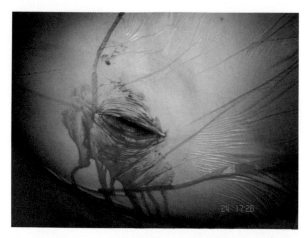

Fig. 10.24 Make a 4–6 cm long stab incision proximal to the tip of the trochanter major, exactly in line with the medullary canal.

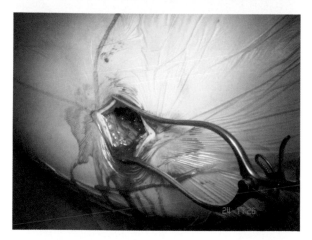

Fig. 10.25 Split the fascia lata longitudinally and divide the fibres of the gluteus maximus muscle.

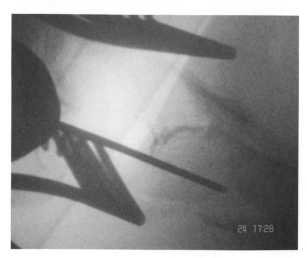

Fig. 10.26 Fluoroscopic control of the nail entry point.

- Routine implant removal is not mandatory.
- Earliest implant removal 1.5 to 2 years post-operatively.

10.4 INTRAMEDULLARY NAILING

Indications

- In adult femoral shaft fractures, intramedullary nailing continues to have the best biomechanical and biological properties and represents the method of choice. Reamed femoral nailing can be performed in Gustilo Type I, II and IIIa open fractures, unreamed femoral nailing in Gustilo Type I to IIIb open fractures.
- Fractures involving the metaphyseal area can be treated by intramedullary nailing, if the locking bolts can control alignment and provide sufficient stability of the metaphyseal fragment. The stability in short metaphyseal fragments can be increased by 'poller screws'.
- Additional intra-articular fractures do not represent a general contraindication for intramedullary nailing. Anatomical reduction and fixation of the intra-articular fragments are required. Then, the insertion of the intramedullary nail must not dislocate the intra-articular fragments.
- Damage control orthopaedic surgery: patients with femoral fractures, who are at high risk of developing post-traumatic systemic complications (e.g. multiple organ failure, ARDS), or haemodynamically unstable patients, should be treated by minimally invasive, rapid fracture fixation with external fixation.
- After primary fracture fixation with an external fixator, intramedullary nailing can be performed, provided the pin sites are clean without signs of infection. If signs of local infection are present, remove the fixator, curette the pin tracts and stabilize the leg in a plaster or in extension until all signs of infection have disappeared.

Pre-operative planning

- See 'General aspects' (p. 179).
- Accuracy of pre-operative planning with templates depends upon the X-ray magnification. Selection of the nail can be based on intraoperative measurements (Fig. 10.23a, b).

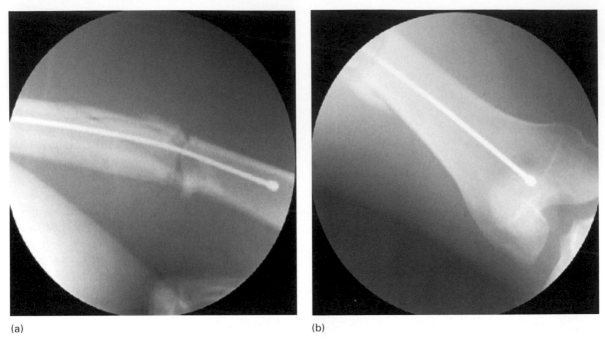

(a)   (b)

Fig. 10.27a, b Insert a long central guide wire and drive it through the fracture into the distal fragment. Insert the guide wire into the centre of the intercondylar notch.

Operative treatment

Anaesthesia

- General anaesthesia preferable, especially in the case of multiple injuries and operations.
- Regional (spinal/epidural) anaesthesia is possible in the case of a single injury.
- Pre-operative prophylactic single shot antibiotics (e.g. 2nd generation cephalosporin).

Table and equipment

- Nail instrumentation set including a complete set of implants.
- Standard radiolucent operating table.
- Image intensifier.
- The authors do not recommend the use of fracture tables, because they are associated with a higher incidence of post-operative rotational deformities and increase the risk of additional iatrogenic soft tissue damage during surgery. Without a fracture table the logistic pre-operative set up in the operation theatre is less time-consuming.

Table set up

- Instrumentation is set up on the side of the operation.
- Image intensifier is set up on the contralateral side.

Patient positioning

- Supine position allows the best control of the alignment. A lateral position provides comfortable access to the piriformis fossa, but fracture reduction and control of alignment is more difficult. A lateral position is favourable in instances such as prophylactic intramedullary nailing of imminent pathologic femoral fractures which do not need reduction.
- In the supine position, the contralateral leg is positioned on a gynaecological leg holder in a flexed position of the hip and knee joint, in order to facilitate easy access of the image intensifier in a lateral direction. Some surgeons position the contralateral leg on the operating table, in order to provide intraoperative comparison of leg length, rotation and alignment.
- The tip of the trochanter major must be visible in 2 directions under the image intensifier.

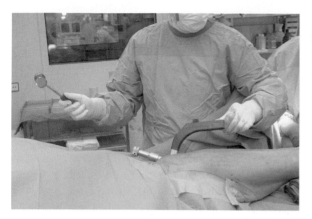

Fig. 10.28 Insert the nail manually into the medullary canal by twisting movements or with slight blows of a hammer.

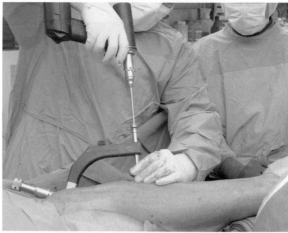

Fig. 10.30 For insertion of the proximal locking bolts, the aiming device is screwed tightly into the internal thread at the proximal tip of the interlocking nail. Then the holes for the bolts are drilled through the aiming device.

distal ends of the bone have to be centred in the X-ray beam and the ruler placed parallel to the diaphysis.

- Alternatively, landmarks can be drawn on the skin using a sterile pen. To determine nail length, the distance is measured by a ruler.
- Optimal nail length can also be determined with a guide wire, which is introduced into perfect intramedullary position at the distal femur. The desired nail length can be calculated measuring the extramedullary length of the guide wire and knowing the total length of the guide wire.

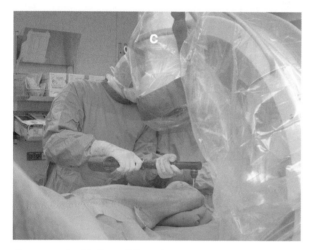

Fig. 10.29 Distal locking of the nail with the 'free-hand technique': the position of the C-arm perfectly aligns with the locking hole. The tip of a radiolucent drill is positioned into the centre of the hole, brought up in line with the image intensifier and driven through the 2 cortices. Before proximal locking, the fracture gap can be closed by 'backstroking' the nail.

- Under unsterile conditions, examination of the contralateral 'lesser trochanter shape sign' is useful.
- Adduction, flexion and internal rotation of the hip joint facilitates an adequate approach to the piriformis fossa and medullary canal.

Implant selection

- A sterile radiolucent ruler permits measurement of the correct implant diameter and nail length. Proximal and

Draping and surgical approach

- Prepare the skin from the gluteal area down to the foot using antiseptic solutions. A common mistake is insufficient draping at the proximal and dorsal gluteal area.
- The draping often detaches from the skin during manipulation of the hip. A trick is to fix the draping to the skin with metal clips.
- For unreamed nailing, make a 2 cm-long stab incision 10–15 cm proximal to the tip of the trochanter major, exactly in line with the medullary canal, under the control of an image intensifier.
- For reamed femoral nailing, the incision has to be a bit larger, in order to protect the soft tissue from the reamer with a protection sleeve (Fig. 10.24).
- Split the fascia lata longitudinally and divide the fibres of the gluteus maximus muscle (Fig. 10.25).

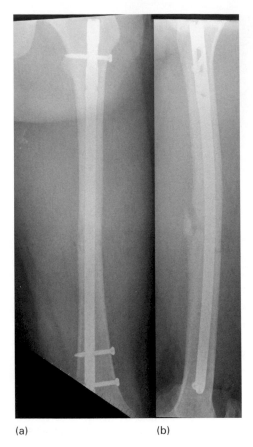

(a)   (b)

Fig. 10.31a,b Post-operative radiographs.

Fracture reduction

- Manual reduction is usually sufficient to reduce fresh fractures. Closed fracture reduction techniques help to preserve osteogenic cells in the fracture haematoma and reduce the risk of infections.
- Delayed fracture reduction or fractures of patients with a very thick soft tissue envelope may require reduction aids:
    - Use temporary Schanz screws, connected by a universal chuck with the T-handle as a 'joystick' to manipulate fragments. Place the Schanz screw unicortically in the proximal fragment, close to the fracture.
    - For the reduction of delayed fractures with shortening, the use of a distractor is helpful. The proximal pin can be placed anteriorly above the lesser trochanter, medial to the entrance point of the nail. The distal pin may be placed medially or laterally into the femur at the proximal border of the patella.

- Owing to indirect fracture reduction, precise control of alignment, rotation and bone length is mandatory.
- Open reduction is reserved for very rare fractures which cannot be reduced.

Implant positioning

- Under the control of the image intensifier, identify the interval between the trochanter major and the piriformis fossa.
- The entry point varies according to the nail design. The entry point for unreamed femoral nails is slightly anterior and lateral to the base of the piriformis fossa. For reamed femoral nails, the insertion is slightly more lateral at the anterior aspect of the medial greater trochanter. If the nail design has much curvature, the entry point has to be more posterior.
- Some nails have a proximal angulation, and can therefore be inserted at the tip of the trochanter major.
- Open the medullary canal with a 3.5 mm guide pin and drive it into the centre of the medullary canal (Fig. 10.26).
- If the position of the guide wire is not perfect, insert a second pin using the initial wire as a reference.
- A lateral entry point can cause varus mal-alignment and iatrogenic fracture of the medial portion of the proximal fragment.
- An inadequate medial position of the entry point can cause osteonecrosis of the femoral head secondary to iatrogenic damage to the vascular arcade around the femoral neck, and can increase stress in the femoral neck.
- For unreamed femoral nails, cut a cylinder of corticocancellous bone with a cannulated cutter. For solid nails, the guide wire has to be extracted.
- If a cannulated nail is used, insert a long central guide wire and drive it through the fracture into the distal fragment (Fig. 10.27a, b). In fractures with translational mal-alignment, bending of the tip of the central guide wire helps to cross the fracture gap. Insert the guide wire into the centre of the intercondylar notch.
- In reamed femoral nailing, use low pressure and sharp reamer heads. The guide wire is not extracted during the change of the reamer heads. Limited reaming until the point of cortical chatter is recommended to avoid heat necrosis. In case of comminuted fractures, push the reamer across the fracture to prevent soft tissue damage.
- Down-size the nail diameter 1.0 to 1.5 mm to the size of the last reamer head.

- The optimal length of the nail can be determined intra-operatively under image intensifier control by a central guide wire, a metal ruler or a nail. For pre-operative measurements based on X-rays, the magnification of the femur has to be taken into account.
- The implant is assembled with the insertion handle and the connection screw.
- Insert the nail manually into the medullary canal by twisting movements or with slight blows of a hammer (Fig. 10.28).
- If solid nails are used, the nail is introduced without a central guide wire, which keeps the fracture reduced. The proximal part of the nail can be used as a 'joystick' to manipulate the proximal fragment and reduce the fracture.
- Drive the nail through the fracture and place the tip of the nail directly into the centre of the intercondylar notch.
- Control alignment, rotation and bone length.
- 'Poller screws': In fractures involving the proximal or distal femur, central placement of the nail and correct alignment may be difficult because of strong muscle pull and wide medullary canals. 'Poller screws' are locking screws or conventional screws, which block an incorrect path of the nail. They can be used as a supplement to correct nail position or mal-alignment, while simultaneously increasing stability in a short fragment after insertion of the nail.
- By the insertion of the nail, distraction of the fracture gap may be produced. Therefore, distal locking is recommended before proximal locking, in order to have the opportunity to 'backstroke' the nail, until the main fragments are reduced and the planned length is achieved.
- For femoral distal locking screw insertion, use the 'free-hand technique'. The position of the C-arm has to align perfectly with the locking hole in the nail. Position the tip of a radiolucent drill into the centre of the hole. Bring up the drill in line with the image intensifier and drive the reamer through the 2 cortices (Fig. 10.29).
- With a measuring gauge, determine the bolt length.
- The locking screws have to pass both cortices.
- Check bone length and rotation before you proceed to lock the nail proximally.
- For insertion of the proximal locking screws, screw the aiming device tightly into the internal thread at the proximal tip of the interlocking nail and drill the holes for the screws (Fig. 10.30).
- Perform proximal and distal locking in case of unreamed nailing. Some nails offer the option to lock

the nail and are therefore rotationally stable, but allow dynamic axial compression. Dynamic locking can be chosen depending on the fracture type and localization, cortical contact at the fracture site, and nail type. If in doubt, static locking is recommended.
- Remove the aiming device. An end cap may be inserted into the internal thread. Disadvantages of the end cap are that the cap may get lost in the soft tissue and the additional cost incurred in using one.

Closure

- Irrigate the wound thoroughly.
- Achieve haemostasis.
- A subfascial drainage is usually not necessary.
- Close fascia lata and the subcutaneous fat with absorbable sutures.
- Close the skin with monofilament non-absorbable sutures.

Post-operative care

- Post-operative radiographs in 2 standard directions (Fig. 10.31a,b).
- Routine post-operative blood laboratory control.
- Physiotherapy on the 1st post-operative day with free active and passive range of motion exercises.
- To prevent post-operative soft tissue contraction or in case of soft tissue contraction, the patient is positioned in the bed with 90° flexed hip and knee joint for the first 3 days.
- Allow post-operative partial weight-bearing (15 kg). The amount of weight-bearing depends on the fracture type, amount of cortical contact at the fracture site, fracture localization, quality of fracture reduction, body weight, and the activity and compliance of the patient. Pain-free loading is an important aspect for increase of weight bearing.
- Post-operative full weight-bearing can usually be allowed in AO type A3 and C2 femoral shaft fractures in case of broad cortical contact at the fracture site, and in some A1–2 and B1–3 fractures of the middle femoral shaft, depending on the cortical contact and fracture localization.

Outpatient follow up

- Serial radiographs at 6 weeks, 3 months, 6 and 12 months to document fracture healing and remodelling.

- Dynamization of statically locked nails is indicated in cases of delayed healing, 3 to 4 months after nailing.
- Nail removal is not a routine procedure. Prerequisites for nail removal are radiographic signs of bony consolidation in 2 standard directions. Implant removal is only recommended in symptomatic patients, i.e. in cases of soft tissue irritation by the implant, and usually not before 1.5 years after trauma.

10.5 FLEXIBLE INTRAMEDULLARY NAILS IN CHILDREN

Introduction

Femoral shaft fractures in infants and young toddlers can be effectively treated with Gallows traction. Healing is rapid and the fracture is stable, even within 2 or 3 weeks. Older pre-school children are small enough to be managed using a combination of traction in a Thomas splint, followed by early application of a hip spica under general anaesthesia. Older children present different problems, since the fracture healing is slower and hip spicas are poorly tolerated by larger children and their fami-

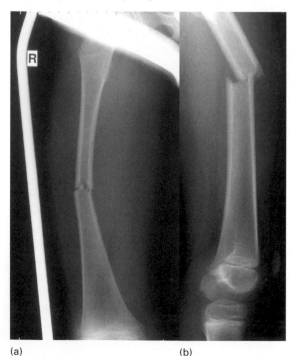

(a)   (b)

Fig. 10.32 (a) An radiograph for site and pattern of fracture; (b) a lateral view may give extra information, but will be difficult to obtain and is not essential in this group of patients.

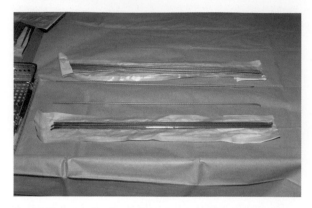

Fig. 10.33 Two nails of each diameter are ideal. Type and availability should be checked.

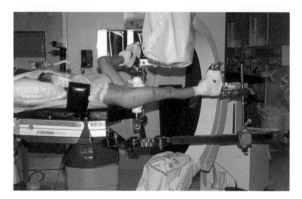

Fig. 10.34 Uninjured leg flexed at hip and knee and abducted fully.

lies. Standard adult techniques for intramedullary nailing will damage the trochanteric physis and also threaten the femoral capital epiphysis blood supply which originates in part from an anastomosis of vessels close to the piriformis fossa at the base of the femoral neck. Internal fixation using a compression plate is possible and works well, but it requires a substantial exposure and leaves a scar in a visible place. External fixation may be used and this is a quick and minimally invasive technique, especially useful for patients is an unstable condition with multiple injuries but it is a technique which has been associated with re-fracture on removal of the device.

Intramedullary fixation using flexible nails is a good alternative technique, especially useful in children of school age and prior to skeletal maturity. The advantages are:

- A minimally invasive technique with little scarring.
- Sufficient stabilization to allow early mobilization and weight-bearing (according to fracture pattern).

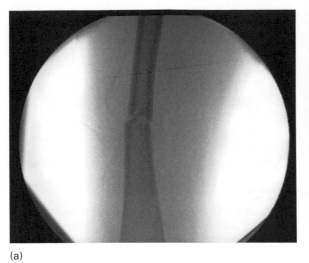

(a)

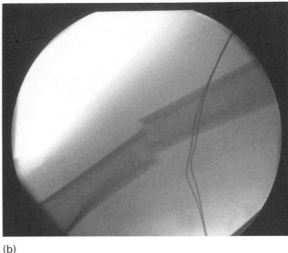

(b)

Fig. 10.35a, b Image intensifier is from the opposite side. Do a 'Trial run' to check access and fracture reduction.

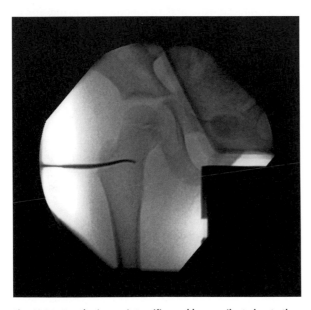

Fig. 10.36 Use the image intensifier and bone spike to locate the trochanteric plate.

- No risk of avascular necrosis of the femoral capital epiphysis.
- No appreciable overgrowth.
- No damage to growth plates.

Indications

- Diaphyseal fracture in the central 50–60% of the femur.

- Age: school age to skeletal maturity.
- Suitable for pathological fractures.

Pre-operative planning

Clinical assessment

- There are often high-energy injuries; check for other injuries.
- Check distal neurovascular function (NB: May have been given a femoral nerve block in the accident department).

Radiological assessment

- Anteroposterior (AP) radiograph for site and pattern of fracture.
- A lateral view may give extra information, but will be difficult to obtain and is not essential in this group of patients (Fig. 10.32).

Operative treatment

Anaesthesia

- General anaesthesia.

Table and equipment

- The fracture table is usually the best. A standard radiolucent operating table may be used for smaller children and if an experienced assistant is available.

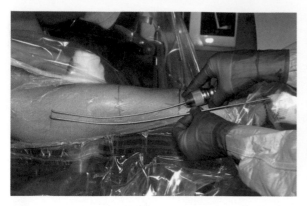

Fig. 10.37 Check nail length against the femur and prebend nails.

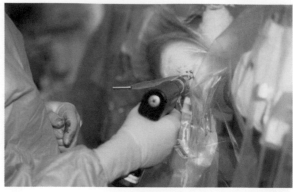

Fig. 10.38 Use a 4.5 drill and guide and drill the metaphysis at the predetermined entry site, 2 cm proximal to the growth plate.

- Two nails of each diameter are ideal. Some nails are of a standard length and are cut to fit. Other manufacturers supply nails of predetermined length and diameter. Type and availability should be checked (Fig. 10.33).
- Image intensifier.

Patient positioning (using fracture table)

- Patient supine. Fracture reduced and affected leg put on traction in slight abduction and in neutral rotation.
- Uninjured leg flexed at hip and knee and abducted fully (Fig. 10.34).
- Image intensifier from opposite side. Do a 'Trial run' to check access and fracture reduction (Fig. 10.35a, b).
- Skin preparation from iliac crest to ankle.
- Adhesive paper drapes around groin and to cover the opposite uninjured leg. Adhesive paper drapes to cover from the ipsilateral shin distally. An adhesive clear plastic drape is a good alternative.

Operative technique

- Use the image intensifier and bone spike to locate the trochanteric plate (Fig. 10.36) and distal growth plates and mark with a skin pen. The nails will enter the metaphysis obliquely and the skin incisions will be more distal than the entry site into the bone.
- To avoid overcrowding of the relatively narrow medullary cavity, select a nail diameter approximately one-third of the diameter of the narrowest part of the canal. Check nail length against the femur and prebend nails (Fig. 10.37). The nails should be the same diameter and bent to the same extent and in the same direction as the prebent tip. There are no firm rules on the amount of bend needed, but a bow of about 3 cm apex to base is

about right. The apex should be situated so that when the wire is fully inserted, it lies at about the level of the fracture.
- Beginning laterally, make a superficial 3 cm incision in the plane of the femur. Divide the fascia lata longitudinally and deepen the incision further using scissors and blunt dissection to avoid bleeding from geniculate vessels.
- Use a 4.5 drill and guide and drill the metaphysis at the predetermined entry site, 2 cm proximal to the growth plate (Fig. 10.38).
- It is difficult to drill an oblique hole and it is best to begin perpendicular to bone and to gently redirect the drill cephalad with the drill spinning, which will minimize the chance of the drill bit breaking (Fig. 10.39a, b).
- Mount the lateral wire in a hand-held chuck and pass into the intramedullary cavity (Fig. 10.40), advancing under image intensifier control across the fracture (Figs. 10.41a, b). Often it helps to use a hammer but beware of buckling of the nail, particularly narrower ones. Sometimes it is preferable to mount the wire with the chuck close to the tip to avoid bucking on insertion but this can be difficult with a prebent wire. In these circumstances the chuck can be backed off by a few centimetres at a time and driven into the bone, with small degrees of bend sequentially introduced using the bone entry site as a fulcrum (Fig. 10.42). If the nail does not easily pass across the fracture then leave it at the level of the fracture and proceed to pass the second nail.
- With the surgeon now standing on the medial side of the knee (Fig. 10.43), a similar approach is made to the medullary canal through the medial metaphysis

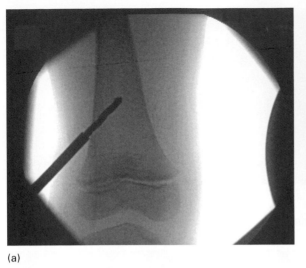

(a)

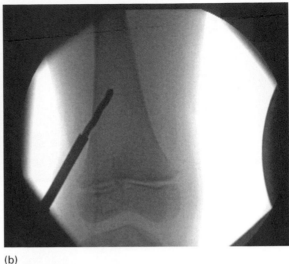

(b)

Fig. 10.39a, b It is difficult to drill an oblique hole and it is best to begin perpendicular to bone and to gently re-direct the drill cephalad with the drill spinning, which will minimize the chance of the drill bit breaking.

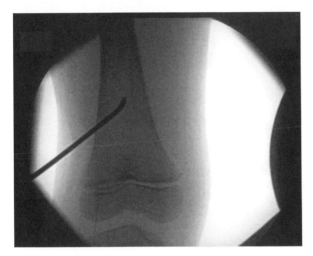

Fig. 10.40 Mount the lateral wire in a hand-held chuck and pass into the intramedullary cavity.

and the second nail passed in a similar way toward the fracture site.

- One or other of the wires is manipulated across the fracture site, followed by the other (Figs. 10.44a, b). This is often the most difficult part of the procedure and an assistant may be needed to manipulate the fracture site. It is often helpful to rotate the tip of the nail, which helps to engage the proximal fragment. If after several attempts, the proximal canal cannot be engaged then it is reasonable to make a 4 cm incision laterally at the site of the fracture site to clear any interposed tissue and assist the reduction and passage of the nail.

- Radiographs in both planes are required to check the nails are intramedullary. The nails are driven proximally using the impaction device for the final few cms (Figs. 10.45a, b).

- The proximal metaphyseal bone is surprisingly hard and the medial nail will not progress beyond the lesser trochanter. The lateral wire usually impacts in the greater trochanter (Fig. 10.46a, b, c).

- The protruding nail should be trimmed to about 1cm and if necessary bent a little to prevent protrusion. Any tendency to protrusion will be more marked when the knee is flexed.

- Nails supplied in predetermined lengths have ends designed to facilitate application of a removal tool. Length selection can be done in theatre using the uninjured leg as a template. If the nail is too long then it can be cut to size after insertion as described above.

- The skin only is closed. The compression bandage can be applied according to need and preference.

- Before the child wakes, the legs should be freed and checked for rotational alignment clinically (Fig. 10.47).

Post-operative care

- For most fracture patterns this technique provides sufficient longitudinal and rotational stability to permit

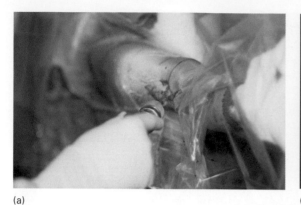

(a)

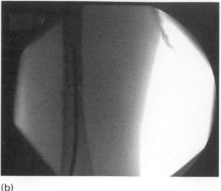

(b)

Fig. 10.41a, b Advancing under image intensifier control across the fracture.

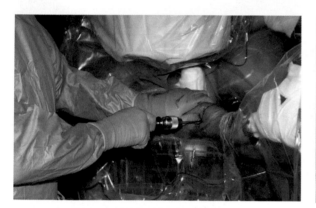

Fig. 10.42 Using the bone entry site as a fulcrum.

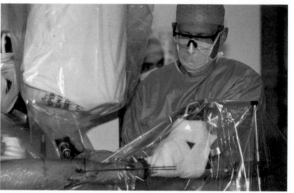

Fig. 10.43 With the surgeon now standing on the medial side of the knee.

mobilization with crutches in a day or two within the limits of discomfort.

- For stable fracture patterns, weight-bearing is permitted. For unstable fracture patterns it is preferable to allow some callus to form before commencing weight-bearing.

Follow up

- Review at 6 weeks for X-rays.
- Review 3 to 6 months later for a further X-ray, with a view to scheduling metalwork removal (Fig. 10.48a, b).

Implant removal

- Only when the fracture is radiologically united.
- In pathological fractures, consider not removing.
- The procedure for removal is straightforward. The special removal tools are particularly useful.
- If the nail is found to be irremovable then it is reasonable to trim any prominence and leave *in situ*.

Acknowledgments

To Mr P. A. Templeton, Consultant Children's Orthopaedic Surgeon for permission to use his case in the photographs.

10.6 APPLICATION OF AN EXTERNAL FIXATOR

Indications

- Damage control orthopaedic surgery: patients with femoral fractures, who are at high risk of developing post-traumatic systemic complications (e.g. multiple organ failure, ARDS), or haemodynamically unstable patients, should be treated by minimally invasive, rapid fracture fixation with external fixation (Fig. 10.49a, b).
- Transfixation of unstable, intra-articular knee fractures, which are not stabilized as a definite treatment in the primary operation.

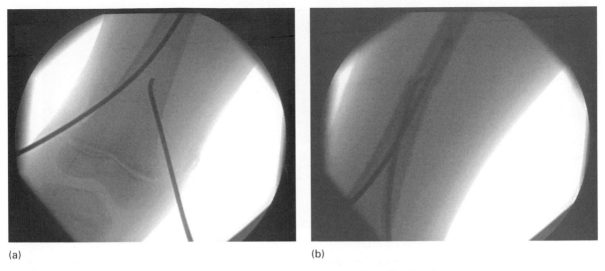

(a)   (b)

Fig. 10.44a, b One or other of the wires is manipulated across the fracture site, followed by the other.

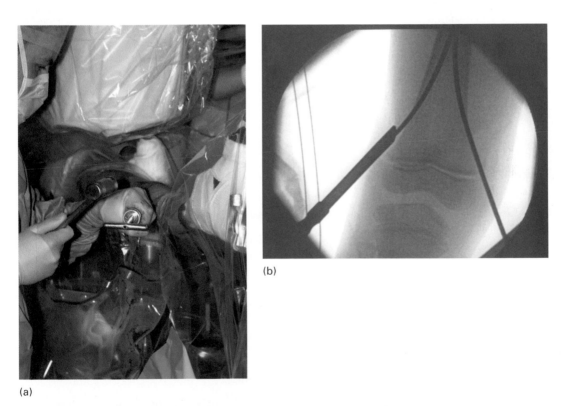

(b)

(a)

Fig. 10.45a, b The nails are driven proximally using the impaction device for the final few centimetres.

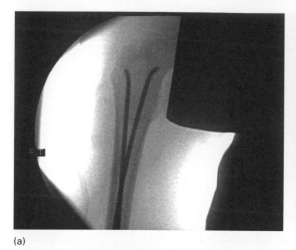

(a)

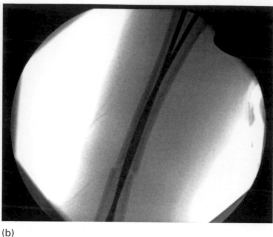

(b)

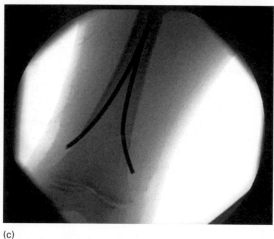

(c)

Fig. 10.46a, b, c The lateral wire usually impacts in the greater trochanter.

- Severe soft tissue damage of open or closed femoral fractures.
- Children's femoral shaft fractures.

Pre-operative planning

- See 'General aspects'. on p. 179.

Operative treatment

Anaesthesia

- General anaesthesia is preferable in multiply injured patients.
- Regional (spinal/epidural) anaesthesia possible in isolated operations of the femur.
- Provide pre-operative prophylactic single-shot antibiotics (e.g. 2nd generation cephalosporin).

Table and equipment

- Monolateral external fixator set including: 5.0 and 6.0 mm diameter Schanz screws.
- Carbon fibre rods or metal tubes (disadvantage: they obstruct X-ray assessment of the fracture).
- Tube-to-tube clamps and pin-to-tube clamps.
- Standard radiolucent operating table.
- Image intensifier.

Table set up

- Instrumentation is set up on the side of the operation.
- Image intensifier is set up on the contralateral side.

Patient positioning

- Supine position.

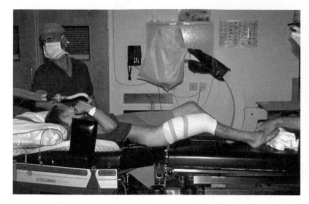

Fig. 10.47 Before the child wakes, the legs should be freed and checked for rotational alignment clinically.

Draping and surgical approach

- Prepare the skin from the gluteal area down to the tibia using antiseptic solutions.
- Via stab incisions, insert the Schanz screws in a posterolateral direction in the plane of the lateral intermuscular septum, in order to minimize transfixation of the vastus lateralis muscle. Consider future approaches of planned secondary procedures.
- Under special circumstances, the Schanz screws can be positioned in a sagittal position, i.e. in patients with transfixed unstable, intra-articular knee fractures, or in polytraumatized patients requiring rapid fracture fixation and long-term respiration with kinetic respiratory therapy.
- For better orientation, the femoral surface is palpated through the stab incision with a small clamp before drilling.

Implant positioning

- Drill holes for the Schanz screws perpendicular to the bone. Some surgeons prefer to place the screws in an oblique direction into the bone, in order to increase bone-implant contact.
- Minimize heat production using low pressure, sharp reamers, and cool water irrigation. Heat damage can cause early loosening of the pins and can increase the risk of pin infections.
- The Schanz screws have to penetrate the full opposite cortex and to protrude some millimetres past it.
- Insert a pair of Schanz screws into each main fragment, and connect them with a short tube.

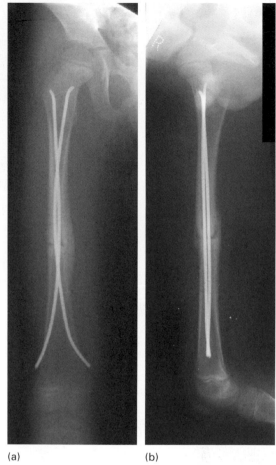

(a)   (b)

Fig. 10.48a, b Review 3 to 6 months later for a further X-ray, with a view to scheduling metal work.

- In case of definite fracture treatment with external fixation, usually 3 Schanz screws in the proximal and distal main fragment are used to increase stability at the fracture site (Fig. 10.50a, b), depending on the patient's weight and the extent of soft tissue damage.
- Soft tissue tension around the pins must be released during surgery by stab incisions.

Fracture reduction

- 'Tube-to-tube' technique: after insertion of a pair of pins in each main fragment, which are each joined by a short tube, the fracture can be manipulated using the two tubes as 'handles'. Fix the 2 tubes by a short third tube with 2 'tube-to-tube' clamps in the desired

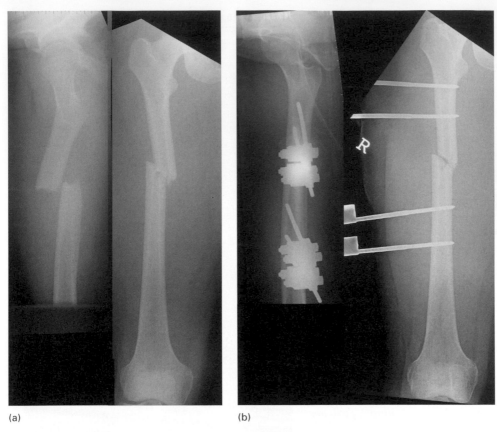

(a)

(b)

Fig. 10.49a, b Primary rapid stabilisation of a femoral shaft fracture of a 21-year-old polytraumatized patient.

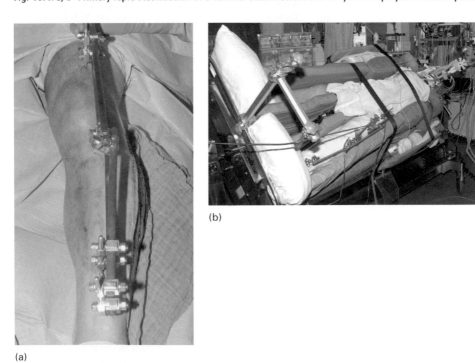

(a)

(b)

Fig. 10.50a, b Under special circumstances, the Schanz screws can be positioned in a sagittal position, i.e. for temporary transfixation of unstable intra-articular knee fractures (with compartment syndrome of the lower leg) or for kinetic respiratory therapy of severely injured patients with thoracic trauma.

fragment position. This technique can be applied without X-ray facility or image intensifier in the operating room. Fracture reduction may be done at a later point in time.

- Tube-to-tube clamps have a better grip on stainless steel tubes than on carbon fibre rods.
- An additional carbon fibre rod between the main fragments increases the stability at the fracture site.

Post-operative care

- Post-operative radiographs in 2 directions.

- Routine post-operative blood laboratory control.
- Physiotherapy with active range of motion exercise and partial weight-bearing (10–20 kg) is allowed on the first post-operative day, depending on the concomitant injuries.

Outpatient follow up

- Serial radiographs in 2 standard directions.
- Intense physiotherapy to maintain knee motion.
- Intense care of the pin sites.

Section III: Fractures of the distal femur

Stefan Hankemeier, Thomas Gosling and Hans-Christoph Pape

10.7 GENERAL ASPECTS

Clinical assessment

- Check for pain, swelling, deformity, shortening and intra-articular effusion.
- Assess neurovascular status of the leg and soft tissue damage of closed fractures.
- Open fractures: do not open dressings placed on the scene in the emergency unit; only open in the operating theatre.
- Assess the local injury severity by the Abbreviated Injury Scale (AIS) and the total severity of injuries with the Injury Severity Score (ISS).
- Check for previous surgery, especially total hip arthroplasty (THA) and total knee arthroplasty (TKA).
- Be aware of typically associated injuries: proximal tibia fracture, patella fracture, ligament ruptures of the knee (posterior cruciate ligament), femoral neck fracture, femoral head fracture, acetabulum fracture.

Radiological assessment

- Order anteroposterior (AP) and lateral radiographs of the knee joint, as well as the femur shaft.
- Perform a CT scan in case of an intra-articular fracture or if an intra-articular extension could not be excluded.
- Classify the fracture according to the AO/ASIF-classification system.

Fixation techniques

- Be aware of damage control (see Fractures of the femoral shaft, General aspects, page 179). Do external femoro-tibial transfixation in these patients. If possible perform preliminary fixation of the intra-articular fragments.

- Definitive stabilization:
  - Type A fractures: retrograde nailing is preferred. Minimally invasive percutaneous plate osteosynthesis (MIPPO) is an alternative but technically much more demanding.
  - Type B fractures: closed reduction and percutaneous screw fixation is preferred.
  - Type C fractures: C1 fractures can be treated either by retrograde nailing or techniques of MIPPO. Minimally invasive percutaneous plate osteosynthesis is preferred in C2 and C3 fractures.
- Specials:
  - Low fracture in osteopenic bone: consider primary TKA.
  - Periprosthetic fracture: use MIPPO.

10.8 MINIMALLY INVASIVE PERCUTANEOUS PLATE OSTEOSYNTHESIS (MIPPO)

Advantages

Preservation of blood supply to the metaphyseal fracture zone with reduced non-union and infection rates.

Implants

- Buttress plates (i.e. condylar buttress plate).
- Condylar screw plates (i.e. dynamic condylar screw).
- Locked screw plates (i.e. less invasive stabilization system).
  - Advantages of locked screw plates: exact contouring of the plate is not necessary; no primary loss of reduction owing to screw tightening; improved stability in osteopenic bone.

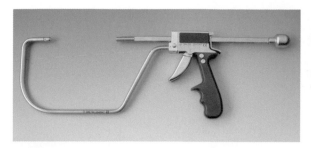

Fig. 10.51 Custom-made reduction clamp.

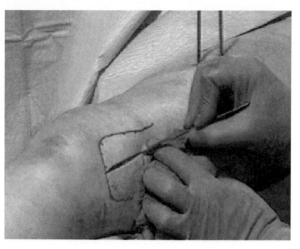

Fig. 10.52 Lateral skin incision for distal femur fractures.

Indications

All type A and C fractures of the distal femur.
Periprosthetic fractures (TKA and THA).

Technique

Operative technique is presented below for the Less Invasive Stabilization System (LISS, Synthes Group).

Pre-operative planning

- Draw all fracture fragments.
- Choose the correct plate length. Use at least 4 (better 5) monocortical screws in the proximal fragment.
- Bone grafting is rarely necessary.
- Plan the position of your lag screws in case of an intra-articular fracture. Do not use lag screws for stabilization of the methaphyseal/ diaphyseal fracture part.

Table and equipment

- Basic fracture set with 4.5 mm cortical screws and 6.5 mm cancellous screws.
- LISS instruments.
- T-handle, Schanz screws, distractor or external fixator.
- Huge reduction clamps (custom-made (Fig. 10.51) or pelvic reduction clamps).
- Herbert screws may be of use in frontal split fractures (Hoffa fracture).
- Additional package of towels.
- Image intensifier.

Staff

- One scrub nurse and at least one assistant surgeon.

Positioning

- Supine position as described for the antegrade femoral nail. With this position lateral image intensifier control is facilitated.
- Check the contralateral leg clinically and radiographically for rotation. Note down the values of external and internal rotation.
- In case of extensive comminution measure the contralateral leg length under fluoroscopic control (distance: cranial border of the femoral head to the lateral joint line). Note down the leg length.
- Examine knee joint stability under anaesthesia.
- Leave the region from the iliac crest to the middle of the tibial shaft free from drapes.

Approach

- For extra-articular fractures and those intra-articular fractures that can be reduced percutaneously, use a lateral approach. Start the skin incision 4–6 cm proximal to the knee joint and end 2–3 cm distal to the knee joint. The incision is in line with the middle of the femur shaft (Fig. 10.52). Split the skin and subcutaneous tissue sharp onto the tractus. Incise the tractus and split it with the scissors in a longitudinal direction (Fig. 10.53). The scissors is introduced retrogradely and the space between tractus and femur is blunt dissected.
- For those intra-articular fractures that cannot be reduced percutaneously use an anterolateral approach. Start the incision 2–3 cm proximal to the cranial part of the patella. End up directly lateral to the tuberosity (Fig. 10.54). Split the lateral retinaculum and

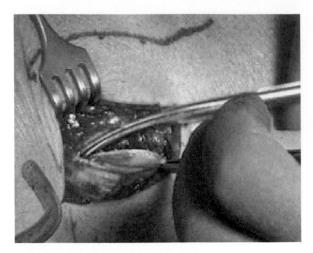

Fig. 10.53 Longitudinal splitting of the tractus.

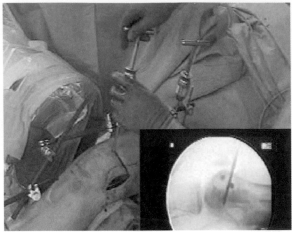

Fig. 10.56 Manipulation of the distal fragment in the sagittal plane with a Schanz screw that can be connected to an external fixator.

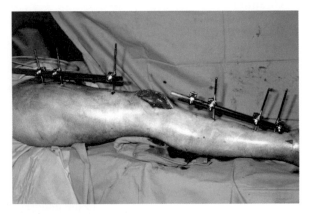

Fig. 10.54 Anterolateral approach in a patient with an intra-articular distal femur fracture and an ipsilateral fracture of the tibial shaft.

reflect the patella medially. Now you have an unrestricted access to the articular part while leaving the metaphysis untouched (Fig. 10.55).

Reduction and fixation

- Always start with the reduction and fixation of the intra-articular fracture part. The distal screws of the LISS have no lag effect and are not for stabilization of the intra-articular fracture. Reduce and fix the fracture according to the general AO/ASIF principles. Make sure that your lag screws will not interfere with the distal part of the LISS.
- Do not go for anatomic restoration of the metaphyseal fracture part. The aim is to restore the alignment of the proximal and distal main fragments, with preservation of the length of the femur.
- Reduce the fracture before application of the LISS.
- Tricks that may be of use for indirect fracture reduction:
  - Put towels under the distal part of the femur to bring the knee into slight flexion. The gastrocnemius, which tends to bring the distal femur into recurvature, is relaxed and the distal main fragment is supported.
  - An external fixator or distractor can be used to restore and retain alignment and length.
  - Additional Schanz screws can be used as 'joysticks' for manipulation of the distal or proximal fragments. These joysticks can be connected to the fixator (Fig. 10.56).

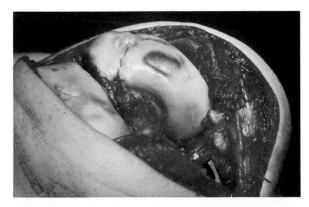

Fig. 10.55 Unrestricted access to the joint after retracting of the patella.

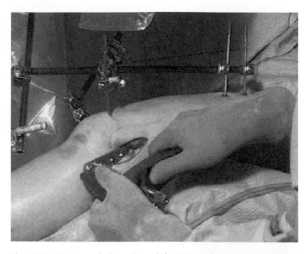

Fig. 10.57 Retrograde insertion of the LISS with the aiming guide.

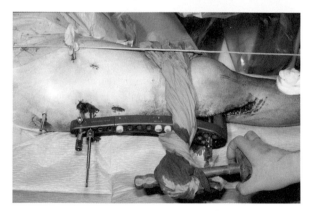

Fig. 10.58 Squeezing of an externally placed towel can be used to manipulate the proximal fragment. This is done under fluoroscopic control of the knee with a cable as varus/valgus indicator that runs through the midpoint of the femoral head and the ankle joint.

- A hammer can be used for pushing; a towel can be used for pulling on the main fragments.
- Check alignment under fluoroscopy in a lateral and anteroposterior (AP) direction.
- Connect the LISS to the aiming guide with the fixation bolt and insert it retrogradely between the periosteum and the vastus lateralis (Fig. 10.57). Retract the LISS slightly distally until its end is 1–2 cm proximal to the joint line.
- Check the correct LISS length under fluoroscopy. At least 4 (better 5) screw holes must be proximal to the fracture.

- Fix the LISS preliminarily with a K-wire distally through the fixation bolt.
- Make a 2–3 cm incision over the most proximal screw hole. Incise the fascia and dissect the vastus muscle bluntly. Connect the second fixation bolt to the most proximal screw hole. With the 2–3 cm incision you can palpate with one finger the position of the end of the plate in relation to the femur. This step is worthwhile, especially for beginners, to prevent an anterior step-off of the LISS with a compromised or no screw hold. After correct positioning of the end of the plate, the LISS is proximally fixed with a second K-wire through the fixation bolt.
- Secure the position of the LISS to the distal part of the femur with the above mentioned clamps.
- Check now again for alignment. For rotational control use the minor trochanter method. For varus/valgus alignment use the cable method. Minor varus/valgus corrections can be done with the LISS in place using the manufacture's traction device or an external towel for squeezing (Fig. 10.58).
- If correct alignment is achieved start to fix the proximal fragment. Use stab incisions for screw placement. Usually 26 mm-screws are used for the shaft. Use the irrigation system to prevent heat necrosis. Be aware that you do not have any reflection of the screw hold during tightening with locked screw devices.
- The length of the distal screws is predicted according to the manufacture's schedule.
- After removing the aiming device check the alignment again. Verify correct rotation by internal and external rotation with the hip flexed to 90°. Compare these values to the contralateral side.

Closure

- Do a thorough irrigation, especially with the antero-lateral approach.
- Use a distal drain.
- Close the fascia resp. retinaculum with strong resorbable sutures. Readapt the subcutis with resorbable sutures. Close the skin in your preferred technique.

Post-operative care

- Perform AP and lateral radiographs with the patella centred. This is best done on the operation table. The patient is under anaesthesia and pain free.

- Start continuous passive motion (CPM) on the first day after the operation especially in intra-articular fractures.
- The drain can usually be removed on the second day.
- Start mobilization on the second day with partial weight-bearing (15 kg).

Outpatient follow up

- Do clinical and radiographic follow up at 6 weeks, 3 months, 6 and 12 months after the operation.
- Order partial weight-bearing for at least 6 weeks in extra-articular fractures and 12 weeks in intra-articular fractures, depending on the radiographs.
- Remove the implant only in case of symptoms after a minimum of 12 months. Try to be as minimally invasive as on implantation.

10.9 RETROGRADE NAILING

Advantages

- Preservation of blood supply to the metaphyseal fracture zone with reduced non-union and infection rates.
- A less demanding technique compared to MIPPO.

Implants

- All types of femoral nails.
- Special retrograde nails preferred.

Indications

- Type A, C1 and C2 fractures of the distal femur.
- Periprosthetic fractures (TKA and THA).
  - TKA: Be sure that the retrograde nail can pass the femoral shield.
  - THA: Avoid stress zones between the tip of the nail and the tip of the hip stem (Fig. 10.59).

Technique

Operative technique is presented for the Distal Femoral Nail (DFN, Synthes Group).

Pre-operative planning

- Estimate nail length and nail diameter on the pre-operative radiographs. The nail tip can be placed distal to the minor trochanter.

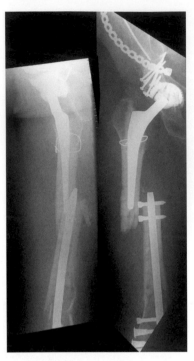

Fig. 10.59 Patient with a distal femur fracture and ipsilateral THA. Stress shielding between the implants lead to fracturing.

- Bone grafting is rarely necessary.
- Plan the position of your lag screws in case of an intra-articular fracture. Do not use lag screws for stabilization of the methaphyseal/diaphyseal fracture part.

Table and equipment

- Basic fracture set with 4.5 mm cortical screws and 6.5 mm cancellous screws.
- DFN instruments.
- T-handle, Schanz screws.
- Additional package of towels.
- Image intensifier.

Staff

- At least one scrub nurse.

Patient positioning

- Supine position as described for the antegrade femoral nail. With this position lateral image intensifier control is facilitated.
- Check the contralateral leg clinically and radiographically for rotation.

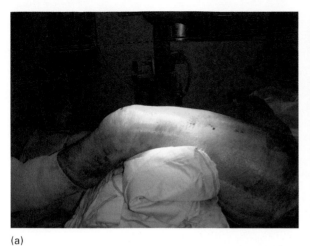

(a)

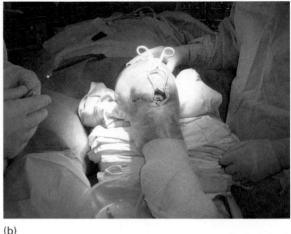

(b)

Fig. 10.60 Length and position of the incision in retrograde nailing.

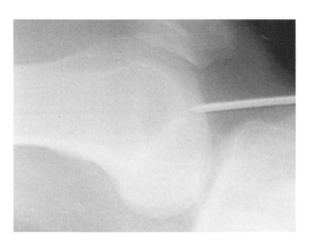

Fig. 10.61 Insertion point in the lateral projection.

- Note down the values of external and internal rotation.
- In case of extensive comminution, measure the contralateral leg length under fluoroscopic control (distance: cranial border of the femoral head to the lateral joint line). Note down the leg length.
- Examine knee joint stability under anaesthesia.
- Leave the region from the iliac crest to the middle of the tibial shaft free from draping.

Approach, reduction and fixation

- In case of an intra-articular fracture start with the percutaneous reduction and lag screw fixation from lateral to medial. Use at least two 6.5 mm cancellous screws. Make sure that these screws do not interfere with the

nail. If you cannot reduce the fracture percutaneously use the anterolateral approach as described for the MIPPO.
- Check the nail length and diameter with the ruler. The nail end should be at least 2 mm underneath the subchondral bone. If possible place the tip proximal to the minor trochanter. With this localization the risk of neurovascular damage is reduced for AP locking.
- Support the distal part of the fracture with several towels until you have a flexion of the knee joint between 25 and 30°. Choose your incision in line with the middle of the femur, which is usually slightly medial to the patellar ligament (Fig. 10.60a,b). The incision should be long enough to pass the drill bit to open the femoral canal. The incision is rarely longer than 3 cm.
- Incise the joint capsule in line with the skin incision.
- Insert the guide wire under fluoroscopic control. The entry point is slightly medial on the AP in extension of the midline of the femur. This line is usually angled 8° to the joint line. In the lateral control the entry point is the beginning of the line of Blumensath (Fig. 10.61).
- Open the femur by passing the drill over the guide wire. We do not recommend reaming of the shaft.
- Push the nail forward until the tip is just distal to the fracture.
- Reduce the fracture. Use the nail to manipulate the distal fragment.
- Additional tricks that may be of use for fracture reduction:
- Put towels under the distal part of the femur to bring the knee into slight flexion. The gastrocnemius, which

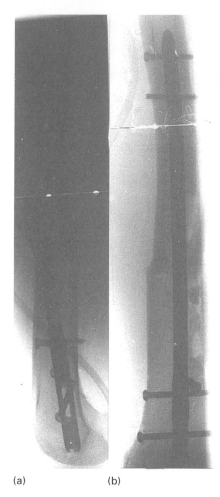

(a)   (b)

Fig. 10.62a, b Medial poller screw to prevent varus mal-alignment.

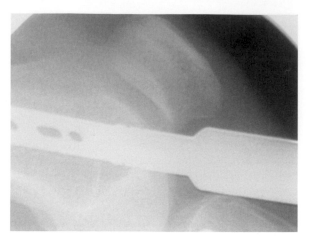

Fig. 10.63 Inserted nail with rings on the insertion device which indicate the nail depth. This nail is much too deeply inserted.

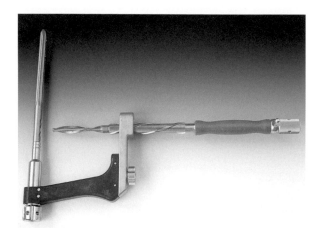

Fig. 10.64 Twisted blade which can be inserted distally over the aiming device to improve stability in osteopenic bone.

tends to bring the distal femur in recurvature, is relaxed and the distal main fragment supported.

- Schanz screws can be used as 'joysticks' for manipulation.
- Valgusation relaxes the iliotibial tractus and eases reduction. With insertion of the nail in the proximal fragment, the shaft straightens around the centric nail.
- A hammer can be used to push the fragments. A towel can be used to pull the fragments.
- Check axial alignment. For varus/valgus alignment use the cable method
- If mal-alignment is present slash the nail back and insert poller screws (Fig. 10.62a, b).
- Be sure that the nail is at least 2 mm underneath the subchondral bone. Most nail designs have marks on their introduction device to verify the nail end (Fig. 10.63).

- If correct alignment is achieved start locking in the distal part using the attached aiming device. In osteopenic bone the twisted blade should be used (Fig. 10.64).
- Check the rotation now using the minor trochanter technique. In case of a trochanter difference the distal fragment can be angulated over the nail until both trochanters have the same shape with the patellal centred.
- If there is no comminution of the fracture check the fracture site under fluoroscopy and push the nail gently forward until the distal and proximal fragments get under slight compression.
- In comminuted fractures check femoral length as described above. Slash the nail forward or backward

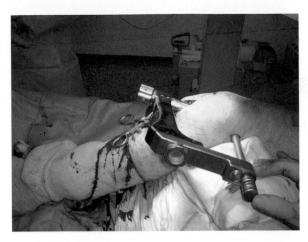

Fig. 10.65 Distal locking.

to achieve the length measured for the contralateral femur.

- Proximal locking is best performed with a radiolucent drill. AP interlocking is much easier in the proximal region than lateral–medial interlocking (Fig. 10.65).

Closure

- Do a thorough irrigation.

- Do not use a drain routinely.
- Only skin closure is necessary.

Post-operative care

- Perform AP and lateral radiographs with the patella centred. This is best done on the operation table. The patient is under anaesthesia and pain free.
- Start CPM on the first day after the operation, especially in intra-articular fractures.
- Start mobilization on the second day with partial weight-bearing (15 kg).

Outpatient follow up

- Clinical and radiographic follow up at 6 weeks, 3 months, 6 and 12 months after the operation.
- Partial weight-bearing for at least 6 weeks in extra-articular fractures and 12 weeks in intra-articular fractures depending on the radiographs.
- Implant removal is only recommended in symptomatic patients. First infiltrate the distal locking screws with local anaesthesia. If the patient becomes pain free remove just the distal locking screws instead of the whole implant. For nail removal, arthroscopic assistance is very useful.

Fractures of the patella

Stefan Hankemeier; Thomas Gosling; Hans-Christoph Pape

11.1 TENSION BAND WIRING

Implants for patellar fractures have to resist high-tensile stress. Tension band wiring transforms distraction forces of the extensor mechanism to compression forces. The wires provide anchorage for the tension band wire and neutralize the rotational forces.

Indications

- Transverse and multifragmental patellar fractures. In case of multifragmental fractures, often a combination of tension band wiring and cortical screws, lag screws, K-wires or cerclage wires is necessary.
- A pair of lag screws can exert high-compression forces to transverse fractures.

Pre-operative planning

Clinical assessment

- Pain, swelling, deformity, haemarthrosis, loss of function.
- Palpate gap between the fragments. Rule out an injury of the quadriceps and patellar tendon.
- Soft tissue injuries like abrasions are common and may require debridement or delayed operation, in order to reduce the risk of infection.
- Assess neurovascular status of the leg.

Radiological assessment

- Analyse fracture geometry by standard anteroposterior (AP) and lateral X-rays, and a tangential patellar view (Fig. 11.1).
- Differentiate between fractures and growth abnormalities (e.g. a bipartite patella is typically found on the proximal lateral quadrant of the patella, usually with sclerotic edges of the fragment in contrast to fractures).
- Rule out an abnormal patellar position caused by isolated quadriceps or patellar tendon ruptures. The Insall index calculates the ratio of greatest patellar length and the distance between the distal patellar pole and the tibial tuberosity. Normal ratio = 1; a ratio <1 suggests a patellar tendon rupture. If in doubt, compare with the lateral view of the contralateral side. Ultrasound reveals the tendon rupture site and haematoma.

Operative treatment

Anaesthesia

- Regional or general anaesthesia.
- Pre-operative prophylactic single shot antibiotics (e.g. 2nd generation cephalosporin).

Table and equipment

- Instrumentation set with 2.0 mm K-wires and 1.25 mm stainless steel cerclage wires.
- Small fragment 3.5 mm cortex screws.
- 4.0 mm cancellous lag screws.
- Radiolucent table.
- Image intensifier.

Table set up

- Instrumentation is set up on the side of the operation.
- Image intensifier is set up on the contralateral side.

Practical Procedures in Orthopaedic Trauma Surgery: A Trainee's Companion, ed. Peter V. Giannoudis and Hans-Christoph Pape. Published by Cambridge University Press. © Cambridge University Press 2006.

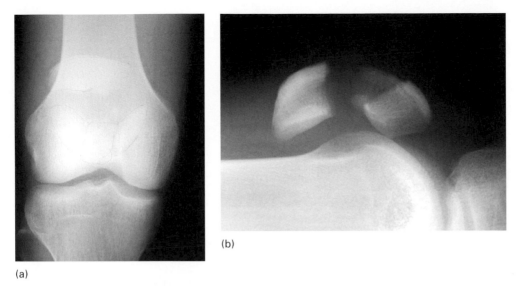

(b)

(a)

Fig. 11.1 (a) The AP X-ray demonstrates the number of fragments and vertical splits in the sagittal plane that are not visible on the lateral X-ray; (b) lateral X-ray demonstrating complete separation of the patella with loss of the extensor mechanism.

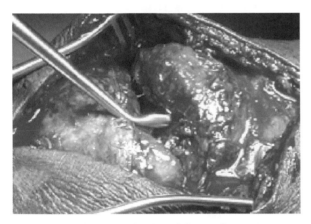

Fig. 11.2 Clear the fracture line from debris to allow an exact reconstruction.

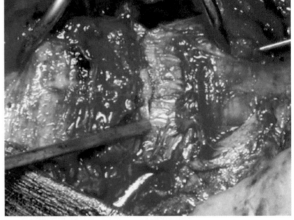

Fig. 11.3 Reduction of the fracture.

Patient positioning

- Supine position.
- An inflated tourniquet may affect the fracture reduction, as the quadriceps muscle is fixed in a shortened position.

Draping and surgical approach

- Prepare the skin over the femur up to the foot with antiseptic solutions.
- Midline longitudinal incision over the patella. Pay attention to crossing infrapatellar branches of the saphenous nerve.

- Alternatively, a parapatellar longitudinal incision can be performed.
- Remove the prepatellar bursa in case of open fractures, injuries of the bursa or pre-existing chronic bursitis.
- Incise the superficial fascia.
- Avoid excessive soft tissue stripping from the bone fragments.

Fracture reduction

- Clear the fracture line from debris to allow an exact reconstruction (Fig. 11.2).
- Irrigate the fracture thoroughly.

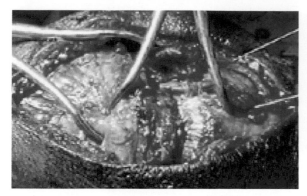

Fig. 11.4 Drill two parallel 2.0 mm K-wires longitudinally in a distance of 25–30 mm through the reduced fragments.

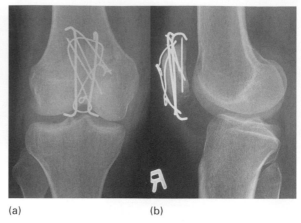

(a)   (b)

Fig. 11.7a,b AP and lateral X-rays during follow up.

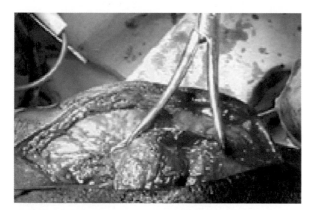

Fig. 11.5 Tighten the cerclage under inspection and simultaneous palpation of the fracture line and the retropatellar surface.

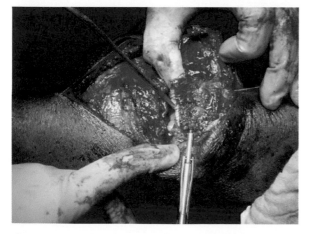

Fig. 11.6 In transverse fractures with further fragmentation of the main fragments, lag screw osteosynthesis can be performed prior to tension band wiring.

- Hyperextension of the knee helps to reduce the main fragments.
- Reduce main fragments with large, pointed, bone reduction forceps (Fig. 11.3).
- The retropatellar surface can be palpated through torn retinacula or through a parapatellar arthrotomy. Exact restoration of the joint surface is essential in order to prevent post-traumatic arthrosis.

Implant positioning

- Drill 2 parallel 2.0 mm K-wires longitudinally in a distance of 25–30 mm through the reduced fragments. The ideal position of the pins is at the anterior half of the patella (Fig. 11.4).
- Push a cerclage wire close to the edge between bone and protruding pin tips/screws. A curved large-bore needle helps to pass through the strong ligamentous insertion. The cerclage wire is to be placed directly on the bone surface, so as to prevent secondary loosening of the wire during post-operative mobilization.
- The cerclage wire can be placed either as a 'figure-of-eight' or as a 'figure-of-zero' at the anterior aspect of the patella. The ends of the cerclage are placed medially or laterally.
- Tighten the cerclage under inspection and simultaneous palpation of the fracture line and the retropatellar surface (Fig. 11.5).
- Shorten and bend the pin tips.
- Push the pin tips into the patella to prevent soft tissue irritation.

- Alternatively, the main fragments are stabilized by two 4.0 mm cancellous lag screws instead of 2 longitudinal K-wires. Lag screws provide better compression and rotational stability.

Implant positioning in other fracture patterns

- In transverse fractures with further fragmentation of the main fragments, lag screw osteosynthesis can be performed prior to tension band wiring (Fig. 11.6). In multifragmentary fractures, a circumferential cerclage prior to tension band wiring may be necessary.
- Control anatomical reduction, e.g. by palpation of the retropatellar surface.
- Control stability of the osteosynthesis by knee flexion.

Closure

- Irrigate the wound and joint. Achieve haemostasis. Suture torn retinacula with absorbable material.
- A drainage may be necessary.
- Close the wound with absorbable subcutaneous sutures and the skin with monofilament non-absorbable material.

Post-operative rehabilitation

- Post-operative standard radiographs in AP, lateral and tangential directions.
- Routine post-operative blood laboratory checks.
- Remove the drainage within 48 hours.
- Physiotherapy is recommended from the first post-operative day onwards, with active assisted motion exercise and continuous passive motion (CPM). The primary post-operative range of movements (ROM) depends on the fracture pattern and bone quality. Usually, 90° flexion is allowed post-operatively.
- Severely comminuted fractures or fractures of osteopenic bone may require delayed mobilization. Isometric quadriceps exercises help to avoid adhesions and to retain quadriceps muscle tone.
- Partial weight-bearing (15 kg).

Outpatient follow up

- Progressive physiotherapy and weight-bearing.
- Radiographs at 6 and 12 weeks post-operatively (Fig. 11.7a,b).
- Implant removal is not mandatory, but can be performed after 12 months.

12

Section I: Fractures of the proximal tibia

John F. Keating

12.1 OPEN REDUCTION AND INTERNAL FIXATION (ORIF) OF A LATERAL TIBIAL PLATEAU FRACTURE

Indications

- Clinical: instability of the knee on valgus testing.
- Radiological: split, central depression or split depression fracture types.
- Joint depression > 3 mm.

Pre-operative planning

Clinical assessment

- Swollen knee.
- Valgus deformity common.
- Common peroneal palsy possible but rare.
- Compartment syndrome – possible but rare.

Radiological assessment

- An anteroposterior (AP) radiograph is most useful to detect fractures and assess degree of joint depression (Fig. 12.1).
- A lateral radiograph is less helpful in determining the degree of depression.
- A CT scan is most useful for additional imaging – mainly indicated in cases where there is doubt about the extent or degree of depression and in complex fractures (Fig. 12.2a,b).

Operative treatment

Anaesthesia

- General anaesthesia preferred – avoid local blocks/ spinal anaesthesia which mask symptoms and signs of compartment syndrome.
- Prophylactic antibiotics at induction.

Equipment

- Standard AO set with reduction clamps and Kirschner wires.
- Radiolucent table with ability to flex at the level of the knee.
- Equipment to harvest bone graft or calcium phosphate cement.

Set up

- Instrumentation on the side of the injured leg.
- Image intensifier on contralateral side.
- Knee flexed at 90° at the outset of the procedure to facilitate exposure (Figure 12.3a,b).
- Knee brought into extension once the fracture is reduced to complete fixation.

Patient position

- Supine position.
- Tourniquet on thigh inflated to 300 mmHg at the start of the procedure.

Practical Procedures in Orthopaedic Trauma Surgery: A Trainee's Companion, ed. Peter V. Giannoudis and Hans-Christoph Pape.
Published by Cambridge University Press. © Cambridge University Press 2006.

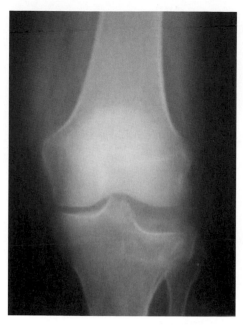

Fig. 12.1 AP view of a split depression tibial plateau fracture.

Draping and surgical approach

- Skin preparation with antiseptic solution.
- Stockinette applied to leg and brought above the level of the knee.
- Large drapes applied below upper level of stockinette.
- U-drape and adhesive transparent drape on skin.
- Longitudinal incision 1cm lateral to midline (Fig. 12.3b).
- Division of skin and subcutaneous tissue in line with the incision.
- Subperiosteal exposure of the proximal aspect of lateral tibial plateau, reflecting muscle from medial to lateral.
- Anterolateral arthrotomy; evacuate haemarthrosis.
- Develop plane between the lateral meniscus and joint capsule by sharp dissection.
- Horizontal incision under anterior horn (Fig. 12.4).

Reduction and fixation technique

- A split component is almost always present – exit anterior.
- Split can be used to access depressed fragments.
- If a pure depression fracture, then an anterolateral cortical window needs to be created.

- Depressed fragments are elevated and maintained with temporary Kirschner-wire fixation.
- Reduction confirmed by direct vision and fluoroscopy (Fig. 12.5a).
- Definitive fixation – either use a lateral plate or multiple screws (Fig. 12.5b).
- Fill significant subchondral defects with bone graft or calcium phosphate cement (Fig. 12.5c, d).

Closure

- Re-attach the lateral meniscus to the joint capsule with interrupted 2/0 Vicryl.
- Closure of capsule with 1/0 Vicryl.
- Closure of subcutaneous tissue with 2/0 Vicryl and skin with staples.

Post-operative rehabilitation

- Mobilize touch weight-bearing for 6 weeks.
- Use hinged knee brace with full extension and 90° of knee flexion for 6 weeks (Fig. 12.6).
- Physiotherapy to restore range of knee motion.

Outpatient follow up

- Review at 2 weeks post-operatively to check the wound, radiograph knee and ensure physiotherapy has commenced.
- Review at 6 weeks with a radiograph to determine if it is appropriate to remove the brace and allow progression to full weight-bearing.
- Review at 3 months and 6 months with radiographs to ensure the patient has progressed to full weight-bearing with restoration of motion.
- Review at 1 year to assess functional outcome and risk of post-traumatic osteoarthritis. Patients with evidence of degenerative change or any loss of reduction need longer term follow up to determine the need for knee joint replacement.

Indications for removal of implants

- Patients with implant-related discomfort.
- Patients with radiographic signs of post-traumatic osteoarthritis developing.
- Implants can usually be safely removed from 9 months post-injury onwards.

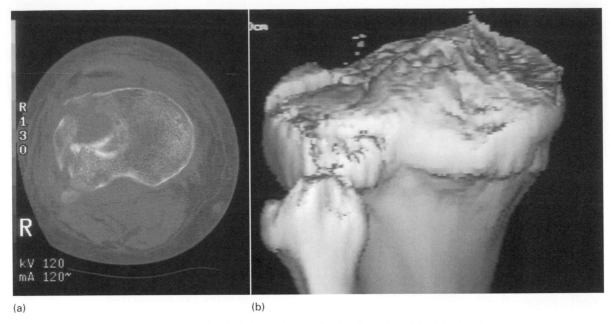

(a)   (b)

Fig. 12.2a,b CT scan and 3-D reconstruction of a tibial plateau fracture showing depression of the lateral plateau.

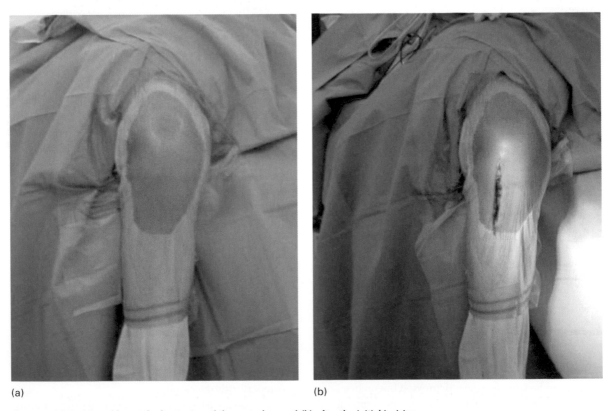

(a)   (b)

Fig. 12.3 (a) Position of leg at the beginning of the procedure and (b) after the initial incision.

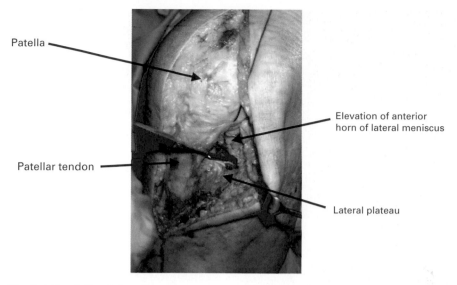

Patella

Patellar tendon

Elevation of anterior horn of lateral meniscus

Lateral plateau

Fig. 12.4 Completion of dissection.

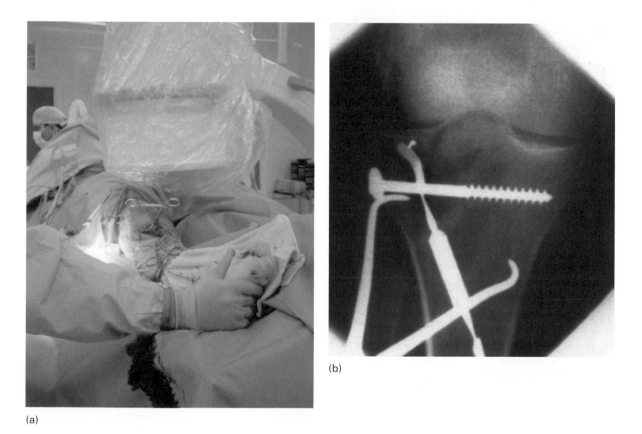

(a)

(b)

Fig. 12.5 (a) Checking reduction and (b) initial fixation with a lag screw and definition of subchondral defect with a dissector.

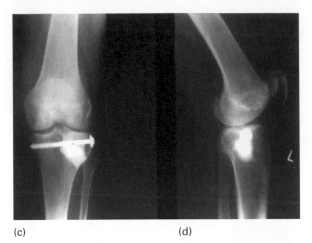

(c)   (d)

Fig. 12.5c, d Completion of fixation with calcium phosphate cement.

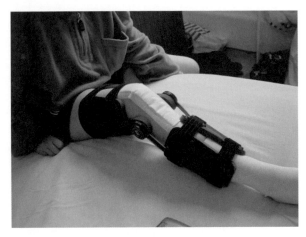

Fig. 12.6 Hinged knee brace to allow early post-operative mobilization.

12.2 OPEN REDUCTION AND INTERNAL FIXATION (ORIF) OF A BICONDYLAR TIBIAL PLATEAU FRACTURE

Indications

- Clinical: instability of the knee on valgus or varus stress testing.
- Radiological: bicondylar tibial plateau fracture with joint depression > 3 mm.
  - Ideally used for articular simple bicondylar fracture patterns – type C1/C2 injuries; can be used for complex articular fractures (type C3) but fine wire, external fixation should be considered as an alternative.

- Minimally invasive surgery with locking plates is now preferred to more radical exposures and conventional plating.

Pre-operative planning

Clinical assessment

- Swollen knee.
- Valgus or varus deformity can occur.
- Common peroneal palsy possible, particularly if there is significant varus deformity which puts the nerve under tension.
- Compartment syndrome – a definite risk with this fracture pattern: incidence 5–10%.

Radiological assessment

- An anteroposterior (AP) radiograph is most useful to detect a fracture and assess the degree of joint depression (Fig. 12.7a).
- A lateral radiograph is needed to help determine distal extent of the fracture (Fig. 12.7b).
- A CT scan is most useful for additional imaging – this should be routine in the majority of these fractures.

Operative treatment

Anaesthesia

- General anaesthesia preferred – avoid local blocks/spinal anaesthesia which mask symptoms and signs of compartment syndrome.
- Prophylactic antibiotics at induction.

Equipment

- Standard AO set with reduction clamps and Kirschner wires.
- Radiolucent table with ability to flex at the level of the knee.
- Equipment to harvest bone graft or calcium phosphate cement.

Set up

- Instrumentation on the side of the injured leg.
- Image intensifier on contralateral side.
- Knee flexed at 90° at outset of procedure to facilitate exposure.

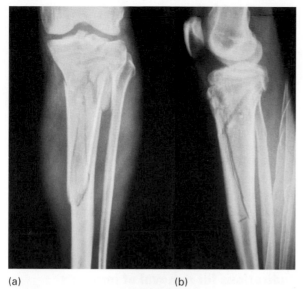

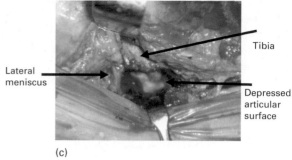

(a)   (b)

(c)

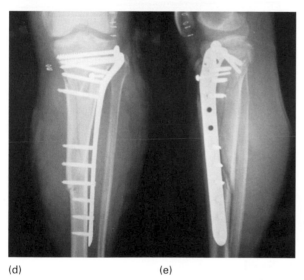

(d)   (e)

Fig. 12.7 (a) Anteroposterior and (b) lateral radiograph of a complex bicondylar tibial plateau fracture; (c) make a horizontal incision under the anterior horn (d) and (e) post-operative view showing the reduction.

- Knee brought into extension once the fracture is reduced to complete fixation.

Patient positioning

- Supine position.
- Tourniquet on thigh inflated to 300 mmHg at start of procedure.

Draping and surgical approach

- Skin preparation with antiseptic solution.

- Stockinette applied to leg and brought above the level of the knee.
- Large drapes applied below upper level of stockinette.
- U-drape and adhesive transparent drape on skin.
- Longitudinal incision 1 cm lateral to midline.
- Division of skin and subcutaneous tissue in line with incision.
- Subperiosteal exposure of the proximal aspect of the lateral tibial plateau, reflecting muscle from medial to lateral.
- On medial side, small stab incisions to apply clamps or insert screws.

- Usual pattern is split depression lateral plateau with single medial plateau fragment.
- Anterolateral arthrotomy; evacuate haemarthrosis.
- Develop the plane between the lateral meniscus and joint capsule by sharp dissection.
- Make a horizontal incision under the anterior horn (Fig. 12.7c).

Reduction and fixation technique

- A split component on the lateral side is almost always present – exit anterior.
- Split can be used to access depressed fragments.
- Elevate fragments – using temporary Kirschner-wire fixation.
- Attach lateral side to medial side with additional Kirschner wires and/or bone reduction clamps.
- Reduction confirmed by direct vision and fluoroscopy.
- Carry out initial fixation with cancellous lag screws in subchondral region.
- Slide plate in along the lateral side via a proximal incision.
- Using traction, reduce the metaphyseal component of the fracture.
- Additional external fixation/femoral distractor can be used if necessary.
- Some plate designs now allow placement of Kirschner wires through plates to help maintain alignment.
- Insert screws into plate above and below fracture (Fig. 12.7d, e).
- A common error is to fix the fracture in a varus position – this overloads medial side of knee.
- Check alignment with the image intensifier.
- Significant subchondral defects should be filled with bone graft or calcium phosphate cement.

Closure

- Re-attach the lateral meniscus to the joint capsule with interrupted 2/0 Vicryl.
- Closure of capsule with 1/0 Vicryl.
- Closure of subcutaneous tissue with 2/0 Vicryl and skin with staples.

Post-operative rehabilitation

- Mobilize touch weight-bearing for 6 weeks.
- Use hinged knee brace with full extension and 90° of knee flexion for 6 weeks.
- Physiotherapy to restore range of knee motion.

Outpatient follow up

- Review at 2 weeks post-operatively to check wound, take radiograph of knee and ensure physiotherapy has commenced.
- Review at 6 weeks with radiograph to determine if appropriate to remove brace and allow progression to full weight-bearing.
- Review at 3 months and 6 months with radiographs to ensure patient has progressed to full weight-bearing with restoration of motion.
- Review at 1 year to determine final outcome and risk of post-traumatic osteoarthritis. Patients with evidence of degenerative change or any loss of reduction need longer term follow up to determine the need for knee joint replacement.

Indications for removal of implants

- Patients with implant-related discomfort.
- Patients with radiographic signs of post-traumatic osteoarthritis developing.
- Timing of implant removal varies with bicondylar fractures.
- Fractures with significant metaphyseal comminution or diaphyseal extension should not undergo implant removal until after 12 months. For more complex patterns of injury, metalwork removal may need to be delayed for 18–24 months post-injury.

12.3 EXTERNAL FIXATION OF BICONDYLAR TIBIAL PLATEAU FRACTURES

Indications

- Clinical: instability of the knee on valgus/varus testing. Significant soft tissue problems that preclude early internal fixation e.g. extensive fracture blisters, marked soft tissue swelling and contusions.
- Radiological: bicondylar tibial plateau fracture with joint depression > 3 mm. Can be used for simple or complex bicondylar fracture patterns. Safer than internal fixation for high-energy type C2/C3 injuries.

Pre-operative planning

Clinical assessment

- Swollen knee.
- Valgus or varus deformity can occur.

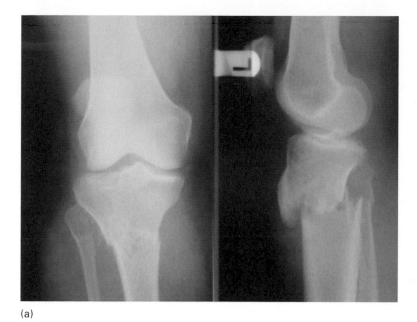

(a)

Fig. 12.8a Type C1 bicondylar tibial plateau fracture.

- Common peroneal palsy possible, particularly if there is significant varus deformity which puts the nerve under tension.
- Compartment syndrome – a definite risk with this fracture pattern: incidence 5–10%.

Radiological assessment

- An AP radiograph is most useful to detect a fracture and assess degree of joint depression.
- A lateral radiograph is needed to help determine distal extent of fracture (Fig. 12.8a).
- A CT scan is most useful for additional imaging – this should be routine in the majority of these fractures.

Operative treatment

Anaesthesia

- General anaesthesia preferred – avoid local blocks/ spinal anaesthesia which mask symptoms and signs of compartment syndrome.
- Prophylactic antibiotics at induction.

Equipment

- Modern external fixator with option of ring or semicircular construction around proximal tibia; alternatively a ring fixator may be used.

- Reduction clamps and Kirschner wires.
- Femoral distractor is a useful addition.
- Radiolucent table with ability to flex at the level of the knee.
- Equipment to harvest bone graft or calcium phosphate cement.

Set up

- Instrumentation on side of injured leg.
- Image intensifier on contralateral side.

Patient position

- Supine position with knee in full extension.
- Tourniquet on thigh. Inflation not required unless open reduction is undertaken.

Draping and surgical approach

- Skin preparation with antiseptic solution.
- Stockinette applied to leg and brought above the level of the knee.
- Large drapes applied below upper level of stockinette.
- U-drape and adhesive transparent drape on skin.
- Minimally invasive surgical approach preferred.
- Minimal access incisions on medial and/or lateral side to facilitate reduction.

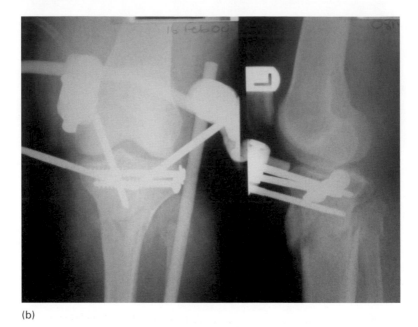

(b)

Fig. 12.8b Post-operative view showing combined internal and external fixation.

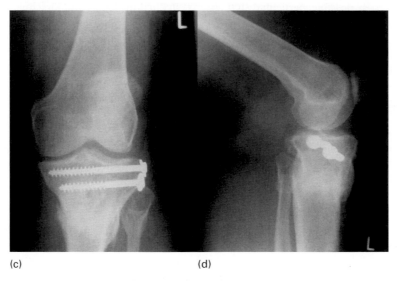

(c)   (d)

Fig. 12.8c,d Final position after frame removal.

Reduction and fixation technique

- Consider a transarticular femoral distractor to assist achieving closed reduction.
- Alternatively the external fixator frame can be fixed to the femoral condyles to aid distraction and reduction.
- Use limited incisions to manipulate fragments and guide reduction.

- Temporary Kirschner wires/reduction clamps to maintain reduction.
- Reduction confirmed by fluoroscopy.
- Apply a cluster of 3 pins distal to the fracture in the tibial shaft.
- Proximally, a ring or semicircle can be used (Fig. 12.8b,c,d).

- Pins or wires can be introduced into periarticular fragments.
- Fine-wire fixation preferred in C3 injuries.
- Pins suitable for type C1/C2 fracture patterns.
- Joint capsule extends 1 cm below plateau – avoid pins/wires proximal to this to minimize risk of septic arthritis.
- Common peroneal nerve is related to fibular neck – this is to be taken into account when placing pins and wires.
- Reduction confirmed by direct vision and fluoroscopy.
- Fill significant subchondral defects with bone graft or calcium phosphate cement.

Closure

- Closure of subcutaneous tissue with 2/0 Vicryl and skin with staples.

Post-operative rehabilitation

- Mobilize touch weight-bearing for 6 weeks.
- Depending on fracture configuration, partial or full weight-bearing.
- Physiotherapy to restore range of knee motion.
- Timing of frame removal varies between 6 and 12 weeks depending on fracture configuration and radiographic evidence of union.

Outpatient follow up

- Review at 2 weeks post-operatively to check wound, radiograph knee and ensure physiotherapy has commenced.
- Review at 6 weeks with radiograph to determine if it is appropriate to remove.
- Brace and allow progression to full weight-bearing.
- Review at 3 months and 6 months with radiographs to ensure patient has progressed to full-weight-bearing with restoration of motion.
- Review at 1 year to assess functional outcome and risk of post-traumatic osteoarthritis. Patients with evidence of degenerative change or any loss of reduction need longer term follow up to determine the need for knee joint replacement.

Indications for removal of implants

- Patients with implant-related discomfort.
- Patients with radiographic signs of post-traumatic osteoarthritis developing.

- Timing of implant removal varies with bicondylar fractures.
- Fractures with significant metaphyseal comminution or diaphyseal extension should not undergo implant removal until after 12 months. For more complex patterns of injury, metalwork removal may need to be delayed for 18–24 months post injury.

12.4 OPEN REDUCTION AND INTERNAL FIXATION (ORIF) OF ANTERIOR TIBIAL SPINE FRACTURES

Indications

- Clinical: evidence of anterior cruciate.
- Radiological: type 2 or type 3 tibial spine fractures with partial or complete displacement.

Pre-operative planning

Clinical assessment

- Assess for signs of anterior cruciate ligament laxity.
- Check other major knee ligaments to rule out associated ligament disruption.

Radiological assessment

- Anteroposterior (AP) and lateral radiographs.
- CT scan may help in doubtful cases to assess the degree of displacement more accurately.

Operative treatment

Anaesthesia

- General anaesthesia preferred – avoid local blocks/spinal anaesthesia, which mask symptoms and signs of compartment syndrome.
- Prophylactic antibiotics at induction.

Equipment

- Facilities for knee arthroscopy.
- 3.5 mm cannulated screws.
- Radiolucent table with ability to flex at the level of the knee.

Set up

- Instrumentation on side of injured leg.
- Image intensifier/arthroscopy screen on contralateral side.

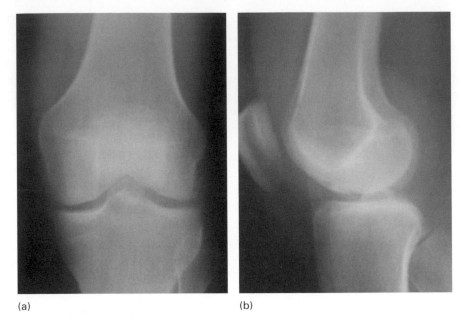

(a)   (b)

Fig. 12.9a,b Avulsion of tibial spine.

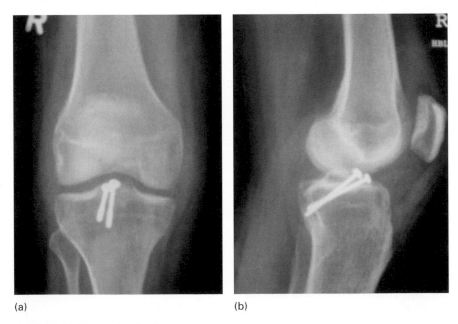

(a)   (b)

Fig. 12.10a,b Position after fixation.

Patient position

- Leg in knee clamp in 70° of flexion.
- Tourniquet on thigh inflated to 300 mmHg.

Draping and surgical approach

- Skin preparation with antiseptic solution.
- Stockinette applied to leg and brought above the level of the knee.
- Large drapes applied below upper level of stockinette.
- U-drape and adhesive transparent drape on skin.
- Diagnostic arthroscopy initially carried out.
- Minimally invasive surgical approach preferred if technically feasible.
- Reduction of fragment using arthroscopic probes.
- Fixation secured using guide wire introduced through patellar tendon portal.
- Fracture fixed with cannulated 3.5 mm screw and washer (Figs. 12.9a,b, 12.10a,b).
- If fracture cannot be reduced arthroscopically then carry out anteromedial arthrotomy.
- Clean and reduce fracture and fix as above with cannulated screws.
- In patients who have yet to reach skeletal maturity screws can be introduced in a more horizontal orientation to avoid the growth plate.

Closure

- Closure of subcutaneous tissue with 2/0 Vicryl and skin with staples.

Post-operative rehabilitation

- Mobilize in hinged knee brace 0–45° of flexion for 2 weeks.
- 0–60° of flexion in weeks 2–4.
- 0–90° degrees of flexion in weeks 4–6.
- Allow weight-bearing as tolerated on fully extended knee.
- Physiotherapy to restore range of knee motion.

Outpatient follow up

- Review at 2 weeks post-operatively to check wound, radiograph knee and ensure physiotherapy has commenced.
- Review at 6 weeks with radiograph, remove brace and allow progression to full range of motion and full weight-bearing.
- Review at 3 months and 6 months with radiographs to ensure the patient has progressed to full weight-bearing with restoration of motion.
- Follow up for 12–18 months may be needed in patients with knee joint stiffness.

Indications for removal of implants

- Patients with implant-related discomfort.
- Patients with significant persistent stiffness, particularly flexion deformity.
- Implants can be removed (usually arthroscopically) from 6 months onwards.

Section II: Fractures of the tibial shaft

Charles M. Court-Brown

12.5 INTRAMEDULLARY NAILING OF THE TIBIA

Indications

- Tibial diaphyseal fractures.

Pre-operative planning

Clinical assessment

- History of mechanism of injury. May be a high-energy injury associated with considerable soft tissue damage.
- History of increasing pain. Suggests compartment syndrome.
- Assess and document neurovascular status of leg.
- Complete physical examination in older patients.
- Careful examination for open wound (20–25% of patients).

Radiological assessment

- Anteroposterior (AP) and lateral radiographs (Fig. 12.11a,b) to identify fracture morphology.
- Look for:
  - Extent of fracture comminution (high-energy injury or osteopenia).
  - Displacement of bone fragments suggesting devital-ization.
  - Bone defects suggesting missing bone.
  - Presence of co-existing proximal or distal fractures.
  - Gas in the tissues (open fracture, anaerobic infection).
  - Previous fracture.

Compartment monitoring

- Use compartment monitoring where possible.
- Place cannula in anterior compartment close to fracture.
- Link to pressure monitoring system.
- Monitor compartment pressure and blood pressure hourly.
- Compartment syndrome when Δ P (diastolic BP – CP) > 30 mmHg.

Operative treatment

Anaesthesia

- Regional (spinal/epidural) and/or general anaesthesia.
- At induction administer prophylactic broad spectrum antibiotic. Usually 2nd or 3rd generation cephalosporin.

Table and equipment

- Locked nailing set. All implants and instruments should be available (Fig. 12.12a,b).
- Nailing table useful. Tibial nailing can be done on a flat table but it is more difficult (Fig. 12.13).
- Image intensifier.

Advantages of a nailing table

- Reduced requirement for surgical assistance.
- Maintains knee at 90° of flexion.
- Maintains traction on tibia.
- Ensures reduced fracture position is maintained.

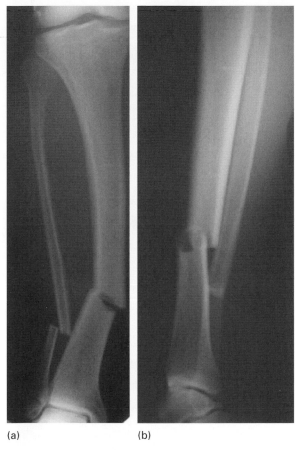

(a)   (b)

Fig. 12.11a,b Anteroposterior and lateral X-rays of a patient involved in a road traffic accident.

Disadvantages of a nailing table

- Open wound debridement is more difficult.
- Less easy to treat 'floating knees' (ipsilateral femoral and tibial fractures).
- Allows application of excessive traction. (Increased incidence of compartment syndrome.)

Table set up

- Scrub nurse and instrumentation on side of operation.
- Image intensifier comes in from the opposite side.
- Ensure adequate room for the operating table and image intensifier.

Draping

- Prepare skin with antiseptic solution from lower thigh to below malleoli (Fig. 12.14).

- Usually use 4 large drapes around the foot and lower thigh and over other the leg. Another large drape is secured to the lateral aspect of the injured leg to ensure sterility when the C-arm is used for lateral imaging.
- Sterile cover over head of C-arm.
- Tourniquet not required.

Surgical approach

- Two common approaches: longitudinal and transverse.
- Longitudinal approach
  - Incision is 8–10 cm from tibial tuberosity to patella.
  - Incision crosses Langer's lines.
  - Risk of damage to lateral geniculate nerve.
  - Easier exposure.
- Transverse approach
  - Incision is 6–8 cm, halfway between joint line and tibial tuberosity.
  - Parallel to Langer's lines (heals better).
  - No nerve damage.
  - Transverse incision recommended.
- Subcutaneous dissection. Make a 1.5–2 cm longitudinal incision, just medial to the patellar tendon, down to bone (Fig. 12.15a,b).

Surgical technique

Initial instrumentation

- Place pointed bone awl on the anterior ridge of tibia, 1 cm below the joint line, in line with the intramedullary canal.
- Push bone awl through the cortex. As the awl enters the cortex, angle the handle downwards to be parallel with the tibia. Failure to do this may cause posterior cortical damage.
- Pass small prebent hand reamer into the proximal intramedullary canal through the proximal tibial metaphysis.
- Pass olive-tipped guide wire down the intramedullary canal.
- As the guide wire is passed down the canal use the image intensifier to check fracture reduction (Fig. 12.16a,b,c). Varus or valgus angulation can be reduced by a laterally or medially applied force.
- If the guide wire is not central in the distal tibia, repass it. If it cannot be centralized use a bent olive-tipped guide wire. Rotate under intensifier control to centralize guide wire.

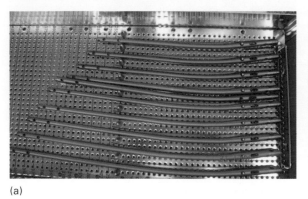

(a)

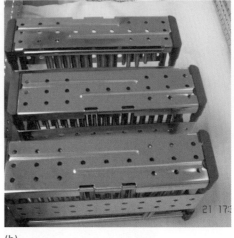

(b)

Fig. 12.12a,b Locked nailing set. All implants and instruments should be available.

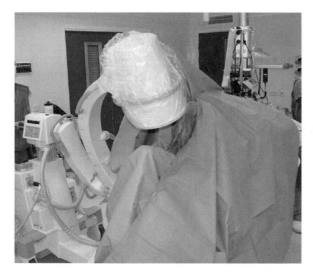

Fig. 12.13 Position of patient on nailing table. Knee is at 90°. The C-arm can visualize all of the tibia.

- The guide wire should be central in AP and lateral planes.

Reaming

- Ream in 0.5 mm increments, making sure fracture is reduced as reamer is passed.
- Ream until there is cortical chatter.
- Ream 1–1.5 mm larger than the proposed nail diameter.
- Use a 9–11 mm nail depending on the canal diameter.

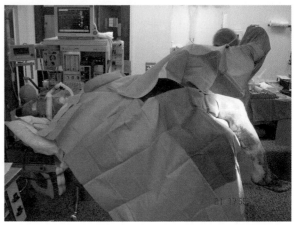

Fig. 12.14 Prepare skin with antiseptic solution from lower thigh to below malleoli.

- Ream slowly with sharp reamers to avoid thermal necrosis and the reamer becoming stuck.
- Ream the full length of the nail (Fig. 12.17a,b).
- If using an unreamed nail take care to ensure the fracture is not distracted.

Nailing

- Change guide wire if required. The necessity to do this varies with different nailing sets.
- Calculate the length of nail. Usually a measuring device is supplied but the guide wire can be measured (Fig. 12.18).

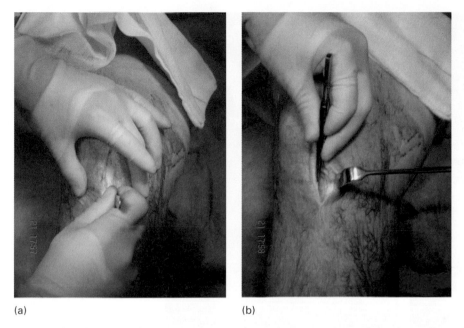

(a)   (b)

Fig. 12.15a,b Subcutaneous dissection, performing a longitudinal incision just medial to the patellar tendon, down to bone.

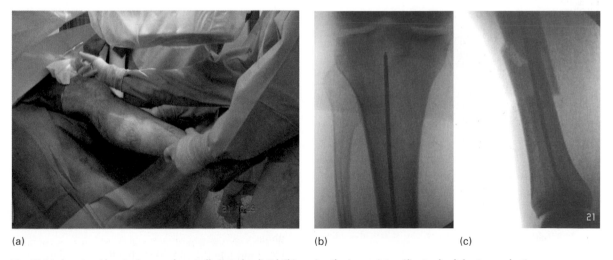

(a)   (b)   (c)

Fig. 12.16a,b,c A guide wire is passed centrally into the distal tibia, using the image intensifier to check fracture reduction.

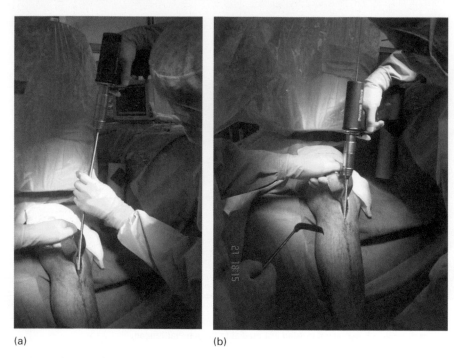

(a)   (b)

Fig. 12.17a,b Ream slowly the full length of the nail with sharp reamers to avoid thermal necrosis and the reamer becoming stuck.

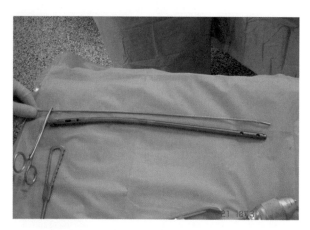

Fig. 12.18 Calculation of nail length.

- Apply nail to introducer making sure the connection is tight.
- Insert the nail into the tibia making sure the nail does not rotate as it is passed down the tibia. This makes distal cross-insertion more difficult.
- Check the fracture is reduced before the nail is passed.
- Bury the nail in the proximal cortex, but only just. You may have to remove it!

- Check nail length on the image intensifier (Fig. 12.19a,b,c).
- Proximal cross screws are inserted with the appropriate jig (Fig. 12.20a,b,c).
- Distal cross screws are inserted with free-hand technique.

Distal screw insertion: free-hand technique

- Align C-arm exactly at 90° to the leg.
- Rotate table and patient if required.
- Adjust image intensifier so the screw holes in the nail appear as perfect circles.
- Insert cross screws from the medial side to avoid the fibula.
- Place sharp point on skin so that it is central in one of the screw holes.
- Make a 1 cm skin incision.
- Replace sharp point on bone to appear in centre of screw hole.
- Make a divot or screw hole in the bone in line with the C-arm (Fig. 12.21).
- Complete screw hole.
- Measure screw length.
- Insert screw(s).

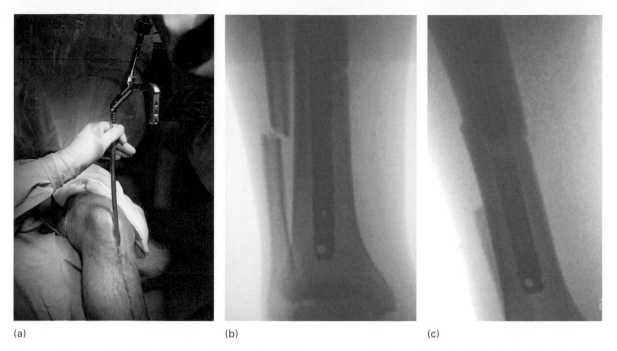

(a)　　　　　　　　　　　　　　(b)　　　　　　　　　　　　　　(c)

Fig. 12.19a,b,c Insert the nail into the tibia making sure the nail does not rotate as it is passed down the tibia. Check nail length on the image intensifier.

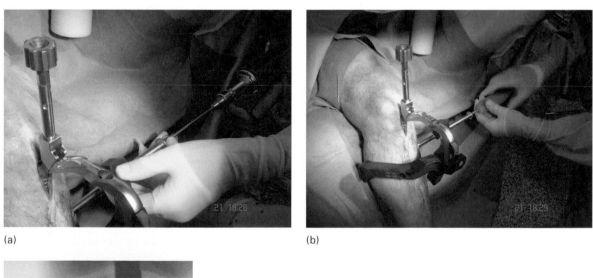

(a)　　　　　　　　　　　　　　　　　　　　(b)

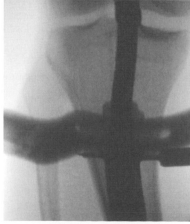

Fig. 12.20a,b,c Proximal cross screws inserted with the appropriate jig.

(c)

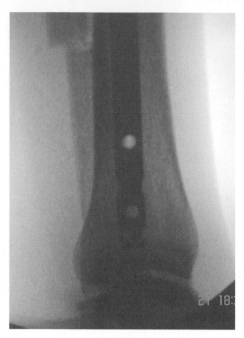

Fig. 12.21 Distal cross screw insertion is usually straightforward. The C-arm and the patient are adjusted to ensure the distal screw holes appear as circles.

Proximal tibial diaphyseal fractures

- Five to 11% of tibial diaphyseal fractures are proximal.
- Usually high-energy, comminuted fractures.
- Varus or anterior mal-alignment is common after nailing.
- Femoral distractor or unilateral external fixator can be used to maintain fracture reduction prior to nailing.
- Blocking (Poller) screws can be used to avoid mal-alignment.
- If closed nailing is difficult use another method.

Distal tibial diaphyseal fractures

- Modern nailing systems have very distal screw holes.
- Fractures within 3–5 cm of the ankle are usually straightforward to nail.
- If an intra-articular fracture is present it should be reduced and fixed with interfragmentary screws prior to nailing.
- In distal fractures the nail must be placed into the distal subchondral bone.
- The distal metaphysis must be fully reamed prior to nail insertion.

Open fractures

- Easy to nail as reduction is under direct vision.
- Same techniques as for closed fractures.
- Good evidence that nailing of open fractures gives good results regardless of the Gustilo grade of the fracture.

Closure

- No subcutaneous sutures are needed although they are often used.
- Staples, non-absorbable sutures, or subcuticular suturing is used (Fig. 12.22a,b).
- Replace compartment; monitor after nailing operation is finished.

Post-operative treatment

- Anteroposterior and lateral X-rays (Fig. 12.23a,b,c,d,e).

Post-operative rehabilitation

- Remove compartment; monitor when compartment pressure stabilizes.
- Two further doses of prophylactic antibiotics.
- Mobilize weight-bearing as tolerated.
- No protective cast is required. This will only cause joint stiffness.
- Physiotherapy may be required, particularly in older patients.

Outpatient follow up

- Follow up at 2 weeks with AP and lateral radiographs of the tibia.
- Thereafter follow up every 4 weeks.
- With reamed tibial nailing there is 96% union in closed fractures.
- Exchange nailing in the remaining 4%.
- Open fractures with bone loss may require later bone grafting.
- Discharge patient after union.

Implant removal

- Mainly removed because of knee pain.
- No other good reason to remove tibial nails.

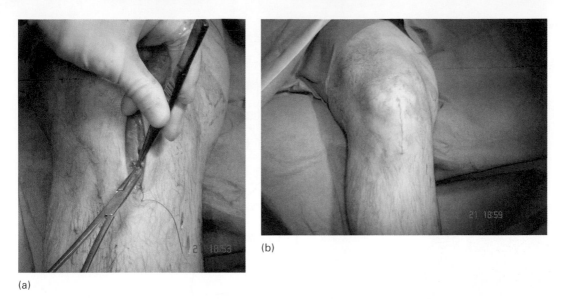

(a)

(b)

Fig. 12.22a,b Staples, non-absorbable sutures, or subcuticular suturing is used.

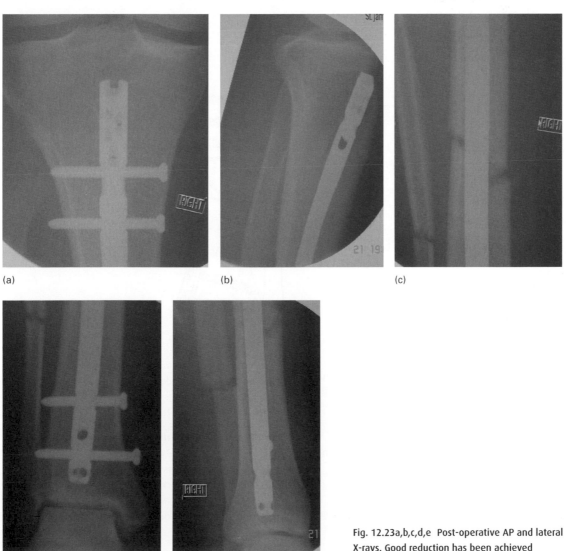

(a)

(b)

(c)

(d)

(e)

Fig. 12.23a,b,c,d,e Post-operative AP and lateral X-rays. Good reduction has been achieved

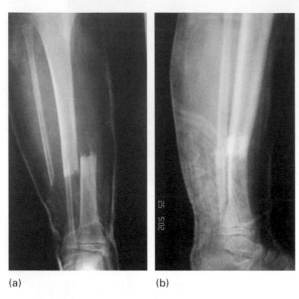

(a)   (b)

Fig. 12.24 Anteroposterior and lateral radiographs to identify fracture morphology.

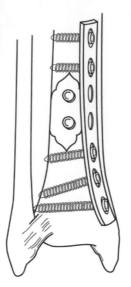

Fig. 12.25 A diagram of interfragmentary screw fixation supplemented by a DCP.

12.6 PLATING OF THE TIBIA

Indications

- Tibial diaphyseal fractures.
- Non-unions and malunions of the tibia.

Pre-operative planning

Clinical assessment

- History of mechanism of injury. May be a high-energy injury associated with considerable soft tissue damage.
- History of increasing pain. Suggests compartment syndrome.
- Assess and document neurovascular status of leg.
- Complete physical examination in older patients.
- Careful examination for open wound (present in 20–25% of patients).
- If plating for non-union, check history of fracture management. In particular check for previous infection.

Radiological assessment

- Anteroposterior (AP) and lateral radiographs to identify fracture morphology (Fig. 12.24a,b).
- Transverse fracture. Use DCP or LC-DCP.
- Spiral fracture or short oblique fracture. Use interfragmentary screws and neutralization plate, DCP or LC-DCP.

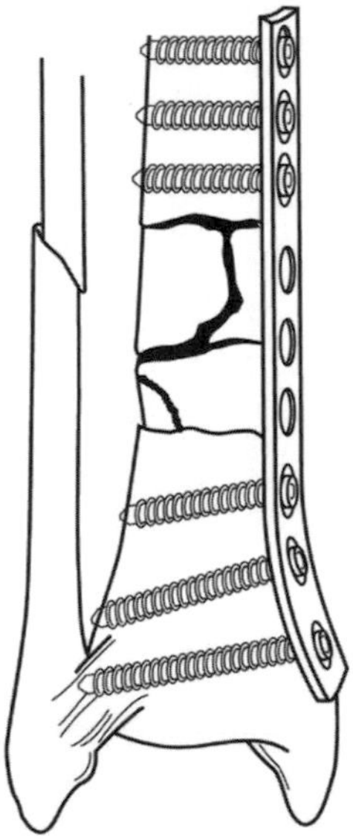

Fig. 12.26 A diagram of bridge plating of a comminuted fracture.

- Wedge fracture. Use interfragmentary screws and neutralization plate, DCP or LC-DCP (Fig. 12.25).
- Comminuted fracture. Use bridge plate (Fig. 12.26).
- Osteopenia. Use a locking plate (LCP) (Fig. 12.27).
- For proximal diaphyseal fractures consider a locked plate, particularly in osteopenic bone.
- Look for:

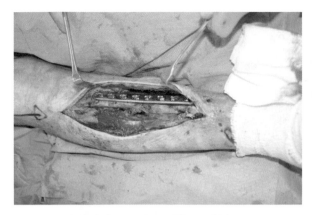

Fig. 12.27 A locked plate used to stabilize a tibial osteotomy undertaken because of malunion.

- Extent of fracture comminution (high-energy injury or osteopenia). May require a bridge plate.
- Displacement of bone fragments suggesting devitalization.
- Bone defects suggesting missing bone. Will require bone graft.
- Presence of co-existing proximal or distal fractures.
- Gas in the tissues (open fracture, anaerobic infection).
- Previous fracture.

Compartment monitoring

- Use compartment monitoring where possible.
- Place cannula in anterior compartment close to fracture.
- Link to pressure monitoring system.
- Monitor compartment pressure and blood pressure hourly.
- Compartment syndrome when ΔP (diastolic $BP - CP$) > 30 mmHg.

Operative treatment

Anaesthesia

- Regional (spinal/epidural) and/or general anaesthesia.
- At induction administer prophylactic broad spectrum antibiotic. Usually 2nd or 3rd generation cephalosporin.

Table and equipment

- Full range of plates including 4.5 mm DCP, 4.5 mm LC-DCP and LCP. LISS system if considering proximal tibial diaphyseal plating (Fig. 12.28).

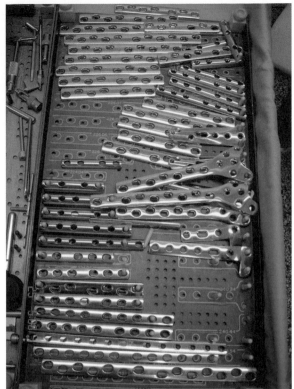

Fig. 12.28 Full range of plates including 4.5 mm DCP, 4.5 mm LC-DCP and LCP. Use LISS system if considering proximal tibial diaphyseal plating.

- Complete instrumentation.
- Flat table.
- Image intensifier required if a minimally invasive technique is used for a proximal diaphyseal fracture.

Table set up

- Scrub nurse and instrumentation on side of operation.
- Image intensifier comes in from the opposite side if required for a minimally invasive technique.
- Ensure adequate room for the operating table and image intensifier.

Draping

- Use a thigh tourniquet.
- Prepare skin with antiseptic solution from lower thigh to hindfoot. If it is thought that bone grafting will be necessary, prepare ipsilateral iliac crest.
- Use appropriate drapes to leave the leg exposed – and the iliac crest if required (Fig. 12.29).

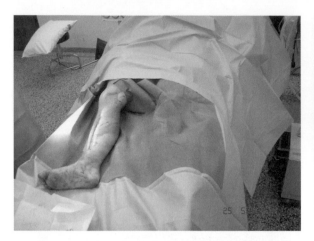

Fig. 12.29 Prepare skin with antiseptic solution from lower thigh to hindfoot. Use appropriate drapes to leave leg exposed.

- Drape the C-arm if a minimally invasive technique is to be used.

Surgical approach

- Use the standard tibial approach. The incision should be placed 1–2 cm lateral to the crest of the tibia. Proximally it curves laterally towards the head of the fibula and distally it curves towards the medial malleolus (Fig. 12.30).
- The length of the incision should be appropriate for length of proposed plate.
- Sharp dissection down to fascia without raising skin flaps.
- Incise deep fascia.
- If plate is being placed on the medial side of the tibia, use sharp extraperiosteal dissection to mobilize skin.
- If plate is being placed on lateral side, use sharp extraperiosteal dissection to mobilize overlying muscle.
- There is no tension side to the tibia. Plate can be place medially or laterally.
- A lateral, submuscular location is preferable – causes less skin irritation.
- Lateral location easier proximally. Medial location easier distally.
- Plates placed extraperiosteally.

Fracture reduction

- The goal is to achieve alignment in all planes.
- Fracture manipulation should be gentle. Avoid devascularization, particularly of loose bone fragments.

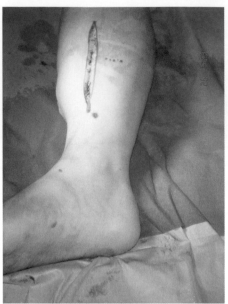

Fig. 12.30 The incision is placed 1 – 2cm lateral to the crest of the tibia. Proximally it curves laterally towards the head of the fibula and distally it curves towards the medial malleolus.

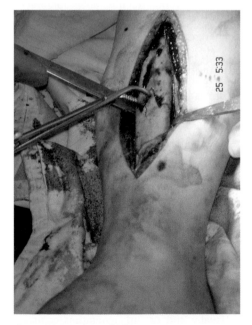

Fig. 12.31 Fracture reduction.

- Direct reduction involves direct digital manipulation of the fracture fragments.
- Direct reduction is useful for simple fracture patterns such as transverse, short oblique, spiral or wedge fractures (Fig. 12.31).

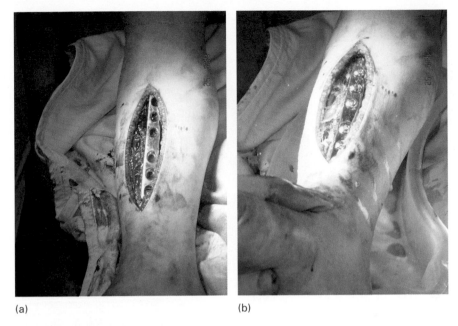

(a)

(b)

Fig. 12.32a,b Positioning of the plate.

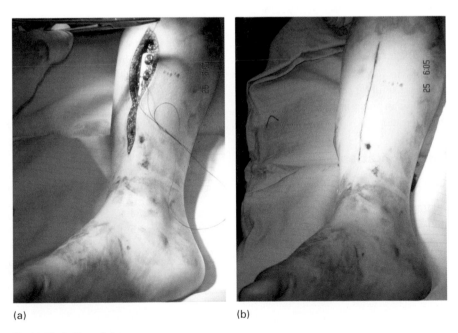

(a)

(b)

Fig. 12.33a,b Wound closure.

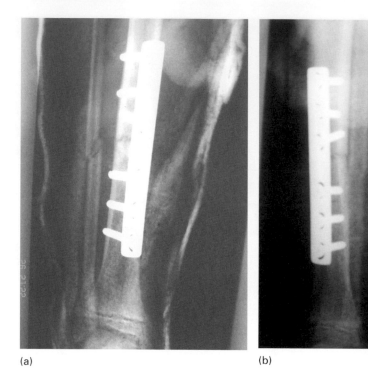

(a)   (b)

Fig. 12.34a,b Post-operative radiographs.

- Indirect reduction involves reduction by traction, either applied manually or with a fracture distractor or unilateral external fixator.
- Indirect reduction is useful for comminuted fractures. For indirect reduction an image intensifier may be useful to check the reduction.

Plate types and application

Interfragmentary screw and neutralization plate

- Initial AO tibial fracture plating technique.
- Direct reduction of simple fracture pattern. Transverse, oblique, spiral or wedge.
- Interfragmentary lagged screw mains reduction and ensures rigid fixation.
- Neutralization plate used to support screw fixation (Fig. 12.25).
- Minimum of screw fixation in six cortices on each side of the fracture.
- Longer plates in osteopenic bone.
- Bone graft used for bone defects.

Dynamic compression plate (DCP)

- Interfragmentary screw not required to achieve fracture compression.

- Fracture is reduced by direct means.
- Plate is secured on one side of the fracture with a screw.
- Eccentric screw is placed in dynamic screw hole on the other side of the fracture.
- Screw is tightened and fracture compressed.
- Same rules governing screw number as with neutralization plate.

Low-contact dynamic compression plate (LC-DCP)

- Same principle as dynamic compression plate but is shaped to minimize. interference with periosteal circulation.
- No proven advantage over dynamic compression plate.
- Use in exactly the same way.

Bridge plate

- Name refers to different mode of use of DCP or LC-DCP.
- Useful for comminuted fractures (Fig. 12.26).
- Indirect fracture reduction by traction.
- Do not disturb comminuted bone fragments. Minimize vascular damage.
- Place longer plate across fracture (usually 8- or 10-hole plate).

- Screws are placed proximally and distally, not into fracture (Fig. 12.32a,b).
- Procedure can be done with a minimally invasive technique using an image intensifier.
- Bone grafting is not required.

Locked plates

- Screws lock into the plates (Fig. 12.27).
- Very useful in osteopenic bone.
- Screws must be placed at 90° to plate.
- Not used much for middle- and lower-third fractures, where intramedullary nailing gives better results.
- Useful in proximal-third fractures.
- Can be inserted using a minimally invasive technique with an image intensifier.
- Technique requires specific plates (LISS) and instrumentation.

Plating for non-union

- Same surgical techniques as for fracture.
- Skin incision may have to be altered because of previous scars or flaps.
- DCP or LC-DCP usually used.
- Bone grafting is not required for hypertrophic non-union after cast management.
- Required for atrophic non-unions and bone defects.

Closure

- No subcutaneous sutures are needed, although they are often used.
- Staples, non-absorbable sutures, or subcuticular suturing used (Fig. 12.33a,b).

- Replace compartment monitor after nailing operation is finished. Anterior compartment is probably decompressed but not the other 3 compartments. Place monitor in another compartment, preferably deep posterior.

Post-operative treatment

- Remove compartment monitor when compartment pressure stabilizes.
- Two further doses of prophylactic antibiotics.
- Mobilize and keep non-weight-bearing for 4–6 weeks (Fig. 12.34a,b).
- Short-leg protective cast or splint is useful for 4–6 weeks.
- At 4–6 weeks increase weight-bearing. Usually full weight-bearing by 10–12 weeks.
- Physiotherapy programme usually required.

Outpatient follow up

- Follow up at 2 weeks with AP and lateral radiographs of tibia.
- Thereafter follow up every 4 weeks.
- Discharge after union.

Implant removal

- Probably no good reason for implant removal.
- Often removed for theoretical reasons such as stress sparing or re-fracture.
- May be uncomfortable if on medial border of tibia.
- If removed avoid strenuous activities for 3 months.

Section III: Fractures of the distal tibia

Peter V. Giannoudis (12.7); Toby Branfoot (12.8)

12.7 OPEN REDUCTION AND INTERNAL FIXATION: PLATING PILON

Indications

- Fractures with >2 mm articular incongruity.
- Fractures with significant displacement of the metaphysis.
- Reconstructable fractures (joint fragments that are large enough to hold small fragment screws).
- Compartment syndrome.
- Adequate soft tissue envelope.

Pre-operative planning

Clinical assessment

- Mechanism of injury (fall from a height, skiing injury, motor vehicle accident, forward fall with a trapped foot).
- Look for associated injuries.
- Thoroughly assess the soft tissue condition.
- Look for the presence of an open injury.
- Assess the neurovascular status of the extremity.
- Look for early signs or symptoms of compartment syndrome.
- Review patient's past medical history and recognize the presence of existing medical conditions (diabetes, osteoporosis, vascular disease) that can modify the plan of treatment).
- Displaced or dislocated fractures must be reduced immediately.

Radiological assessment

- Standard high-quality anteroposterior (AP), lateral, 45° external rotation and mortise views of the ankle.

- CT scan: provides information regarding the fracture pattern, the number and location of the cortical fragments, the extent of articular comminution and the amount of articular displacement (Fig. 12.35a,b,c).

Timing of surgery

- Open fractures are treated on an emergency basis.
- Generally it is determined by the condition of the soft tissues.
- Simple fractures or fractures with minimal soft tissue injury can be definitively stabilized in 6–8 hours.
- For other types of fractures a 6–12 day delay is preferable.
- The use a joint bridging external fixator with elevation of the limb in the meantime is mandatory.

Operative treatment

Anaesthesia

- Spinal or general anaesthesia.
- Prophylactic antibiotics as per local hospital protocol (e.g. 2rd generation cephalosporin).

Table and equipment

- Flattened 1/3 tubular plates or modified 3.5 mm cloverleaf plates or 3.5 mm LC-DC plates can be used.
- Standard osteosynthesis set as per local hospital protocol.
- An image intensifier.

Table set up

- The instrumentation is set up on the side of the operation and at the foot of the operating table.

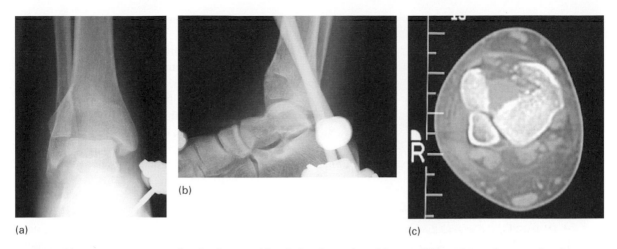

(a)

(b)

(c)

Fig. 12.35 (a) Anteroposterior X-ray of a pilon fracture with a displaced anterolateral fracture; (b) lateral X-ray demonstrating the impaction of the anterior lateral surface; (c) CT scan of the fracture.

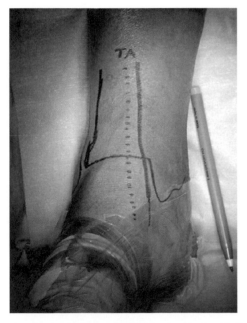

Fig. 12.36 An anteromedial incision is placed medially to the palpable tibialis anterior tendon. It is important when performing this approach that the tendon sheath will not be violated.

- Image intensifier is from the contralateral side.
- Position the table diagonally across the operating room so that the operating area lies in the clean air field.

Patient positioning

- The patient is positioned supine on a radiolucent table.
- Place a pneumatic tourniquet and inflate if needed.

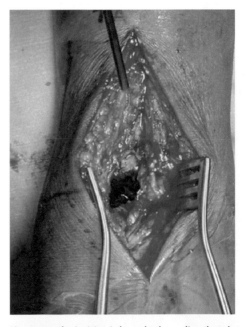

Fig. 12.37 The incision is brought down directly to bone, medial to the tibialis anterior tendon sheath; a large void is seen adjacent to the talar articular surface caused by the impaction of the anterior articular surface.

Draping and surgical approach

- Prepare the skin over the lower leg, ankle and entire foot with the usual antiseptic solutions (aqueous / alcoholic povidone–iodine). Prepare skin between toes thoroughly.
- Apply standard draping around lower leg in calf region.

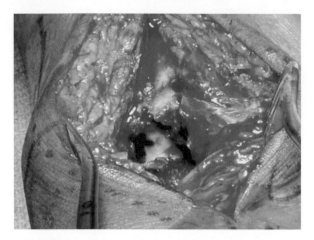

Fig. 12.38 A no-touch technique is utilized with self-retaining retractors, allowing access to the intra-articular displacement. The two articular fragments, including the impacted articular fragment, are visible with medial retraction of the plafond.

- Apply tape around toes to minimize the risk of infection.
- Palpate the tibialis anterior tendon and using a skin marker draw the anteromedial incision line medially to the tendon over the skin, starting proximally, slightly lateral to the anterior tibial crest and curving distally to the medial malleolus (Fig. 12.36).
- Incise the skin, taking care not to violate the tendon sheath.
- Bring down the incision directly to bone creating full thickness flaps (Fig. 12.37).
- Using self-retaining retractors (no-touch technique) access the intra-articular displacement. The 2 articular fragments, including the impacted articular fragment, can be visualized with medial retraction of the plafond (Fig. 12.38).
- Identify the impacted articular surface that must be reduced.

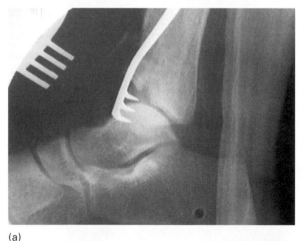

(a)

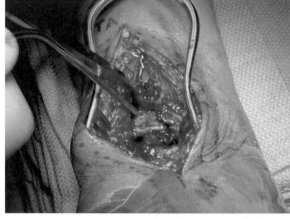

(b)

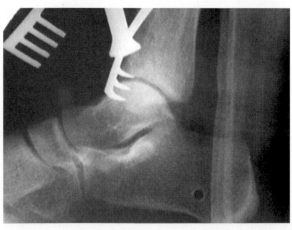

(c)

Fig. 12.39a,b,c Reduction is normally performed by placing a curved osteotome above the attached cancellous bone of the articular segment and forcefully manipulating the fragment distally against the talus as a template.

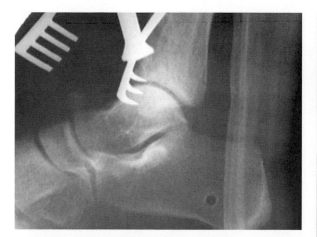

Fig. 12.40 A bone tamp can be used to support the articular surface against the talus while fixation is performed, typically with a lag screw or push plate.

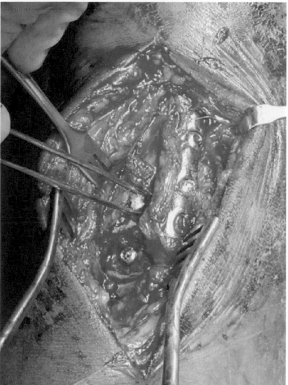

Fig. 12.42 A pointed reduction clamp will then be used to reduce the anterolateral fragment to the reconsrtructed anteromedial portion of the joint, which has been reconstructed. A percutaneous screw and an anterolateral push plate is then used to support the reduction.

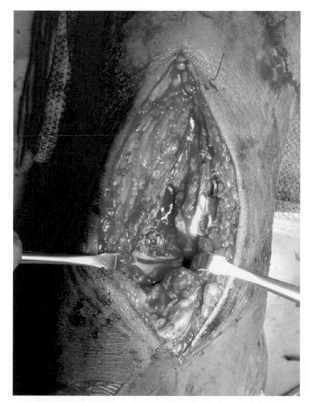

Fig. 12.41 The joint is now well reconstructed anteriorly and medially. A lag screw has been used to fix the anterior impacted fragment and a medial push plate has been used to support the anteromedial cortical rim.

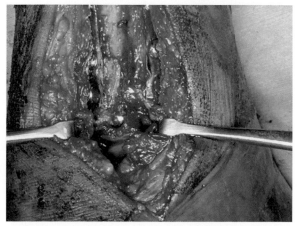

Fig. 12.43 The reduction is anatomic and supported with two low profile plates, one medially and one anterolaterally.

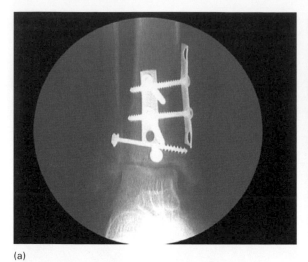
(a)

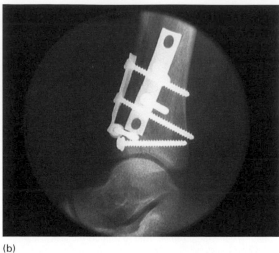
(b)

Fig. 12.44 Anteroposterior and lateral radiographs demonstrating good alignment and fixation of the plafond fracture.

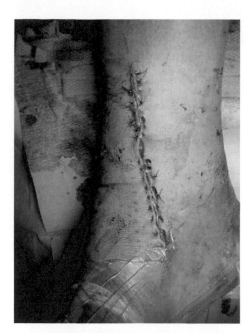

Fig. 12.45 Closure is performed in layers, being careful to protect the tibialis anterior paratendon and soft tissue sleeve. The closure should be performed with vertical mattress sutures of Donati without tension. If any tension is present, relaxing incisions or a pie-crusting technique should be utilized.

- Place a curved osteotome above the attached cancellous bone of the articular segment and manipulate the fragment distally against the talus, which is used as a template (Fig. 12.39a,b,c).
- Use a bone tamp to support the articular surface against the talus (Fig. 12.40).

- Once the articular surface has been restored, use a lag screw to fix the anterior impacted segment.
- Place a medial push plate to support the anteromedial cortical rim (Fig. 12.41).
- With the help of a pointed reduction forceps reduce the anterolateral fragment to the reconstructed anteromedial portion of the joint.
- Place a percutaneous screw and an anterolateral push plate to support the reduction (Fig. 12.42).
- The reduction is anatomic and supported with 2 low-profile plates, 1 medially and 1 anterolaterally (Fig. 12.43).
- Use fluoroscopic images to verify axial alignment, length and joint congruency (Fig. 12.44).

Closure

- Leave the anterior tibial fascia open.
- Repair the capsule and close the wound in layers using 2.0 Vicryl and 4.0 nylon Donati sutures for the skin.
- If any tension is present, relaxing incisions or a pie-crusting technique should be utilized (Fig. 12.45).

Post-operative treatment

- Two more prophylactic doses of antibiotics are administered.
- Apply a posterior splint with the foot in 90° dorsiflexion.
- Elevate the limb for a time period of 48 hours.
- Carefully assess the neurovascular status of the extremity.

- Begin ankle motion only when the surgical wound has sealed and the soft tissue condition has improved.

Outpatient follow up

- Review in clinic after 2 weeks with X-rays on arrival and monthly afterwards.
- Allow ambulation with crunches only after swelling diminution and wound healing.
- After 2 weeks begin active range of motion.
- Toe-touch weight-bearing is instituted for 8 weeks.
- Full weight-bearing is allowed between 3 and 4 months post-operatively.

Implant removal

- Rarely indicated.
- After 12 months if there is soft-tissue irritation.

12.8 CIRCULAR FRAME FIXATION FOR DISTAL TIBIAL FRACTURES

Indications

Circular frames are used to stabilize:

(a) Partial articular pilon fractures.
(b) Complete articular pilon fractures.
(c) Extra-articular distal tibial fractures.

Pre-operative planning

Clinical assessment

- History of high-energy trauma to the lower leg, typically a fall from a significant height or a high-speed road traffic crash.
- Pain and swelling around the distal tibia and ankle.
- Assess and document the soft tissues of the lower leg and foot (consider the involvement of plastic surgeons).
- Assess and document neurovascular status of the leg.
- Because these are a result of high-energy trauma a careful and full examination for other injuries must be made:
  - locally (e.g. LisFranc or calcaneal fractures) or
  - generally (e.g. compression fractures around the knee, pelvic fractures, compression fractures of the thoraco-lumbar spine after a fall from a height).

Radiological assessment

- Anteroposterior (AP) and a lateral radiograph of the whole tibia.
- Anteroposterior radiograph and a lateral view of the distal tibia and foot, centred on the ankle joint, to demonstrate the fracture geometry.
- CT scan of the fracture to:
  - assess the extent of joint surface damage
  - demonstrate the major fracture fragments requiring reduction/fixation
  - plan surgical approaches for percutaneous or limited open reduction and fixation (Fig. 12.46a,b).

Operative treatment

Anaesthesia

- Regional (spinal/epidural) and/or general anaesthesia.
- At induction, administer prophylactic antibiotic as per local hospital protocol (e.g. 3rd generation Cephalosporin).

Table and Equipment

- Circular frame instrumentation (e.g. Ilizarov or Taylor Spatial Frame) including appropriate sizes of rings (radiolucent if possible) and a foot-plate, plain & olive fine-wires and half-pin fixation options.
- Small-fragment fixation screws (cannulated if desired).
- Large and small clamps for percutaneous reductions.
- Large (approximately 10 × 20 cm) and small (approximately 5 × 10 cm) towel / bolster rolls to elevate and support the leg.
- A radiolucent table table, which for taller patients may require an extension to ensure adequate operative space without radio-opaque bars etc compromising surgery.
- Thigh tourniquet (not usually inflated before the operation starts).
- An image intensifier and a competent radiographer.

Table set up

- The instrumentation is set up on the side of the operation.
- Image intensifier C-arm is from the contralateral side.
- Image intensifier screen is either on the contralateral side at the level of the patient's shoulder, or beyond the patient's feet.

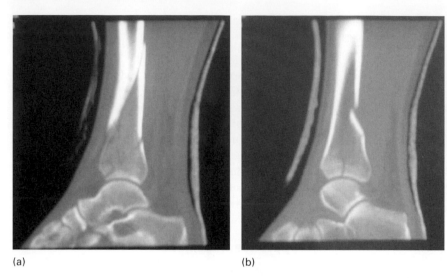

(a)   (b)

Fig. 12.46a,b CT scan of the fracture.

Patient positioning

- Supine with adequate extension of the table below the foot for surgery.
- Ensure uninterrupted C-arm view of the whole tibia and foot before draping.

Draping

- Prepare the skin over the whole foot and tibia to above the knee using usual antiseptic solutions (aqueous/alcoholic povidone–iodine).
- Apply transparent, plastic, adherent 'isolation' drape (or small glove) over forefoot/toes if required.

Surgical approach

- Fracture reduction:
  - Pre-construct a basic 3-ring frame using rings sized for the patient's leg, planning for a single ring at the level of the fracture and 2 rings proximally, one just above the level of the fracture and one 15–20 cm proximally (this may be a 5/8ths ring to allow for better knee flexion if quite proximal).
  - Add an additional half-ring or footplate below the distal ring for attachment of a calcaneal distraction wire.
  - Ensure there is a sufficient spare rod/strut length to allow for distraction and adjustment of final ring positions.

- Apply the frame to the injured leg, and pass a single plain calcaneal wire parallel to the ankle joint, which is then tensioned across the distal foot ring.
- Wires should be sharp and passed through the skin by pressure only, not rotating on the drill, to minimize the chances of neurovascular injury. Passing them through bone should be done by drilling slowly and without excessive pressure to minimize heating and burning the bone. Frequent pauses, long enough to allow the wire tip to cool, may be required. Repeated passes through cortical bone should not be made with a progressively blunter wire – a new sharp wire should be used. This is especially important when passing wires through the tibial diaphysis in young patients as the cortical bone is thick and dense.
- Once through the bone, ideally the wire should be pushed or hammered through, rather than drilled, to minimize risk to soft tissue structures. Muscles and tendons should ideally be under tension when the wire is passed through that compartment, to minimize subsequent problems of tethering. This will require the assistant to move the foot between dorsi- and plantar-flexion.
- Pass a second single plain 'reference' wire, perpendicular to the tibial shaft, at the level of the proximal ring to which this is tensioned.
- Apply distraction across the fracture/ankle joint using this frame to achieve as much reduction as

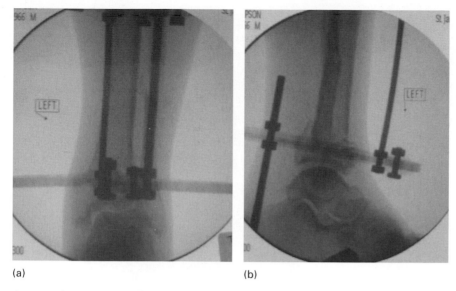

(a)   (b)

Fig. 12.47a,b Intraoperative fluoroscopic images.

possible of the fracture by ligamentotaxis under image intensifier guidance in the AP and lateral planes – the medial and posterior columns usually reduce well, the anterolateral fragment often does not (Fig. 12.47a,b).

- Using small incisions (avoiding injury to tendons and neurovascular structures by limited open exploration), guided by the pre-operative radiographs and CT as well as image intensification, use small instruments (K-wires, Macdonald's, small-fragment set periosteal elevators, small punches, etc.) to reduce the major metaphyseal fragments to anatomical alignments and restore the joint surface as much as the extent of injury allows.
- 'Perfect' reduction of the diaphyseal components may not be necessary, provided restoration of length and anatomical alignment of the joints is achieved.
- Percutaneous screws (solid or cannulated) can be used (under image intensification guidance) to secure the major metaphyseal fragments to each other. Remember that 'crossed olive wires' can provide alternative/additional stabilization, especially in the coronal plane.
- Fracture stabilisation:
  - The distal ring position should be adjusted on the rods to lie just above the ankle joint – a wire fastened to the distal surface of this ring should lie 9–12 mm from the joint surface to ensure it is clear of the joint capsule.

- In some complex and/or distal fractures it may not be possible to stabilize the fracture without intra-articular wires (and the risk of septic arthritis) – this may be a relative indication to consider bridging the metaphysis to the ankle.
- Fixation of the 2 proximal rings would normally be with 4 plain wires, 2 on each ring, usually the transverse and 'medial face' wires illustrated in standard 'safe corridor' atlases. In tall and/heavy patients additional wires should be considered. Maximal crossing angles should be achieved if possible to enhance the stability of the frame. Wires should normally be tensioned to approximately 1300 N to maximize frame stiffness.
- Six mm half-pins may be used instead of, or in addition to, fine wires. At best (i.e. when clamped directly to the ring rather than elevated on a post or Rancho blocks that can cantilever) a 6 mm half-pin is equivalent to 1 wire. Using 5 mm half-pins and/or 3-hole (or more) Rancho blocks markedly reduces the half-pin stiffness and thus additional fixation will be required to reach the equivalent of 4 wires.
- Distal fixation on the distal ring would ideally be with 4 wires: 2 attached directly to the ring, plus 2 'flying' wires off the ring. Olive wires may enhance the stability and help with the reduction of fragments. The addition or substitution of wires with half-pins (6 mm diameter if possible) may be appropriate – sometimes the only way adequate stability can be

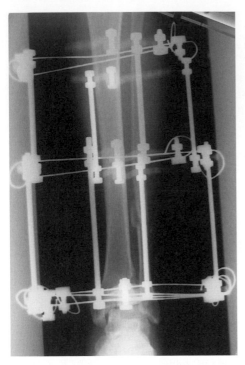

Fig. 12.48 Post-operative radiograph of a circular frame application.

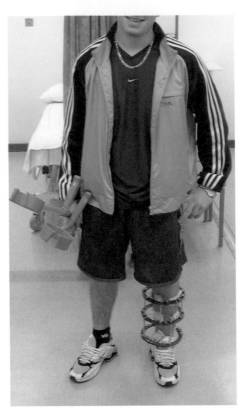

Fig. 12.49 Patient mobilization with progressive full weight bearing.

achieved. Wires can bypass internal fixation screws under image intensifier guidance usually without difficulty.

- If satisfactory levels of stability on the metaphysis can be achieved the distal calcaneal fixation can be removed. If inadequate stability (owing to poor bone quality, extensive comminution, low level of the fracture, etc.) is achieved, bridging fixation to the calcaneum should be retained and an additional calcaneal wire should be passed. Further stabilization of the forefoot may be appropriate.
- In cases where extensive chondral damage has occurred to the ankle joint surfaces, consider bridging the ankle and maintaining ankle distraction (possibly with a hinged construct) to allow for optimal cartilage healing.

Closure

- Close larger skin incisions with 2-layer closure, e.g. 2/0 Vicryl for deep layers and 3/0 Monocryl for skin.
- Close small 'stab' incisions with a skin suture only.

- Use subcuticular and absorbable sutures where possible to minimize problems and patient anxieties of removing sutures from within the frame.
- Apply pin-site dressings after cleaning – 2 layers of padded absorbable sponge (e.g. Alevyn from Smith & Nephew) with firm compression from a clip – will minimize subsequent problems of pin-site infection.

Post-operative rehabilitation

- Two further doses of prophylactic antibiotics.
- Routine bloods, and radiographs of the whole tibia, and of the distal tibia centred on the ankle joint (Fig. 12.48).
- Provide adequate analgesia to encourage early rehabilitation and independence, avoiding NSAIDs if possible.
- Redress the pin sites at 48 hours after cleaning with alcoholic chlorhexidine, and then weekly thereafter.
- Encourage early ankle motion (if fixation allows) and prevent equinus contracture using a Theraband loop.

- Mobilize touch- or partial-weight-bearing (depending on strength of fixation and the frame applied, and being pragmatic about what a patient can realistically achieve) at the earliest opportunity and tailor physiotherapy to meet individual needs and demands.

Outpatient follow up

- Review at 2 weeks, 4–6 weeks, 8–10 weeks and 12–14 weeks with check radiographs to look for:
  - Maintenance of fracture reduction.
  - Radiological evidence of healing.
  - Progressive physical rehabilitation towards weight-bearing without aids and full knee and ankle joint function.
  - Progressive functional return to independence in activities of daily living, mobility, employment, etc. (Fig. 12.49).
  - Satisfactory pain control.
  - Satisfactory pin-site care – treat pin-site infections if they occur initially by optimizing (and reinforcing) pin-site care protocols, and giving a short course of oral antibiotics (e.g. flucloxacillin 500 mg 4 times daily for 7 days).

- Expect significant radiological and clinical evidence of progress towards healing at 8–10 weeks – if there is no evidence of this, consider actions to enhance healing such as cyclical compression–distraction, iliac crest bone grafting, ultrasound, etc.
- Clinically (i.e. the patient is weight-bearing independently without walking aids) and radiologically (i.e. callus is spanning previous fracture gaps) anticipate the fracture to have nearly united at 10–16 weeks (significant diaphyseal components take longer than purely metaphyseal injuries). At this point dynamize the frame by destabilizing the construct across the fracture site (e.g. removing the footplate and wires, some connecting rods or wires, etc.).

Implant removal

- Review the patient 2–4 weeks later. If there is further progress towards clinical and radiological union, the frame may be removed – in the operating theatre under anaesthesia or in clinic, according to local practice and patient preference.
- No removal of internal fixation is indicated unless there is good evidence of soft tissue irritation or other problems.

13

Fractures of the ankle

Christopher C. Tzioupis and Peter V. Giannoudis

13.1 OPEN REDUCTION AND INTERNAL FIXATION (ORIF) FOR BIMALLEOLAR ANKLE FRACTURES

Indications

- None of the existing classifications is adequate alone to dictate the treatment strategy.
- Fractures with talar displacement.
- Almost all bimalleolar fractures.

Pre-operative planning

Clinical assessment

- Mechanism of injury: direct or, more commonly, by indirect rotational, translational and axial forces.
- Soft tissue swelling, ecchymosis, tenderness.
- Look for associated injuries.
- Assess neurovascular integrity of the extremity.
- Obtain a careful patient history.
- Evaluate age, osteoporosis and systemic conditions.

Radiological assessment

- High-quality anteroposterior (AP) and lateral radiographs (Fig. 13.1a,b).
- Mortise view: AP in 20° internal rotation.
- CT scan: for evaluation of posterior malleolus.
- Assess: degree of fragment displacement, quality of bone.

Timing of surgery

- Dictated by the soft tissue condition.

- Before the development of soft tissue swelling or blisters.
- Delayed ORIF when soft tissue injury resolves.

Operative treatment

Anaesthesia

- Spinal or general anaesthesia.
- Prophylactic antibiotics as per local hospital protocol.
- Application of a pneumatic tourniquet to the upper thigh.

Table and equipment

- AO small fragment set.
- 3.5 mm cortical and 4.0 cancellous screws.
- Standard osteosynthesis set as per local hospital protocol.
- A radiolucent table.
- An image intensifier and a competent radiographer.

Table set up

- The instrumentation set is at the foot end of the table.
- Image intensifier is from the contralateral side.

Patient positioning

- The patient is positioned supine with a bolster underneath the buttock of the affected side (Fig. 13.2).

Practical Procedures in Orthopaedic Trauma Surgery: A Trainee's Companion, ed. Peter V. Giannoudis and Hans-Christoph Pape. Published by Cambridge University Press. © Cambridge University Press 2006.

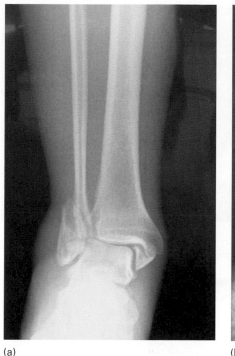

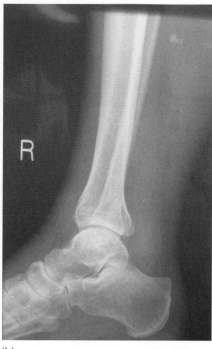

(a)   (b)

Fig. 13.1 a,b Anteroposterior and lateral views of a bimalleolar fracture of the right ankle.

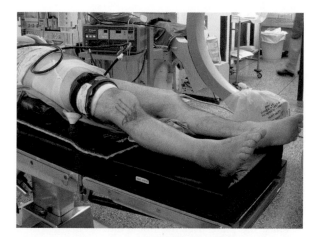

Fig. 13.2 The patient is positioned supine with a bolster underneath the buttock of the affected side.

Draping and surgical approach

- Prepare the skin over lower leg, ankle and entire foot with usual antiseptic solutions (aqueous/alcoholic povidone–iodine). Prepare skin between toes thoroughly.

- Draw the skin incision plane using a skin marker (Fig. 13.3a,b).
- Apply standard draping around lower leg in calf region.
- Apply tape around toes to minimize the risk of infection.

Lateral malleolus

- Make a longitudinal incision over the distal fibular shaft.
- Care should be taken not to damage the superficial peroneal nerve (anteriorly) or the sural nerve (posteriorly).
- Avoid subcutaneous flaps (Fig. 13.4).
- Incise just anterior to the peroneal tendons and musculature and retract them posteriorly.
- Visualize the fracture site and the talar dome (Fig. 13.5).
- Irrigate and use suction to inspect for articular damage.
- Periosteal stripping must be kept to a minimum.
- Use pointed reduction forceps to reduce the fracture, placing it perpendicular to the fracture plane (Fig. 13.6).
- If the fracture is sufficiently oblique and with a good bone stock, place a 3.5 mm lag screw perpendicular to the fracture line, from anterior to posterior (Fig. 13.7a,b).

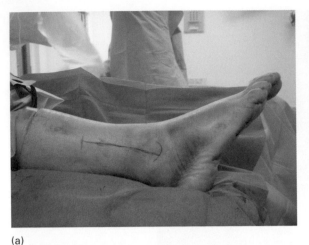

(a)

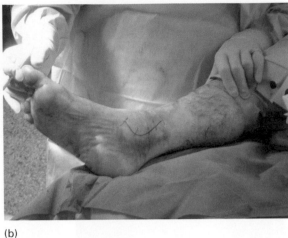

(b)

Fig. 13.3a,b Skin incision planes drawn with a skin marker over the fibula and the medial malleolus.

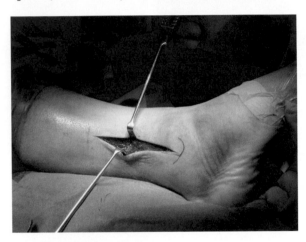

Fig. 13.4 Longitudinal incision over the distal fibular shaft avoiding subcutaneous flaps.

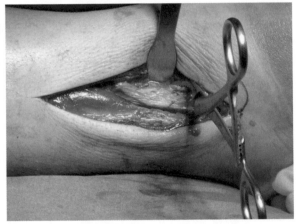

Fig. 13.6 After irrigation and minimum periosteal stripping, reduction of the fracture.

- Use intraoperative fluoroscopic views to verify maintenance of reduction.
- Precontour a 1/3 tubular neutralization plate (concave above the plafond and convex above the lateral malleolus).
- Place the plate over the fibula and secure it with a clamp, avoiding loss of reduction (Fig. 13.8a,b).
- Use intraoperative fluoroscopic views to verify maintenance of reduction.
- Using the offset drill guide, first drill a hole in the plate hole proximal to the fracture line.
- Identify the screw length with the depth gauge.
- Prepare the screw hole with a 3.5 mm tap.
- Secure the plate, with a screw in the plate hole.
- On the opposite site of the fracture place a second screw in a similar fashion (Fig. 13.9a,b).

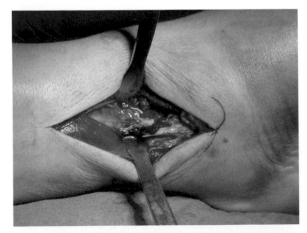

Fig. 13.5 After incision and retraction of peroneal tendons and musculature, exposure of the fracture plane.

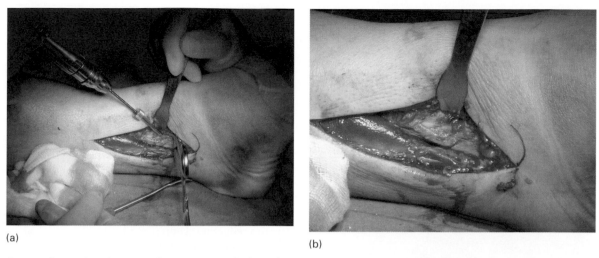

Fig. 13.7a,b Insertion of a 3.5 mm lag screw perpendicular to the fracture line, from anterior to posterior.

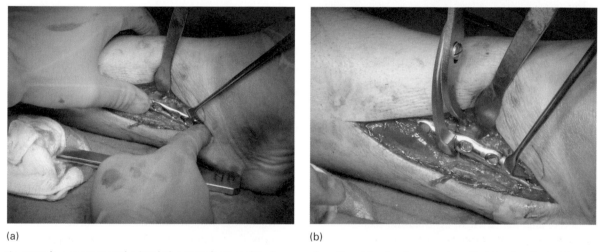

Fig. 13.8a,b A precontoured 1/3 tubular neutralization plate (concave above the plafond and convex above the lateral malleolus) is placed over the fibula and secured with a clamp.

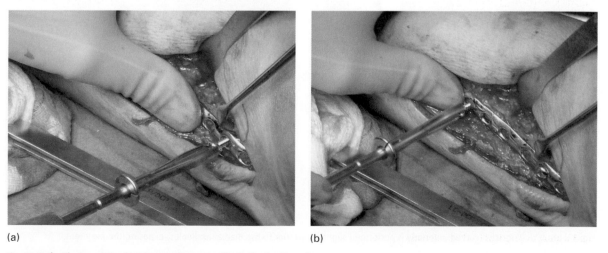

Fig. 13.9a,b Placing of the first two screws, opposite to the fracture plane.

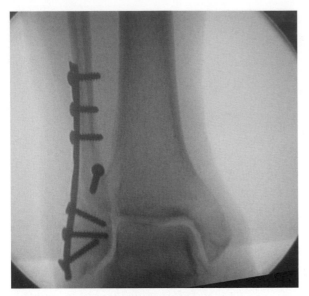

Fig. 13.10 Confirmation of restoration of alignment, length of fibula and accurate screw positioning with fluoroscopic images.

- Ensure reduction maintenance with fluoroscopic control.
- Secure the plate, placing the rest of the screws.
- Below the plafond level one can use cortex screws without tapping, or untapped fully threaded 4.0 cancellous screws.
- Take care not to penetrate the articular surface in the distal lateral malleolus.
- Obtain AP and lateral radiographs confirming restoration of alignment, length of fibula and accurate screw positioning (Fig. 13.10).

Medial malleolus

- Make an incision slightly posterior to the medial malleolus, in line with the tibia, and curve it anteriorly distally to form a 'J' incision.
- Retract the skin with the subcutaneous tissue to preserve the blood supply to the area.
- Protect the saphenous vein and nerve.
- Expose the fragment medially and anteriorly (Fig. 13.11a,b).
- Using a periosteal elevator or a curette, remove the interposed periosteum from the fracture site.
- Using a pointed reduction forceps grasp the medial malleolus and reposition it, maintaining the reduction with a reduction clamp (Fig. 13.12).
- Stabilize the fragment temporarily with K-wires or a 2.5 drill bit (Fig. 13.13).
- Evaluate reduction with AP and lateral fluoroscopic views.
- Definite stabilization is achieved with two 4.0 mm partially threaded cancellous bone lag screws inserted perpendicular to the fracture plane (Fig. 13.14).
- Ensure that the screws have not crossed the articular surface at the interior of the joint.
- The thread should pass fully beyond the fracture plane, staying in the dense bone of the distal tibia metaphysis (Fig. 13.15).

Closure

- Irrigate the wound thoroughly and achieve haemostasis.

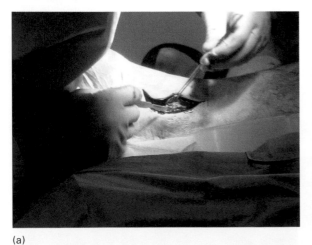

(a)

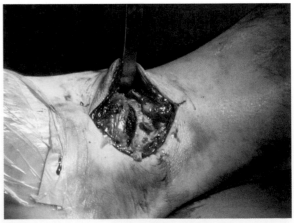

(b)

Fig. 13.11a,b A 'J' incision curved anteriorly is performed slightly posterior to the medial malleolus, exposing the fragment.

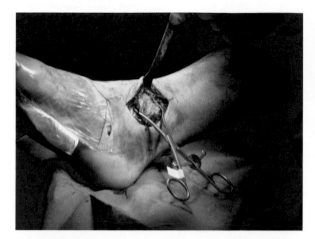

Fig. 13.12 Using a pointed reduction forceps the medial malleolus is repositioned.

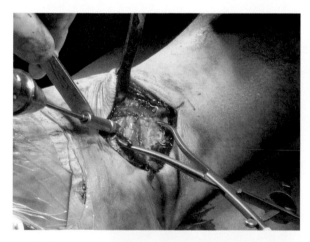

Fig. 13.13 Fragment stabilization using a drill bit.

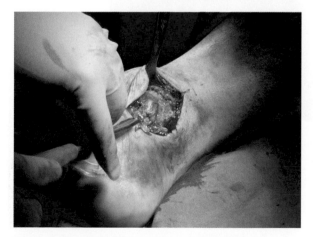

Fig. 13.14 Permanent fixation with two partially threaded 4.0 mm cancellous bone lag screws.

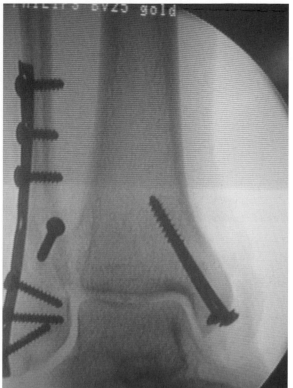

Fig. 13.15 Intraoperative fluoroscopic image confirming the correct placement of cancellous lag screws and the restoration of articular congruity.

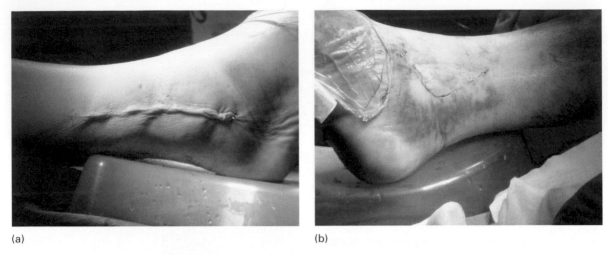

(a)   (b)

Fig. 13.16a,b Skin closure with 3/0 subcuticular monofilament suture.

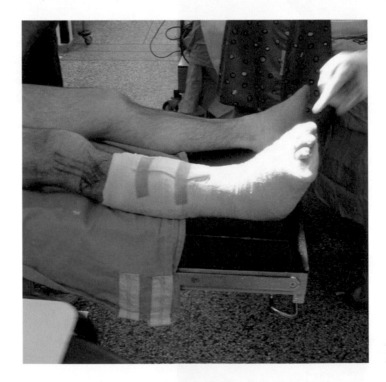

Fig. 13.17 Application of a short-leg posterior plaster splint with the foot at 90°.

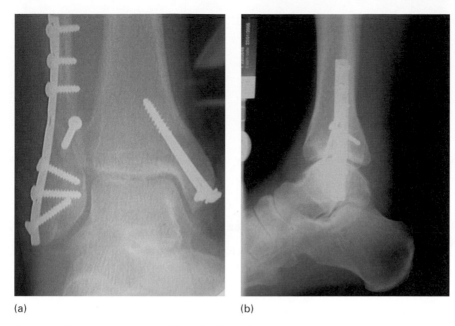

(a) (b)

Fig. 13.18 a,b Post-operative AP and lateral radiographs.

- Leave the fascia open.
- Close subcutaneous fascia (2.0 PDS/Vicryl).
- Skin closure – 3/0 subcuticular monofilament suture (Fig. 13.16a,b).

Post-operative treatment

- Apply a short-leg posterior plaster splint with the foot at 90° (Fig. 13.17).
- Assess neurovascular status of the extremity.
- Obtain post-operative AP and lateral radiographs (Fig. 13.18 a,b).
- Early active movement of toes at 24–48 h after the surgery.

Outpatient follow up

- Review at 2 weeks, 6 weeks and 12 months with radiographs on arrival.
- At 2 weeks allow protected partial weight-bearing.
- At 6 weeks encourage active mobilization.
- Start full weight-bearing after 6 weeks if radiographs are satisfactory.
- Ascertain complete fracture healing with radiographs after 12 weeks.
- Discharge from the follow up after clinical and radiological evidence of fracture healing.
- Review again at request of the general practitioner.
- Consider implant removal if there is soft tissue irritation after 1 year.

Fractures of the foot

Martinus Richter

14.1 OPEN REDUCTION AND INTERNAL SCREW FIXATION FOR TALAR NECK FRACTURES

Indications

- Open reduction and internal screw fixation (ORIF) is used to stabilize a displaced talar neck fracture (Fig. 14.1).

Pre-operative planning

Clinical assessment

- Swelling, neurovascular status, stability.
- Be aware of compartment syndrome (see below). If suspicion for compartment syndrome exists, pressure measurement should be performed (for example with the Intracompartmental Permanent Pressure Monitoring System, Stryker™ Corporation, Santa Clara, CA, USA). Fasciotomy is indicated, if there is a difference of less than 30 mmHg between diastolic blood pressure and compartment pressure.
- Be aware of associated fractures in the adjacent foot and ankle (Fig. 14.1a,b).

Radiological assessment

Three standard views:

- Mortise view of the ankle (20° internal rotation).
- True lateral ankle view.
- Anteroposterior (AP) view of the talar neck and head (15° internal foot rotation, 15° caudo-cranial X-ray angle); Canale view.
- CT Scan.

Classification

- Talar neck fractures are classifed according to Hawkins, and Canale and Kelly (who added Type IV, Fig. 14.2).

Operative treatment

Anaesthesia

- Regional (spinal/epidural/popliteal) or general anaesthesia.
- Prophylactic antibiotics as per local hospital protocol (e.g. 3rd generation cephalosporin).

Table and equipment

- 3.5 mm standard cortical and cancellous screws, steel or titanium alloy.
- Standard osteosynthesis set as per local hospital protocol.
- A radiolucent table.
- An image intensifier and a competent radiographer.

Table set up

- The instrumentation set is at the foot end of the table.
- Image intensifier is from the contralateral side.

Patient positioning

- Supine position.
- Tourniquet use not recommended because of increased risk of ischaemic wound necrosis.

Practical Procedures in Orthopaedic Trauma Surgery: A Trainee's Companion, ed. Peter V. Giannoudis and Hans-Christoph Pape. Published by Cambridge University Press. © Cambridge University Press 2006.

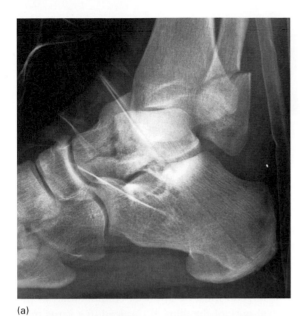

(a)

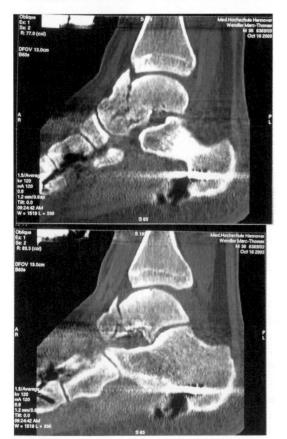

(b)

Fig. 14.1 Talar neck fracture Hawkins III with incomplete talar head fracture and associated ankle facture: (a) lateral radiograph with the talar body still dislocated in the ankle and subtalar joint; (b) CT scan after closed reduction.

Type	HAWKINS
I	
II	
III	
IV	

Fig. 14.2 Hawkins Classification of talar neck fractures according to the number of joints involved.

Draping

- Prepare the skin over lower leg, ankle and entire foot with usual antiseptic solutions (aqueous/alcoholic povidone–iodine). Prepare skin between toes thoroughly.
- Apply standard draping around lower leg in calf region.
- Apply tape around toes to minimize the risk of infection.

Approach

- Anteromedial approach is standard for most talar neck fractures (Fig. 14.3). A combined anteromedial and

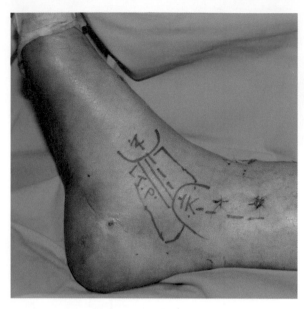

Fig. 14.3 Anteromedial approach to the talar neck. Stab incisions from tibial nailing (broken line: incision; T.P.: tibialis posterior tendon; N: navicular; IK: medial malleolus).

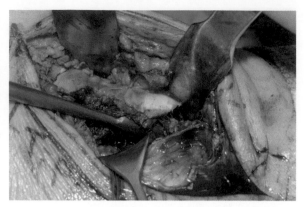

Fig. 14.4 Talar neck fracture Hawkins III through medial approach. Fracture displaced with a raspatorium for cleaning.

anterolateral approach to the neck of the talus should be used if reduction and internal fixation through the standard anteromedial approach is insufficient.

- The anteromedial approach is performed from the anterior aspect of the medial malleolus to the dorsal aspect of the navicular tuberosity (Fig. 14.3).
- The dissection is made down to the bone, just dorsal to the posterior tibial tendon.
- Disruption of the deltoid ligament should not be performed, because it will violate some of the remaining blood supply to the body of the talus.
- The fracture can be visualized and subsequently mobilized through this incision to allow removal of fracture haematoma and to begin mobilizing the fracture (Fig. 14.4).
- Dissection of soft tissues at the talar neck dorsally or plantarly should not be performed to avoid disrupting the blood supply any further.

Open reduction and internal fixation

- Fracture comminution is frequently present on the medial neck of the talus, and visualization of the lateral aspect of the neck can provide a more accurate gauge of the adequacy of reduction because there is rarely comminution laterally (Fig. 14.4).

- The fracture is reduced under direct visualization.
- The surgeon must be aware of comminution of the medial neck of the talus. It can lead to a varus malreduction of the neck of the talus that may increase inadequate rigid supination.
- The fracture site often demonstrates a diastasis or gap if the fracture is malpositioned in varus positions. Once provisional reduction is performed, it should be temporarily stabilized with 2.0 mm Kirschner wires.
- After provisional pin stabilization, the clinical alignment of the foot should be assessed to ascertain that no tendency toward varus or supination occurs. Intraoperative lateral, anteroposterior (AP) and Canale fluoroscopic views should be obtained to assess the quality of reduction.
- If reduction is adequate, fully threaded titanium screws may be placed for definitive fixation.
- Medial comminution is frequently present. Therefore, lag screw fixation typically is not used, because it may displace the fracture into varus. A minimum of 2 screws should be placed across the fracture site.
- A hard, cortical ridge of bone may be present along the dorsal aspect of the Sinus tarsi that allows for excellent fixation with 1 or 2 screws inserted from the lateral neck of the talus across the fracture site (Figs. 14.5, 14.6a,b).
- Titanium screws allow for post-operative magnetic resonance imaging (MRI) of the talus to assess for presence of avascular necrosis. Stainless steel screws may also be used, but with MRI scanning, signal abnormalities adjacent to the screws are expected and preclude visualization of part of the talus.
- If the fracture is located in the distal neck of the talus, the head of the screw should be countersunk into the

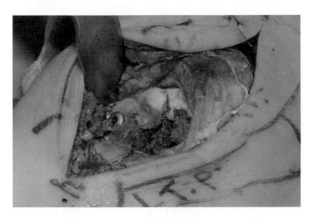

Fig. 14.5 Talar neck fracture Hawkins III through a medial approach. Fracture after open reduction and internal fixation with 2 fully threaded 3.5 mm titanium screws (screws on top). One screw was used for fixation of the talar head fracture (screw on bottom). Medial plantar comminution beneath the talar dome (bottom right).

head of the talus. As an alternative, a different method of fixation such as a polylactic acid (PLA) bioabsorbable screw (Bionix Implants, Inc., Blue Beil, PA, USA), Herbert screw (Zimmer Corp., Warsaw, IN, USA), or Acutrak screw (Acumed, Beaverton, OR, USA), can be used in an antegrade direction. Although placement of the screws from the posterolateral approach from the posterior tuberosity of the talus into the head has been shown to provide good mechanical stability, it is a more difficult approach, and fracture reduction may be more challenging.

Closure

- Irrigate the wound thoroughly and achieve haemostasis.
- Close subcutaneous fascia (2.0 PDS/Vicryl) over a drain (12F).
- Skin closure – stainless steel surgical staples or monofilament non-absorbable sutures.
- Apply splintered lower leg cast.

Post-operative rehabilitation

- Remove drains and cast in 48 hours.
- Mobilize 15 kg partial weight-bearing at the earliest, and tailor physiotherapy to meet individual needs and demands.

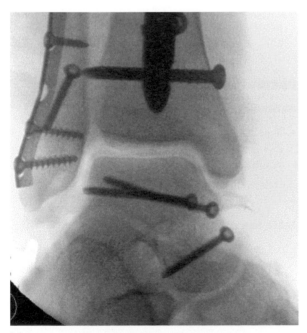

(a)

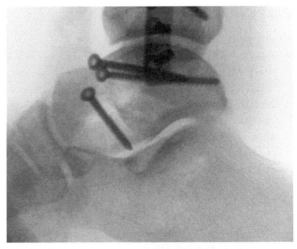

(b)

Fig. 14.6 Talar neck fracture Hawkins III after open reduction and internal fixation with 2 fully threaded 3.5 mm titanium screws (screws on top). One screw was used for fixation of talar head fracture (screw on bottom). Tibial nailing and plate fixation of fibula for accompanying fractures: (a) AP view; (b) lateral view.

Outpatient follow up

- Review at 6 weeks with radiographs.
- Start full weight-bearing after 6 weeks if radiographs are satisfactory.
- Ascertain complete fracture healing with radiographs after 12 weeks.
- Discharge from the follow up after clinical and radio-logical evidence of fracture healing.
- Review again at request of the general practitioner.
- Review after 1 year with radiographs to rule out head necrosis.
- Implant removal is rarely indicated.

14.2 OPEN REDUCTION AND INTERNAL PLATE FIXATION FOR OS CALCIS FRACTURES

Indications

- Open reduction and internal plate fixation (ORIF) is used to stabilize intra-articular calcaneus fractures Sanders Type II and III (Fig. 14.7).

Pre-operative planning

Clinical assessment

- Swelling, neurovascular status, stability.
- Be aware of compartment syndrome (see below). If suspicion for compartment syndrome exists, pressure measurement should be performed (for example with the Intracompartmental Permanent Pressure Monitoring System, Stryker™ Corporation, Santa Clara, CA, USA). Fasciotomy is indicated, if there is a difference of less than 30 mmHg between diastolic blood pressure and compartment pressure.
- Be aware of associated fractures in the adjacent foot and ankle.

Radiological assessment

- Four standard views:
  - (1) Dorsoplantar view of the foot (20° caudo-cranial X-ray angle).
  - (2) Lateral view of the hindfoot (Fig. 14.8a).
  - (3) Axial view of the calcaneus (Fig. 14.8b).
  - (4) Broden's view (45° internal foot rotation, 20° caudo-cranial X-ray angle).
- CT Scan.

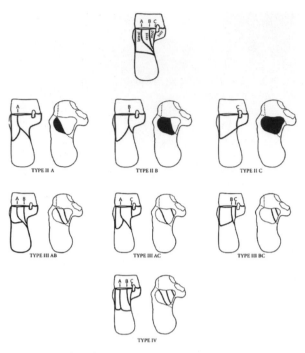

Fig. 14.7 Sanders classification.

Classification

- Sanders classification: CT based, coronal view of posterior joint facet, number and course of joint fracture lines (Fig. 14.8c).

Operative treatment

Anaesthesia

- Regional (spinal/epidural/popliteal) or general anaesthesia.
- Prophylactic antibiotics as per local hospital protocol (e.g. 3rd generation cephalosporin).

Table and equipment

- 3.5 mm cortical screws, steel or titanium alloy, standard osteosynthesis set as per local hospital protocol.
- Calcaneus plate.
- A radiolucent table.
- An image intensifier and a competent radiographer.

Table set up

- The instrumentation set is at the foot end of the table.
- Image intensifier is from the contralateral side.

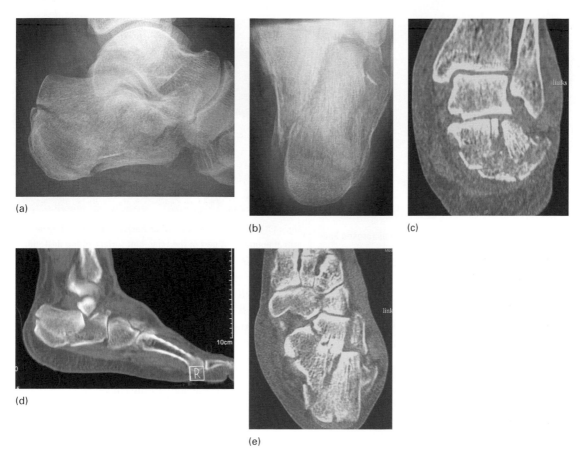

Fig. 14.8 Calcaneus fracture type Sanders III AB: (a) lateral radiograph; (b) axial radiograph; (c) CT, coronar view through posterior facet; (d) CT, parasagittal view; (e) CT, horizontal view.

Patient positioning

- The patient is placed in the lateral decubitus position, with the affected side up.
- Tourniquet use not recommended.

Draping

- Prepare the skin over lower leg, ankle and entire foot with usual antiseptic solutions (aqueous/alcoholic povidone–iodine). Prepare skin between toes thoroughly.
- Apply standard draping around lower leg in the middle between knee and ankle.
- Apply tape around toes.

Approach

- Extensile lateral approach (Figs. 14.9, 14.10).
- A curved incision is designed with vertical and horizontal limbs.

- The vertical limb is oriented halfway between the posterior aspect of the peroneal tendons and the anterior aspect of the Achilles tendon.
- At the superior margin of this incision, the sural nerve passes in the subcutaneous tissue.
- The horizontal limb of the incision parallels the plantar surface of the foot and is inclined slightly at the anterior margin.
- The sural nerve crosses at the junction of the middle and distal third of the horizontal limb of the incision. The sural nerve is very closely associated with the subcutaneous tissue above the peroneal tendons.
- The incision should be brought sharply to bone on its vertical limb and on the curved portion of the incision and then carried more superficial distally to the area of the peroneal tendons.
- Careful dissection should be performed near peroneal tendons and in the area of the sural nerve. The skin is dissected and raised as a full-thickness flap from the

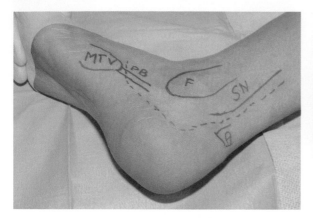

Fig. 14.9 Extensile lateral approach to the calcaneus (broken line: approach; F: fibula; SN: sural nerve; A: achilles tendon attachment; MT V: 5th metatarsal; PB: peroneus brevis tendon).

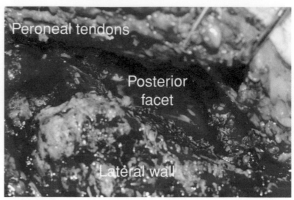

Fig. 14.11 Sanders III AB calcaneus fracture through extensile lateral approach. A part of the talar joint surface of the posterior facet is visible.

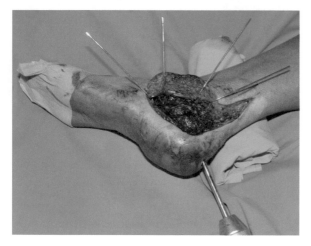

Fig. 14.10 Extensile lateral approach to the calcaneus. Fasciocutaneus flap after elevation and retention with 1.8 mm K-wires in talar body, fibula, navicular and cuboid. Insertion of a 5 mm Schantz screw in the upper tuber fragment for reduction manoeuvres.

periosteum of the calcaneus and should include the calcaneofibular ligament.

• The subtalar joint can be seen as the flap is raised. Four 1.6 mm Kirschner wires (navicular, cuboid, talar neck, fibula) are placed to maintain retraction of the flap without excessive tension (Fig. 14.10). The Kirschner wires (K-wires) are advanced into the bone by approximately 1.5 cm, and bent to provide soft tissue retraction.

• The lateral aspect of the calcaneus is displaced in a more lateral and distal position to its native position

and tends to block visualization of the joint until the fracture is reduced.

• After exposing the subtalar joint, the organizing haematoma and small fracture fragments are removed by suction, irrigation, and use of a pituitary rongeur. The lateral aspect of the posterior facet typically is depressed into the body of the calcaneus. Depression of the posterior facet initially allows improved visualization of the anterior process.

Open reduction and internal fixation

• There are multiple steps to reducing and fixing a displaced fracture.

• First, the surgeon should insert a 5 mm Schantz screw in the tuber through a posterior stab incision. This allows easier reduction for all steps described below (Fig. 14.10).

• The lateral wall fragment should be opened and the impacted posterior facet fragments should be lifted up. These should then be reduced and held with a Kirschner wire. Next, one or two 3.5 mm fully threaded lag screws should be inserted to fix the posterior facet fragments (Fig. 14.11).

• After the medial wall and the anterior process are reduced, reduction of the posterior facet can be performed. The posterior facet cannot be reduced properly until the front of the medial part of the posterior facet is elevated to its proper height. The relationship between the anterior calcaneus and the tuberosity is reduced medially and plantarly.

• Then, reduction of Boehler's angle (normal, 25–40°), calcaneus length (normal, 70–90 mm) and tuber position in the sagittal plain (avoid varus) should be achieved with traction at the Schantz pin. Temporary retention with 1.6–2.0 mm K-wires with transfixation of subtalar joint for increased stability follows. Hindfoot varus, i.e. varus of the tuber should be avoided.

- The entire anterior process is typically elevated toward the talus. To reduce the remaining fractures to the anterior process, the anterior process can be retracted plantar-ward. A Langenbeck retractor or a laminar spreader is therefore placed between the lateral aspect of the talar head and the anterior process of the calcaneus.
- Insertion of the calcaneus plate.
- Many different plates can be used for treatment of calcaneus fractures. The preferred plate should have a low profile, particularly in the area of the peroneal tendons. The plate should be stiff enough to correct varus alignment, and it should have a superior limb that prevents depression of the posterior facet. Tongue-type fractures require the plate to prevent rotation of the tongue fragment. This can be accomplished with a traditional Y-shaped plate augmented with a screw from dorsal to plantar or by use of one of the more recently designed plates that allows multiple screws to be placed in the tongue fragment anteriorly and posteriorly. The main aspect of the plate MUST NOT be bent. Plate bending is only allowed around the posterior facet (Fig. 14.12). If the calcaneocuboid joint is involved, reduction and temporary K-wire fixation prior to insertion of the plate is necessary.
- For a tongue-type fracture, i.e. a horizontal fracture through the calcaneal tubercle, an additional screw from the top of the tuberosity towards the bottom is recommended (Fig. 14.13a).
- Intraoperative dorsoplantar, lateral, axial and Broden's fluoroscopic views should be obtained to assess the quality of reduction and internal fixation Fig 14.13b, c, d.

The main goals of the ORIF are:

- Anatomic reduction of the posterior facet and lag screw fixation.
- Restoration of Boehler's angle (normal, 25–40°), calcaneus length (normal, 70–90 mm) and orientation of tuber in sagittal plane (avoid varus).

Closure

- Irrigate the wound thoroughly and achieve haemostasis.

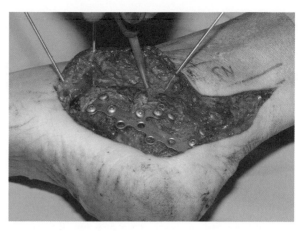

Fig. 14.12 Sanders III AB calcaneus fracture after application of the plate. Before application of the plate the fracture in the anterior process through the calcaneocuboid joint was reduced and temporarily fixed with two 1.8 mm K-wires. Then, reduction of Boehler's angle (20–40° normal), calcaneus length and tuber position in the sagittal plain was achieved with traction at the Schantz pin. Temporary retention with 1.6–2.0 mm K-wires with transfixation of the subtalar joint for increased stability followed. Chisel in the posterior facet.

- Close subcutaneous fascia (2.0 PDS/Vicryl) over a drain (12F).
- Skin closure – monofilament non-absorbable sutures.
- The sutures should start at the 2 ends of the incision and should be placed in a manner to allow absolute tension-free closure at the corner of the incision (Fig. 14.14).
- Stainless steel surgical staples or intracutaneous sutures should not be used because of the critical soft tissue conditions.
- Apply splintered lower leg cast.

Post-operative rehabilitation

- Remove drains and cast in 48 hours.
- Mobilize 15 kg partial weight-bearing at the earliest and tailor physiotherapy to meet individual needs and demands.

Outpatient follow up

- Review at 6 and 12 weeks with radiographs.
- Start full weight-bearing after 12 weeks if radiographs satisfactory.
- Discharge from the follow up after clinical and radiological evidence of fracture healing.
- Review again at request of the general practitioner.

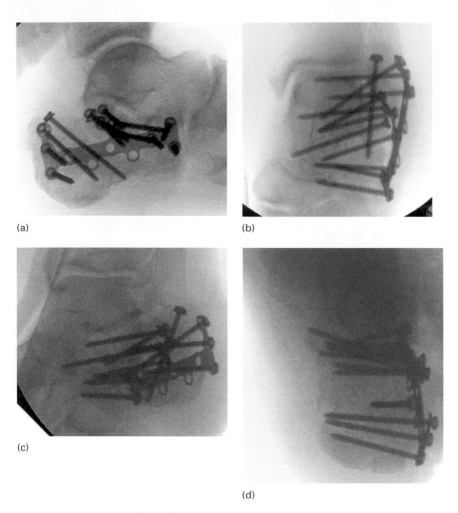

(a)

(b)

(c)

(d)

Fig. 14.13 Intraoperative radiographs of a Sanders III AB calcaneus fracture after open reduction and internal fixation: (a) lateral view – note the screw running from the top of the tuber to the bottom, for the tongue-type fragment; (b) dorsoplantar view; (c) Broden's 20° view; (d) axial view.

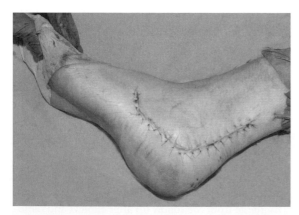

Fig. 14.14 Sanders III AB calcaneus fracture after wound closure. Note the absolute tension-free condition at the corner of the incision.

- Review after 1 year with radiographs to rule out development of osteoarthritis.
- Implant removal can be considered if there is soft tissue irritation.

14.3 OPEN REDUCTION AND INTERNAL SCREW AND K-WIRE FIXATION FOR LISFRANC FRACTURE DISLOCATIONS

Indications

Open reduction and internal screw and K-wire fixation is used to stabilize:

(a) Lisfranc dislocation after unsuccessful closed reduction.

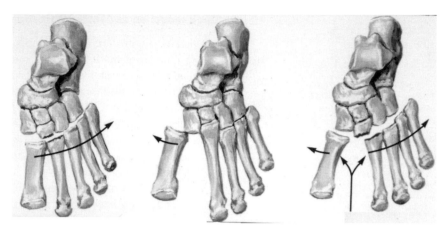

Fig. 14.15 Quenu and Küss classification : homolateral (left), isolated (middle), divergent (right).

(b) Lisfranc fracture–dislocation after unsuccessful closed reduction.

Pre-operative planning

Clinical assessment

- Swelling, neurovascular status, stability.
- Be aware of compartment syndrome (see below; incidence up to 25%). If suspicion for compartment syndrome exists, pressure measurement should be performed (for example with the Intracompartmental Permanent Pressure Monitoring System, Stryker™ Corporation, Santa Clara, CA, USA). Fasciotomy is indicated, if there is a difference of less than 30 mmHg between diastolic blood pressure and compartment pressure.
- Be aware of associated fractures.

Radiological assessment

- Three standard views:
  (1) Dorsoplantar view of the foot (20° caudo-cranial X-ray angle).
  (2) Exact lateral view of entire foot.
  (3) Oblique view of entire foot (foot 45° internal rotation).
- Stress views if there is anatomic reduction but a suspicion of instability.
- CT scan.

Classification

Quenu and Küss classification (Fig. 14.15); later modified by Hardcastle and Myerson.

Operative treatment

Anaesthesia

- Regional (spinal/epidural/popliteal) or general anaesthesia.
- Prophylactic antibiotic as per local hospital protocol (e.g. 3rd generation cephalosporin).

Table and equipment

- 3.5 mm cortical and cancellous screws, 1.0–2.5 mm K-wires, steel or titanium alloy, standard osteosynthesis set as per local hospital protocol.
- A radiolucent table.
- An image intensifier and a competent radiographer.

Table set up

- The instrumentation set is at the foot end of the table.
- Image intensifier is from the contralateral side.

Patient positioning

- Supine position.
- Tourniquet use not recommended.

Draping

- Prepare the skin over lower leg, ankle and entire foot with usual antiseptic solutions (aqueous/alcoholic povidone–iodine). Prepare skin between toes thoroughly.
- Apply standard draping around lower leg in the middle between knee and ankle.

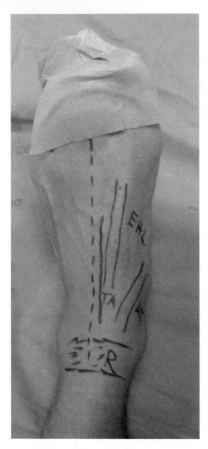

Fig. 14.16 Dorsal median approach to the Lisfranc joint (broken line: approach; R: retinaculum, EHL: extensor hallucis longus tendon; TA: dorsalis pedis artery; AT: tibialis anterior tendon.

- Apply tape around single toes (better for reduction manoeuvres).

Approach

- A long dorsal median incision is used in the majority of the open procedures. Incision between 2nd and 3rd ray, starting at the level of the ankle and ending at metatarsophalangeal joint level (Fig. 14.16).
- Be aware of the dorsal pedis artery that is located between the 1st and 2nd ray.
- Isolate and mobilize extensor hallucis longus and extensor digitorum tendons. Mobilization of tendons allows shifting of tendons towards medial and lateral.
- Extensor retinaculum is left intact.
- Dorsal aspect of Lisfranc joint is placed beneath extensor tendons.
- Leave dorsal joint capsule intact.

Open reduction and internal fixation

- Open reduction starts at the 2nd metatarsal. The second metatarsal fits between the medial and lateral cuneiform as a keystone. There must be no gap, especially between the base of the 2nd metatarsal and the medial cuneiform. Check reduction fluoroscopy. For anatomic reduction, resection of soft tissue might be necessary. Internal fixation with 1.8–2.0 mm K-wire running retrograde dorsal of 2nd metatarsal base to intermedium cuneiform.
- Open reduction of 1st metatarsal follows. For internal stabilization between 1st metatarsal and medial cuneiform, a 2.0 mm K-wire or a 3.5 mm fully threaded cortical screw is appropriate.
- Open reduction and internal fixation of 3rd to 5th ray requires K-wire fixation crossing the Lisfranc joint. Sometimes additional transfixation between lesser metatarsals is necessary to achieve enough stability (Fig. 14.17).
- A primary arthrodesis should be performed in cases with massive or irreconstructable articular damage. The clinical outcome is better after primary than after secondary arthrodesis. Arthrodesis of parts of the Lisfranc joint shows better results than arthrodesis of the entire Lisfranc joint. For arthrodesis the dorsal capsule of the joint should be opened and the remaining cartilage removed. Internal fixation should be performed with 3.5 mm fully threaded cortical screws for all rays that are fused.

Closure

- Irrigate the wound thoroughly and achieve haemostasis.
- Close subcutaneous fascia (2.0 PDS/Vicryl) over a drain (12F).
- Skin closure – stainless steel surgical staples or monofilament non-absorbable sutures.
- When a primary skin closure is not possible, the skin defect should be covered with artificial skin. Within 1 or 2 weeks a secondary skin closure is normally possible and a skin graft is mostly not necessary.
- Apply jigsaw lower leg cast.

Post-operative rehabilitation

- Remove drains in 48 hours.
- Apply closed lower leg cast when swelling has improved.

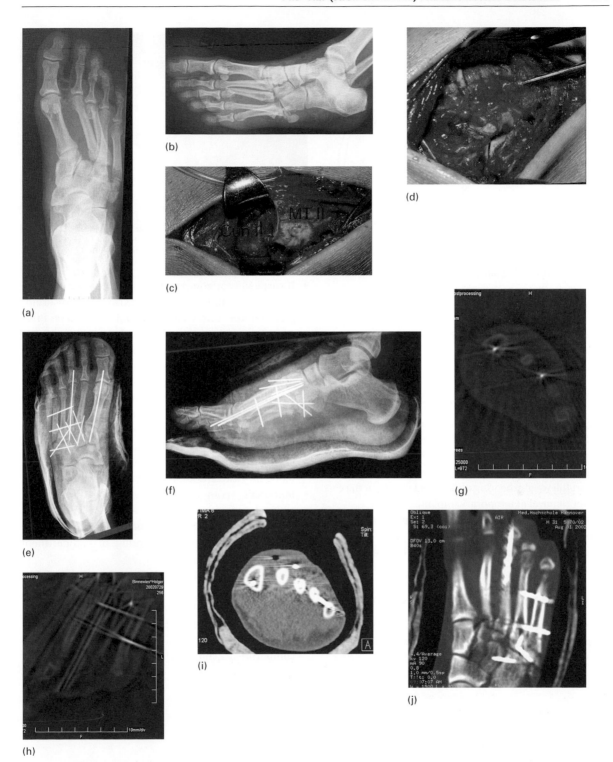

Fig. 14.17 Homolateral lateral Lisfranc fracture–dislocation of 1st–5th ray; metatarsal 3-neck fracture. Closed reduction and internal K-wire fixation with temporary transfixation of metatarsal 5 to metatarsal 3 and 4. Intraoperative evaluation of reduction with three-dimensional X-ray aquisation (ISO-C-3D, Siemens Inc., Germany); (a) and (b): Pre-operative radiographs; (c): intraoperative view before reduction with base of 2nd metatarsal dislocated; (d): intraoperative view after reduction of 2nd metatarsal and internal fixation with 2 mm K-wire; (e) and (f): Post-operative radiographs; (g) and (h): three-dimensional X-ray aquisation with ISO-C-3D; (i) and (j): post-operative CT.

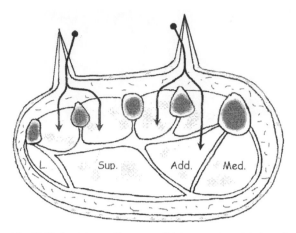

Fig. 14.18 Fasciotomy. (Sup.: superficial compartment; L: lateral superficial compartment; Add.: adductor compartment; Med.: medial compartment; no designation, interosseous compartments).

- Mobilize 15 kg partial weight-bearing at the earliest and tailor physiotherapy to meet individual needs and demands.

Outpatient follow up

- Review at 6 and 12 weeks with radiographs.
- Remove cast and implants that were inserted for temporary transfixation at 6 weeks if radiographs are satisfactory.
- Start full weight-bearing after 6 weeks without the cast after removal of temporary implants.
- Discharge from the follow up after clinical and radiological evidence of fracture healing.
- Review after 1 year with radiographs to rule out post-traumatic osteoarthritis.

Compartment syndrome – fasciotomy

- Compartment syndrome of the foot is an emergency. Fasciotomy for compartment syndrome must be performed without delay.

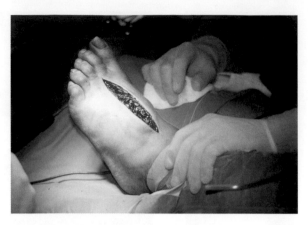

Fig. 14.19 Fasciotomy through one dorsal incision.

- If suspicion for compartment syndrome exists, pressure measurement should be performed (for example with the Intracompartmental Permanent Pressure Monitoring System, Stryker™ Corporation, Santa Clara, CA, USA). Fasciotomy is indicated if there is a difference of less than 30 mmHg between diastolic blood pressure and compartment pressure.
- Specific pressure measurement recommended (for example with the Intracompartmental Permanent Pressure Monitoring System, Stryker™ Corporation, Santa Clara, CA, USA). The indication for a fasciotomy is a difference of less than 30 mmHg between diastolic blood pressure and compartment pressure.
- Imminent compartment syndrome is treated with elevation to heart level, intensive cooling, maintenance/elevation of blood pressure for sufficient circulation and monitoring of compartment pressure.
- Technique fasciotomy (Figs. 14.18, 14.19): 1 or 2 dorsal incisions. Two dorsal incisions are only recommended if needed for further surgical treatment (for example for ORIF in a Lisfranc fracture–dislocation). The skin bridge between incisions is at least 5 cm. All compartments should be incised.

Part IV

Spine

Fractures of the cervical spine

Peter Millner

15.1 APPLICATION OF A HALO AND HALO-VEST FOR CERVICAL SPINE TRAUMA

Indications

Halo devices are used in a variety of trauma settings, including:

- Reduction of cervical spine facet subluxations and dislocations (usually via axial traction applied through the halo).
- Stabilization of undisplaced cervical spine fractures.
- Post-reduction stabilization of cervical spine fractures, subluxations and dislocations.
- Temporary stabilization of a cervical spine injury, prior to definitive surgical treatment, or to facilitate safe transfer of the patient to a specialist spinal centre.

If the patient is physically able to mobilize, the halo can be attached to a 'vest'. The vest may be a custom-made plaster or fibre-glass orthosis, or one of the readily available 'off-the-shelf' devices. Several orthopaedic implant manufacturers market combinations of haloes and vest orthoses, in a range of sizes. The most useful halo and vest devices contain no ferrous components and are therefore MRI-compatible, permitting scanning of the patient after application.

Pre-operative planning

Most halo and halo-vest systems are available as pre-packed kits containing all of the necessary implants and tools for halo application and subsequent attachment of the halo to a detachable vest. A careful check of the manu-facturer's kit inventory against the kit components and instruments should be done in every case; do not assume that even a pre-packed kit will be complete! If the halo is to be used for ambulatory cervical spine stabilization, a suitably-sized orthosis (vest) is selected. Standard anti-septic skin preparation solutions should be available. If not supplied in the halo kit, a small pointed scalpel will also be needed.

- Measure head circumference using a tape measure and select the smallest possible halo size (Fig. 15.1).
- The halo selected should permit an air gap of approx-imately 10 mm between the inner aspect of the halo and the largest circumference of the skull, measured as shown on the diagram (Fig. 15.2).

Anaesthesia

- The cervical spine must be protected from further injury at all times, and this may require manual in-line immobilization by an assistant.
- Local or general anaesthesia can be used, according to circumstances and the overall status of the patient.
- In a conscious patient, 1% or 2% lignocaine with adrenaline (epinephrine) should be used.

Positioning and set up

Most modern haloes are an incomplete ring, deficient posteriorly, and these can be fitted to the patient with a hard cervical collar still in place. Older variants of halo, consisting of a complete ring, may require removal of a cervical collar and slight elevation of the head from the

Practical Procedures in Orthopaedic Trauma Surgery: A Trainee's Companion, ed. Peter V. Giannoudis and Hans-Christoph Pape.
Published by Cambridge University Press. © Cambridge University Press 2006.

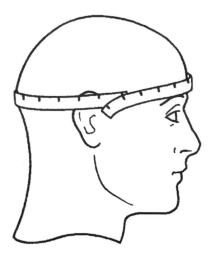

Fig. 15.1 The maximum circumference of the head is measured, just above the eyebrows and ears.

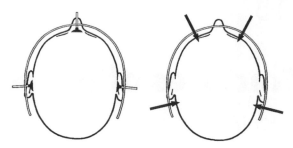

Fig. 15.3 (a) The halo is placed by the surgeon, and held in the correct position by three temporary positioning pins; (b) the definitive halo pins are placed though the screw holes of the halo and into the skull at the previously cleaned and anaesthetised 'safe zones'. Sequential tightening of diametrically opposed halo pins maintains equilateral clearance between the halo and the skull.

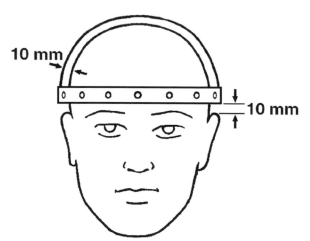

Fig. 15.2 The halo is positioned such that there is approximately 10 mm of clearance above the ears and the eyebrows, with a similar gap between the halo and the skull.

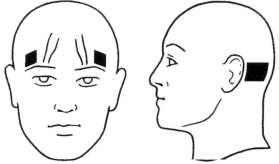

Fig. 15.4 The safe zones for pin insertion are shaded. Anteriorly, an area 10 mm above the lateral third of the eyebrow will avoid the cutaneous nerves and frontal sinuses medially, and will be over the relatively thick plate of bone at the fronto-temporal junction. Posteriorly, the safe zone lies over the thick bone of the external occipital protruberance, avoiding branches of the occipital nerve posteriorly, and branches of the auricular nerves more anteriorly.

table or bed to ensure that the halo can be placed behind the occiput.

- The patient is placed in the supine position on a trolley, bed or operating table. At least one assistant is required, to maintain in-line cervical immobilization, and the more help that is available, the better! The surgeon stands at the top of the table or bed, looking down towards the patient's feet.

Application of halo

The surgeon holds the halo to ensure that the pin sites will be in the correct positions. Three temporary positioning pins, with detachable soft contact pads in lieu of sharp points, are placed through the halo screw holes at approximately equal distances around the skull and tightened to ensure equilateral placement of the halo from the skull surface. The gap between halo and skin should be approximately 10 mm (Figs. 15.2, 15.3).

The optimal positions for halo pin site insertion are shown in Fig. 15.4:

- Anteriorly: 10 mm above the lateral third of the eyebrow (junction between frontal and temporal bones).
- Posteriorly: external occipital protruberance, just below maximal circumference of skull.

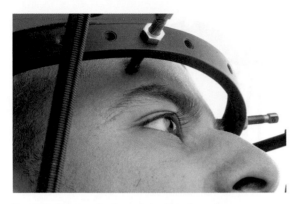

Fig. 15.5 Anterior pin placement within the safe zone.

- Correctly placed anterior pins will therefore avoid injury to the supra-orbital and supra-trochlear cutaneous nerves, or penetration into the sinuses (Fig. 15.5).
- The anterior pins always leave visible scars, and where possible the patient should be warned of this in advance.
- The sites of pin site insertion are cleaned with antiseptic agent; the 2 anterior pin sites are usually in the bare skin of the forehead, whilst it may be necessary to shave the 2 posterior pin sites.
- With the patient's eyes tightly closed, 1–2 ml of lignocaine is injected at each of the 4 pin insertion sites, down to bone. If the eyes are not tightly closed at the time of pin insertion, the patient will not be able to close them subsequently, owing to the 'tenodoesis' effect of the pins on the orbicularis muscles.
- A small pointed scalpel blade is used to incise the skin entry point at each of the 4 proposed pin sites.
- A halo pin is then inserted through the appropriate screw hole of the halo at each of the 4 pin sites, taking care to ensure that the halo position is not lost.
- Initially, the pins are tightened manually using 'finger and thumb' only. Manually stretching the skin around the pin using finger and thumb as the pin is inserted will minimize cosmetic problems from skin puckering.
- Once the pins are 'finger-tight', torque screwdrivers are used for final tightening (usually supplied as part of pre-packed kit). Diametrically opposite pins should be tightened against each other, either simultaneously by the surgeon and an assistant using 2 screwdrivers, or sequentially by the surgeon using a single screwdriver, alternating between diametrically opposite pins in steps of 1 inch-pound torque.
- The maximum torque applied to each pin is 6–8 inch-pounds. Locking nuts are then placed over each halo

pin, and these are tightened with a spanner to lock the halo pins within the halo.
- The temporary positioning pins are removed.
- Once secured in place, the halo can be attached to the vertical posts of a thoracic or thoraco-lumbar orthosis; this constitutes the so-called halo-vest (Fig. 15.6a,b).
- Alternatively, traction can be easily applied through the halo, giving excellent control of head and neck positions in all planes. Reduction of subluxed or dislocated facet joints, or gradual correction of deformity can be achieved by the judicious use of halo-traction; the patient must be monitored closely and regularly for any signs of neurological deterioration. Once a vest orthosis has been attached to the halo, further adjustments to optimize the alignment of the cervical spine can be performed in the erect (sitting) position.
- After any reduction manoeuvres using traction, or after a change of spinal alignment within a halo-vest, check radiographs should be performed in both the frontal and sagittal plane.
- Any change in neurological status following a new manoeuvre, such as increasing traction weight, should result in reversal of the offending manoeuvre e.g. reduction in the level of applied traction, and immediate radiographic checks. Persistence of altered neurology and/or signs of further deformity or displacement mandate an urgent MRI scan of the cervical spine.

Post-operative treatment

- Pin sites should be cleaned daily, to remove crusted blood and serous exudates. Each pin site should be checked for tightness after 48–72 hours; this is done by temporarily loosening the locking nuts, and with the aid of a torque-limiting screwdriver. The maximum torque applied should be no more than 8 inch-pounds. Loose or obviously infected pin sites should be treated by insertion of a new halo pin at an adjacent position through the halo, followed by removal of the loose/infected pin.
- The duration of halo immobilization will depend on several factors, such as co-existing injury or morbidity, and the exact nature of the cervical spine condition. Most injuries treated by halo immobilization will require no more than 3 months of such external stabilization. Stability at the level of the injury can be assessed dynamically, if necessary, by temporarily detaching the halo from its attachment to the vest orthosis, followed by supervised active flexion and extension lateral radiographs.

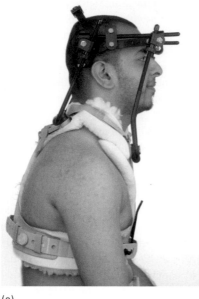
(a)

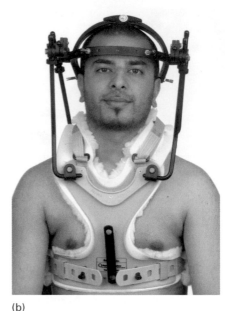
(b)

Fig. 15.6a,b The completed halo-vest orthosis.

- Removal of the halo pins is occasionally followed by bleeding from the pin site; this will usually settle with direct pressure for a few minutes. The skin at the pin insertion site, particularly anteriorly, will often adhere to the periosteum of the skull and this can cause an unsightly, tethered scar. Vigorous massage over the insertion site, after pin removal, will usually break down these adhesions; however, this can be extremely uncomfortable for the patient, who may prefer to have a scar rather than pain.

15.2 OPERATIVE POSTERIOR STABILIZATION OF THORACO-LUMBAR BURST FRACTURES

Indications

- Operative versus non-operative management of thoraco-lumbar burst fractures remains a controversial issue within the spinal surgery fraternity.
- Some surgeons argue that neurological injury with imaging evidence of significant bone retropulsion – 'canal compromise' – is an absolute indication for surgery.
- Others argue that the neurological deficit in such cases is a consequence of the instantaneous transfer of energy at the moment of injury, and that surgical decompression of retropulsed bone from the spinal canal is irrelevant, as the neurological insult has already occurred.
- The degree of comminution and kyphotic deformity is often quoted as a strong relative indication for operative management, to minimize the risk of late kyphotic deformity and possible late neurological deterioration.
- However, few spinal surgeons would argue against operative stabilization for the multiply injured patient with a burst fracture, and this is probably the least contentious of all indications for surgical intervention.

Posterior stabilization, using short segment pedicle screw fixation with or without fusion, is a relatively quick and simple technique in experienced surgical hands. Performed as an emergency procedure, such stabilization can reduce kyphotic deformity and effect an indirect decompression of the spinal canal via ligamentotaxis. Subsequent nursing care, mobilization and rehabilitation of a polytrauma patient are greatly facilitated by such treatment, which reduces the likelihood of structural instability and potential for new or additional neurological injury.

- More severe injuries may not be rendered completely stable in the long term by posterior stabilization alone; in such instances, additional anterior decompression and/or reconstruction may be necessary, to produce a circumferential fusion.

- However, as a damage-limitation and first-aid manoeuvre, posterior stabilization is a useful initial step.

It is rare for anterior surgery to be indicated or performed as an emergency, particularly in the polytrauma setting. Indeed, some surgeons regard emergency anterior surgery as contraindicated, in view of the potential for haemorrhage and possible deleterious effects upon respiratory function, where a transthoracic or transdiaphragmatic approach is required for access. The need for anterior decompression and/or reconstruction is often only apparent after provisional posterior stabilization, and can usually be done as a semi-elective procedure if necessary.

- The reader is referred to the load-sharing classification, described by McCormack *et al.* in 1994 (Table 15.1). This classification is based upon post-stabilization imaging parameters such as degree of comminution, kyphotic correction and apposition of bone fragments, to predict the need for supplementary anterior surgery after initial posterior surgery (short-segment pedicle screw fixation).
- However, most spinal surgeons agree that fracture morphology alone cannot dictate the need for a specific management plan; other factors are equally important, such as co-morbidities and patient-informed choice.

Pre-operative planning

- Burst fractures are often the result of high-energy trauma and, as such, management of associated life-threatening conditions along the principles of Advanced Trauma Life Support (ATLS) protocols will often take precedence over investigation and management of any thoracolumbar spine injury.
- Clinical examination will focus upon any neurological deficit, and any signs of structural spinal injury such as tenderness, swelling, bruising or open wounds along the spine.
- Documentation and timing of examination findings is a vital part of assessment, particularly with respect to any evolving or de novo neurological deficit. Static neurological deficits almost certainly represent neurological insult from the moment of injury.
- In contrast, the development of new neurological deficits after hospital admission may signify an unstable fracture–dislocation rather than a burst fracture;

Table 15.1. The load-sharing classification, based upon CT scans after posterior surgery

Parameter	Score
Degree of comminution in sagittal plane	
< 30%	1
30–60%	2
60%	3
Apposition in axial plane	
Minimal displacement	1
>2 mm displacement, <50% cross-section of vertebral body	2
>2 mm displacement, >50% cross-section of vertebral body	3
Correction of pre-operative deformity	
Kyphosis correction <4°	1
Kyphosis correction 4–9°	2
Kyphosis correction >9°	3

Total score:

7 points or more → anterior surgery (reconstruct anterior column)

6 points or less → posterior surgery alone

(McCormack, T., Karaikovic, E. E. and Gaines, R. W. The load-sharing classification of spine fractures. *Spine*, 1994; **19**(15):1741–4.)

alternatively, an expanding epidural haematoma can give rise to a similar picture of progressive neurological deficit.

Radiological assessment

- Plain radiographs should include good-quality frontal and lateral films, and in the presence of a visible abnormality such as a fracture, the *entire* spinal column should be vizualised; this is vital since there is a significant incidence of a second, discontinuous spinal injury in such circumstances (Fig. 15.7a,b).
- If the patient's condition permits, a CT scan with multiplanar re-formatting can yield useful information on fracture morphology and this may help to determine the treatment strategy (Fig. 15.8). For example, a near-normal CT scan, with no appreciable deformity and no evidence of canal compromise, may strengthen the argument for non-operative management in a neurologically intact patient; the same scan appearance in a paraplegic patient would form an indication for an urgent MRI scan, to look for signs of cord disruption or extradural compression, perhaps from haematoma.

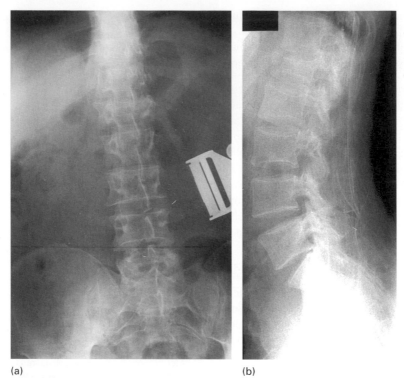

(a)   (b)

Fig. 15.7 (a): Frontal (AP) radiograph of a simple burst fracture of L1; (b): lateral radiograph of a simple burst fracture of L1.

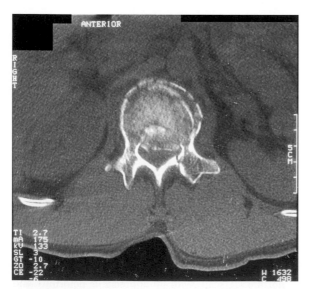

Fig. 15.8 Axial CT scan of a simple burst fracture of L1 (same case as Figure 1).

- Cases of neurological progression after admission to hospital are rare, provided patients are appropriately immobilized with spine protection at all times.

Rarely, an urgent decompression is indicated and this is usually because of neurological deterioration secondary to bleeding and cord compression from epidural haematoma.

Anaesthesia

- Posterior stabilization of a thoraco-lumbar burst fracture is always performed under general anaesthetic.
- Prophylactic antibiotics are given at induction of anaesthesia, according to local protocols; the same applies for anti-thrombosis prophylaxis, which can be via mechanical methods e.g. calf pumps, or pharmacologically e.g. low molecular weight heparin. In cases where major deformity correction is planned, particularly in the neurologically intact patient, spinal cord monitoring is advisable.

Table, positioning and set up

- The patient will be face-down, in the prone position, and so great care must be taken to protect the eyes from pressure (Figs. 15.9, 15.10).

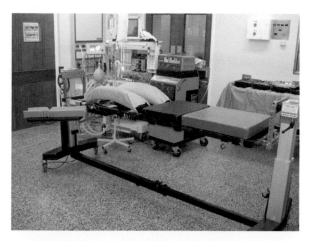

Fig. 15.9 Operative set up for posterior stabilization.

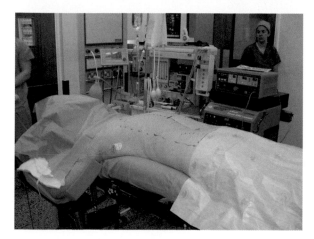

Fig. 15.10 Patient positioning and draping for posterior stabilization.

- Ideally, a radiolucent operating table is used, such as an OSI table; the carbon-fibre construction permits circumferential radiography of the spine with an image intensifier.
- Some form of padded support frame is also used to ensure that the abdomen can hang free, such as a Wilson frame; this has a variable radius of curvature, allowing lordosis or kyphosis of the spine and will facilitate deformity correction, as well as minimizing bleeding secondary to raised intra-abdominal pressure and distension of epidural and paraspinal veins.
- The patient's arms, if possible, are secured to padded extension boards, with the shoulders abducted away from the sides of the table (and hence out of the way of the image intensifier beam). All possible pressure

points, such as knees, ankles, etc. should be protected from external pressure, by careful positioning and the use of appropriate padding.
- The set up will be described for a right-handed surgeon, who will be most comfortable operating from the prone patient's left side. Sterile drapes should be applied to the image intensifier.
- The image intensifier is placed behind the surgeon, on the patient's left, and the height of the operating table adjusted to permit the C-arm to swing underneath the patient, for lateral views; frontal views are taken in standard fashion. To allow the C-arm to swing into the cross-table lateral position, and remain sterile, a large drape is secured along the right-hand side of the patient, hanging down to floor level.
- The scrub nurse, instrument tray and the assistant surgeon are on the patient's right side, across from the surgeon. All personnel within the operating theatre should wear protective lead gowns until completion of X-ray guided procedures.
- Lead gowns with separate shoulder straps are preferred, since these can be released and removed intra-operatively and without the need for de-scrubbing and re-scrubbing.

Table and equipment

- There are a multitude of pedicle screw systems available and suitable for posterior spinal fracture stabilization; one of the best known and simplest is the AO USS Fixator Interne. Whatever system is chosen, the instrumentation and implant set must be checked to ensure that all necessary tools and implants are readily available.

Draping/surgical approach

- The spinal midline is marked using a permanent marker pen, to outline the readily palpable spinous processes. Usually, the site of the fracture is evident from bruising and/or swelling, but the exact level can be confirmed with the image intensifier, if necessary.
- Antiseptic skin preparation is applied e.g. povidone, and then the operative field is isolated with surgical drapes and an adhesive plastic drape directly over the planned wound (Fig. 15.10).
- The skin and deep fascial incisions are made in the midline, from the cephalic end of the spinous process above the vertebral fracture level, to the caudal end of the spinous process below the fracture level, Thus, for

an L1 burst fracture, the spine is exposed from the top of the T12 spinous process down to the bottom of the L2 spinous process.

- The erector spinae muscles are elevated from the spine over the area of planned instrumentation, just lateral to the facet joints, to expose the junction of pars interarticularis, transverse process and base of the superior articular process; this point marks the insertion site for a pedicle screw. The exact topography of the pedicle screw insertion point, and the trajectory of the screw, will depend on the exact level in the spine to be instrumented.

Instrumentation

- A screw track is prepared on each side at each vertebra to be instrumented, using a pedicle starter awl followed by a pedicle probe; alternatively, an oscillating drill can be used, although manual probing is usually easy.
- The image intensifier is used to check the position of the pedicle awl and probe in both the frontal and sagittal planes, to ensure concentric screw placement within the pedicle.
- A small hook-probe can be used to 'feel' the proposed screw track, and confirm that the pedicle wall has not been breached (particularly medially, i.e. into the spinal canal).
- Pedicle screws of appropriate diameter and length are then inserted bilaterally at the level above and below the injured level. Typically, 6 mm or 7 mm diameter screws are used, although narrower screws may be necessary in small patients, or in the mid-thoracic region.
- The left-hand screws are then connected to a rod of appropriate length, and the procedure repeated on the right-hand side.
- Kyphosis can be corrected and loss of vertebral body height can then be restored, or at least improved, by a variety of manoeuvres depending upon the type of instrumentation used.
- Simply lowering the Wilson frame will often allow a degree of kyphosis correction by gravity.
- Using the AO USS (Fixateur Interne) system, and long-stemmed Schanz screws, lordosis can be restored by approximating the superficial (free) ends of the cephalic and caudal screws together.
- Loss of vertebral body height can be reversed by subsequent distraction of the Schanz screws along the connecting rods, before final tightening of the secur-

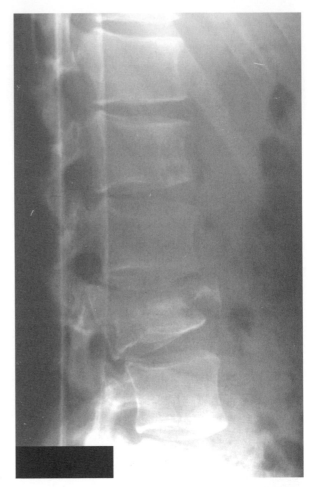

Fig. 15.11 Pre-operative lateral radiograph of a comminuted lumbar burst fracture of L3.

ing clamps. This manoeuvre will also effect an indirect decompression of any retropulsed bone fragments from the spinal canal, via ligamentotaxis.

- Most instrumentation systems available on the market will permit some deformity correction by similar means (Figs. 15.11, 15.12, 15.13).
- Care should be taken during the 'lordosis' manoeuvre to prevent inadvertent compression of the posterior wall of the injured vertebra; this will lead to further retropulsion of bone into the spinal canal, and loss of vertebral height.
- This complication can be prevented by the use of a rod clamp or small detachable C clamps which can be placed on the connecting rods between the Schanz (or similar) screws, blocking excessive 'shortening' of the screws along the rod during lordosization.

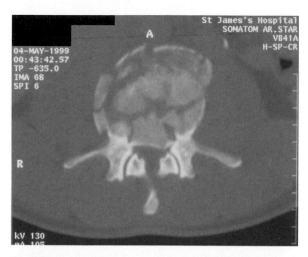

Fig. 15.12 Axial CT scan of a comminuted burst fracture of L3 (same case as Figure 15.11).

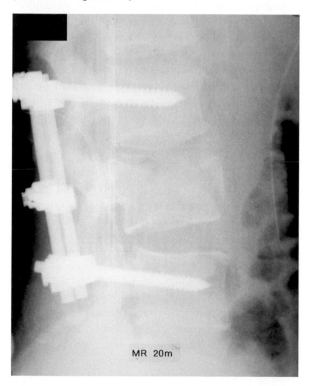

Fig. 15.13 Post-operative lateral radiograph of a burst fracture after posterior stabilization (same case as Figures 15.11 and 15.12).

- Intra operative X-rays with the image intensifier should confirm reduction of the fracture, in the form of restoration of vertebral body height, and normal sagittal profile. The rods are usually cross-linked with a short rod and clamp system; this increases the mechanical sta-

bility of the construct greatly, particularly with respect to torsional loads.

- Depending on the fracture configuration and the patient's overall status, some surgeons will elect to merely stabilize the fracture, without any further procedure at this point, and with a view to metalwork removal once the fracture has healed – usually at least 9 months after surgery.

- Others will carry out a posterolateral fusion procedure, with autograft or bone graft substitute; this can be done over the entire instrumented area, i.e. a two-level fusion, or can be confined to one level only – usually the superior level, as most burst fractures involve the superior half of the vertebra.

- Yet others will carry out a transpedicular bone-grafting procedure under X-ray control, in an effort to fill the vertebral body 'void' created by the reduction manoeuvre and prevent late kyphotic collapse and/or breakage of implants.

- Whatever approach is taken, some degree of recurrent anterior collapse must be expected, even with transpedicular grafting and a posterolateral fusion. The tendency for late collapse, often with screw breakage, is greater with increasingly severe damage to the anterior supporting structure.

- Thus, as outlined by McCormack *et al.*, gross comminution, displacement (loss of apposition) and kyphotic collapse of the vertebral body – the anterior column – is associated with late failure of fixation and recurrent deformity.

- In such circumstances, supplementary anterior surgery is advised, at a suitable time after the initial posterior stabilization (Fig. 15.14).

- Clearly, this can be done as a combined posterior/anterior procedure under the same anaesthetic, if the conditions permit, or as a delayed procedure, if the patient is physiologically unstable.

Closure

- All implant clamps are checked for tightness.
- A standard wound drain is placed in the midline, brought out through the muscles and deep fascia, exiting the skin well lateral to the midline wound.
- If possible the muscles are approximated to the midline soft tissues (interspinous ligaments) and to each other using a heavy gauge absorbable suture e.g. No. 1 PDS. The subcutaneous fat is closed with 2/0 PDS or similar, and the skin is closed according to local preference.

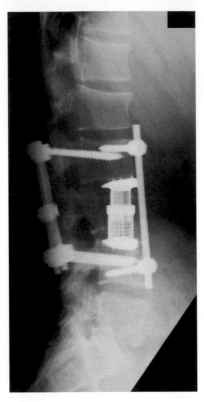

Fig. 15.14 Same case as Figures 15.11, 15.12 and 15.13 after anterior column reconstruction with telescoping cage, bone graft and anterior fixation.

Post-operative treatment

- Antibiotics are continued for 2 further doses, unless continuation is indicated for other reasons.
- The wound drains are removed at 24 hours. Other injuries permitting, the patient is nursed as upright as possible, with the spine fully supported; there should be no 'air-gap' between the bed and the patient's back.
- Mobilization with the help of physiotherapy is commenced as soon as the patient is free of drains and other rate-limiting co-morbidities.
- Fractures with minimal comminution, minimal loss of apposition and minimal kyphosis – i.e. relatively stable injuries with intact anterior load-sharing structures – can be actively mobilized within a removable thoraco-lumbar orthosis. In these patients, the orthosis should be retained for 3–6 months, and core stabilization exercises should commence once fully mobile and the wound healed, usually 3–4 weeks post-surgery.
- Fractures deemed to be less stable, in terms of loss of anterior load-sharing capability, may lead to consider-

ation of anterior surgery, either as a primary or delayed procedure

Follow up

- After hospital discharge, patients should be reviewed 4–6 weekly, with radiographic reviews in the form of erect frontal and lateral X-rays.
- Possible complications to be on guard for are late kyphotic collapse with metalwork failure, and non-union; this latter complication is usually associated with complete burst fractures with herniation of the disc into the vertebral body, or split or pincer-type fractures, where a segment of vertebral body is rendered avascular.
- Full return to contact sport and heavy manual labour is not advisable until fusion is confirmed (if fusion has been performed) or until metalwork has been removed (if simple stabilization performed). Implant removal in non-fused cases is advised at 9–12 months post-stabilization.
- Once fusion has occurred, or implants removed (and wound then re-healed), most patients can be discharged from medical follow up; for most, this will be at 12–15 months after the initial surgery. A small proportion will need further investigation for back pain, and some of these will require revision surgery, including anterior surgery.

15.3 OPERATIVE ANTERIOR STABILIZATION OF COMPLEX THORACO-LUMBAR BURST FRACTURES

Indications

Rarely, anterior surgery (decompression and/or anterior column reconstruction) is performed as the primary treatment. Usually, such surgery follows initial posterior stabilization and deformity correction, either immediately or as a delayed, secondary procedure. The indications for anterior surgery are discussed earlier.

Pre-operative planning

- The need for anterior surgery is usually dictated by radiographic parameters suggesting a high risk of late kyphotic collapse or non-union.
- Where posterior surgery is contraindicated, such as major posterior soft tissue injury, anterior stabilization may be the initial surgical strategy.

- Where no significant neurological compression is evident, either clinically or radiologically, it may be sufficient to plan for a limited corpectomy alone, merely to create enough space for a strut graft or fusion cage.
- The degree of kyphotic deformity should be measured on lateral radiographs or re-formatted sagittal plane CT scans. The size of any interbody deficit after corpectomy and disc excision above and below the injured level should be measured, allowing for correction of any kyphus, since this will determine the size of any strut graft harvest or fusion cage.
- The advent of telescopic fusion cages, e.g. AO Synex cage, has simplified the necessary inventory required for reconstruction. If a cage is to be used, a range of suitable sizes and sagittal profile can be ordered in advance of the operation.
- Where time permits, bowel preparation should be initiated, since this will make retraction of the peritoneal sac and contents much easier for exposure of fractures below diaphragm level (T12 or L1 downwards).

Anaesthesia

- The surgical approach may be purely transthoracic for injuries above T12, or may require a transthoracic, transdiaphragmatic and extraperitoneal approach for injuries at T12 or L1; injuries at L2 or below may be approached without transgressing the pleura or diaphragm.
- Unless there is a significant right convex scoliosis associated with the fracture, the left side is by far the easiest access, avoiding the need for liver retraction.
- The anaesthetist should pass a double-lumen endotracheal tube if a transthoracic route is necessary. This will permit selective collapse of the left lung and will greatly facilitate the exposure.
- Routine antibiotic and thromboembolic prophylaxis is used. If not already performed as part of emergency management, the bladder should be emptied via an indwelling catheter, and a nasogastric tube should be passed to empty the stomach and protect against gastric distension.
- Spinal cord monitoring may be a useful adjunct to surgery, particularly in the neurologically intact patient with radiological signs of severe canal encroachment by retropulsed bone.
- Central venous access is advisable and should be via the great veins on the left side (subclavian or internal jugular).

Table, positioning and set up

- The patient will be in the lateral decubitus position, left side up.
- A standard operating table may be used and if possible, the table should be hinged or 'broken' to adduct the lower limbs downwards from the ribcage; this increases the distance between the costal margin and the iliac crest.
- Alternatively, if posterior stabilization has not preceded the anterior surgery, a table with a mechanical bridge can be used to arch the spine and achieve the same access; this is rarely necessary, and may be inadvisable in severely comminuted and unstable injuries.
- Positioning posts are placed at strategic points to stabilize the patient in the lateral decubitus position, and these should be well padded.
- Care should be taken to ensure no pressure is applied to boney prominences such as the malleoli or fibular neck. The dependent lower limb (usually the right leg) is flexed, and separated from the uppermost leg with a pillow; the uppermost leg is extended.
- A permanent marker pen is used to outline the line of the incision; the tenth rib is selected for a thoraco-abdominal approach, and is easily palpated. For higher levels of injuries, the rib above the fractured level is usually marked, and this will afford good access if the rib is excised. In cases of doubt, e.g. in the obese patient, an image intensifier should be used to localize the injured level.
- Finally, if an iliac crest graft is planned, the anterior iliac crest and anterior–superior iliac spine is marked (Figs. 15.15, 15.16).
- The surgeon usually stands behind the patient's back; the scrub nurse can be on the same side as the surgeon, whilst the image intensifier can be placed ready, if necessary, on the opposite side (behind the assistant).
- Sterile drapes should be applied to the image intensifier, which can usually only provide a cross-table frontal view of the spine; intra-operative imaging is rarely required.

Incision/approach

The left thoraco-abdominal approach (transthoracic, transdiaphragmatic and extraperitoneal) to L1 will be described:

- The skin overlying the left 10th rib is incised down to deep fascia, overlying the rib, and then curved obliquely downwards at the costal margin, towards the

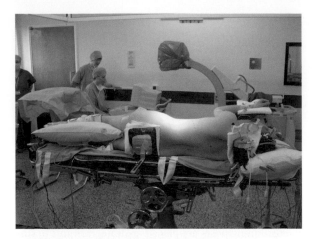

Fig. 15.15 Lateral decubitus position for anterior thoraco-abdominal approach.

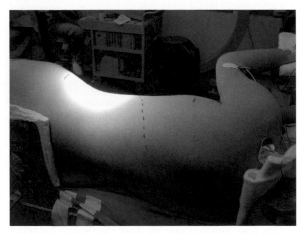

Fig. 15.16 Left thoraco-abdominal approach, showing line of skin incision (line of tenth rib) and markings to identify the iliac crest.

umbilicus but falling short of the lateral margin of the rectus sheath.

- Over the rib, the incision is deepened through muscle (latissimus dorsi, serratus anterior and external oblique) with a diathermy and through the rib periosteum, staying in the middle of the rib to avoid injury to the intercostal neurovascular bundle running in the groove below the rib.
- Distally and medially, the external oblique muscle is split in line with its fibres, and the deeper layers (internal oblique and transverses abdominus) are incised with diathermy.
- Below the costal margin, the peritoneal sac is bluntly dissected free from the lateral abdominal wall musculature and the undersurface of the diaphragm, and retracted medially with a hand-held retractor or swab on a stick.

- The 10th rib is exposed subperiosteally along its length, and then removed by cutting the rib at the costochondral junction and close to the costovertebral junction.
- The parietal pleura under the bed of the rib is then incised, to enter the left hemithorax; if a double-lumen endotracheal tube has been used, the left lung can now be selectively occluded and collapsed.
- Sharp division of the costal cartilage will leave this as an important landmark during wound closure. After stripping of the peritoneum from its undersurface, the diaphragm is divided approximately 2 cm from its costal origin, placing paired marker sutures along the line of division to facilitate later repair.
- A rib spreader retractor is then inserted and opened, care being taken to retract the left lung and peritoneal sac (and contents) away from the retractor blades.
- Blunt dissection from lateral to medial with a swab will expose the lumbar spine; the fractured level is usually self-evident.
- It is usually necessary to divide the left crus of the diaphragm between stay sutures from its vertebral attachment before completing the peripheral incision of the diaphragm medially, and through the aortic hiatus to complete the direct path between thoracic and abdominal cavities.
- The greater splanchnic nerve and sympathetic trunk can be directly visualized and laterally retracted without division; occasionally, it is necessary to ligate and divide segmental vertebral vessels or ascending lumbar veins.
- The retroperitoneal adventitia is easily mobilized from the front of the spine with a swab.
- The parietal pleura overlying T12 and above must be split with scissors upwards after elevation from the underlying structures (including the segmental vessels and sympathetic trunk).
- Blunt dissection with the finger or a swab on a stick will expose the vertebral bodies from T12 to L2 circumferentially, around to the bases of the transverse processes.
- The psoas major origin from the lumbar intervertebral disc can be elevated by a combination of blunt and bipolar diathermy dissection, taking care not to penetrate the adjacent intervertebral foramen; a stay suture can be used to retract the mobilized psoas laterally.

Instrumentation

- Corpectomy, either total or partial, begins with excision of the discs and endplates at T12/L1 and

L1/L2. If complete decompression is the aim, the foramen at the respective levels are identified, and the disc removed piecemeal from posterolateral to anteromedial, until the epidural space and dural sac is identified.

- Bone fragments at L1 are then removed piecemeal with rongeurs and curettes to complete the corpectomy. The posterior vertebral body wall can be left intact, along with the contralateral (right) portion of the vertebra, if a complete corpectomy is not required; sufficient bone should be removed to permit strut graft or cage placement.
- Care should be taken not to breach the endplates at T12 or L2, to avoid excavation of the underlying vertebral bodies and weakening of the load-bearing surfaces for the graft or cage.
- The height of the corpectomy defect is measured with a small ruler or measuring callipers; if there has a been a prior posterior stabilization, this will be a relatively fixed height. Without prior posterior surgery, the interbody defect can be maximized by a combination of interbody distraction, using a spreader, and by pressure directed forwards over the posterior spine surface, to create lordosis.
- A suitably sized strut graft is harvested from the anterior iliac crest or, alternatively, a suitable cage is selected. Telescopic cages make this aspect of the procedure much easier, since there is no need for 'on-table trimming' of either a graft or static cage.
- The cage or graft is then carefully placed into the defect, ensuring a stable position without overhanging the endplates at T12 or L2 (particularly posteriorly, into the epidural space) and any distraction or lordosis force relaxed.
- A telescopic cage can now be distracted to ensure a tight fit. If there is any doubt about the integrity or stability of the graft or cage, supplementary anterior fixation should be inserted to compress T12 to L2; a simple single rod and vertebral-body screw contact may suffice where posterior stabilization already exists, or may not be necessary at all. For stand-alone anterior stabilization, a plate or double-rod system is advisable, and there are several appropriate systems available commercially e.g Kaneda device; AO Ventrofix.
- The bone debris from the injured level can be used to supplement bone grafting around the strut or cage and this is usually sufficient to avoid the need for additional harvest of autologous cancellous bone. Any bone graft should be placed circumferentially around the strut or cage, avoiding the posterior aspect.

- Many surgeons will perform an intraoperative radiograph at this point, to ensure correct cage or graft placement prior to closure.

Closure

- A large-bore (28–32 gauge) intercostal tube drain is inserted through the chest wall into the thoracic cavity, at least 1 rib space above the excised 10th rib level.
- Some surgeons prefer to drain the retroperitoneum separately, although bleeding is usually minor and is tamponaded by the peritoneal sac.
- The psoas muscle may need to be approximated to its origin, and the divided left crus is sutured together carefully with PDS.
- The parietal pleura over the spine can often be repaired with a running PDS or Vicryl suture, although minor defects are unimportant.
- The divided diaphragm is carefully repaired, from posteromedial to anterolateral, preferably with a few interrupted PDS sutures supplemented by a running suture; the stay sutures will facilitate matching of the divided edges.
- The 10th costal cartilage is easily sutured together, followed by suture repair of the thoracotomy portion of the wound; a rib approximator will appose the free edges of parietal pleura and intercostals muscles together.
- Care should be taken to avoid inclusion of the neurovascular bundle within the suture line.
- The chest and abdominal wall musculature are then sutured in layers, and the chest drain secured in place with a strong retaining suture.
- The chest drain is attached to a container with an underwater seal.

Post-operative treatment

- Post-operative spine and chest radiographs are performed at the earliest opportunity.
- Antibiotics are given for 24 hours post-operatively, unless there is a further indication for continuation.
- The nasogastric tube should remain on free drainage until the inevitable ileus has resolved, identifiable as passage of flatus and/or return of bowel sounds; once bowel activity returns, oral intake can resume, initially with fluids only. If fluids are tolerated without nausea or copious nasogastric drainage, the nasogastric tube is removed, usually 24–48 hours after surgery, and normal diet is introduced.

- The chest drain tube remains until the lung is seen to be fully inflated on a chest X-ray, and drainage subsides to less than 100 mls in a 24-hour period.
- The dependent lung – in this case, the right lung – is prone to major atelectasia, secondary to under-ventilation in the lateral decubitus position. Aggressive chest physiotherapy is usually all that is necessary.
- Rarely, unrecognised injury to the cisterna chyli or thoracic duct will manifest itself as a post-operative chylothorax or drainage of lymph via the chest tube or retroperitoneal wound drain. This can usually be managed non-operatively, by continued intercostal drainage and parenteral nutrition.
- Removal of central venous access lines should precede chest drain removal, whenever possible. Once liberated from drains, etc. the patient is mobilized as for posterior stabilization. With combined posterior and anterior stabilization/reconstruction, there is usually little need for external support with an orthosis.
- Post-discharge follow up is as for posterior stabilization.

Part V

Tendon injuries

Reconstruction of tendons

Peter V. Giannoudis (16.1), Caroline McGuiness and
Simon Knight (16.2)

16.1 ACHILLES TENDON REPAIR

Indications

- Controversy regarding this injury as to whether surgical repair or cast immobilization is the most appropriate method of treatment.
- Healthy, vigorous young adults.
- Athletes.
- According to patient's age, activities, medical history.

Pre-operative planning

Clinical assessment

- Mechanism of injury: mechanical imbalance, degenerative changes, high-energy disruptions, lacerations at the posterior distal tibia aspect.
- Obtain a detailed patient's history.
- Usually sudden onset of pain, audible snap, patient unable to weight bear, unable to toe-raise at the affected site.
- Only leg weakness in chronically ruptured tendon.
- Oedema, bruising, ankle swelling.
- Clinically palpable gap that may be obscured by swelling.
- Perform Thompson's test, O'Brien test.
- Compare the affected leg with the contralateral limb.
- Be alert for longstanding ruptures.

Radiological assessment

- Radiographs: only to diagnose associated bony abnormalities.

- High-resolution ultrasonography: produces an acoustic vacuum.
- MRI: to evaluate associated intra-articular injuries and neglected tears.

Operative treatment

Anaesthesia

- At induction administration of prophylactic antibiotics as per local hospital protocol.
- Spinal or general anaesthesia.

Table set up

- The instrumentation set is at the foot end of the table.

Patient positioning

- The patient is placed in prone position.

Draping and surgical approach

- Prepare the skin over lower leg, ankle and entire foot with usual antiseptic solutions (aqueous/alcoholic povidone–iodine). Prepare skin between toes thoroughly.
- Apply standard draping around lower leg in calf region.
- Apply tape around toes to minimize the risk of infection (Fig. 16.1).
- Extend the wound edges longitudinally, taking care not to damage the sural nerve (Fig. 16.2).
- Proximally search for the central end of the ruptured tendon and pull it downwards (Fig. 16.3).

Practical Procedures in Orthopaedic Trauma Surgery: A Trainee's Companion, ed. Peter V. Giannoudis and Hans-Christoph Pape.
Published by Cambridge University Press. © Cambridge University Press 2006.

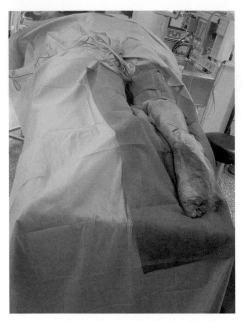

Fig. 16.1 The patient is placed in the prone position with standard draping applied around the lower leg in the calf region and tape around toes to minimize the risk of infection.

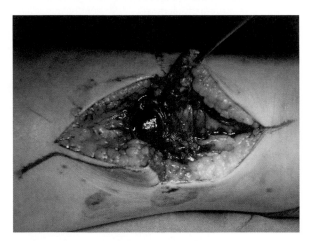

Fig. 16.2 Extend the wound edges longitudinally, taking care not to damage the sural nerve.

- Place 2 separate double loops of a No. 5 non-absorbable tension suture using a modified Kessler stitch into the proximal and distal ends of the ruptured tendon, producing an 8-strand repair (Fig. 16.4).
- Approximate the ruptured ends of the tendon (Fig. 16.5a,b).
- Plantarflex the foot up to 5°, flex the knee at 30° and whilst observing the contralateral limb tie the sutures, approximating the ruptured ends (Fig. 16.6).

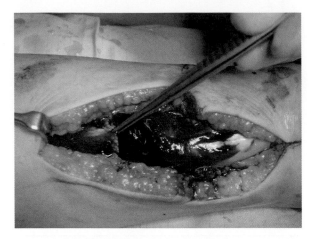

Fig. 16.3 Proximally search for the central end of the ruptured tendon and pull it downwards.

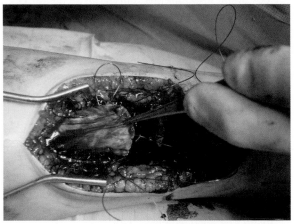

(a)

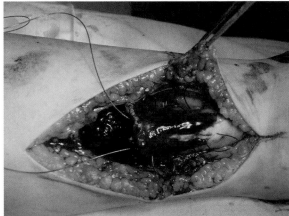

(b)

Fig. 16.4 a,b Placing of 2 separate double loops of a No. 5 non-absorbable tension suture using a modified Kessler stitch into the proximal and distal ends of the ruptured tendon.

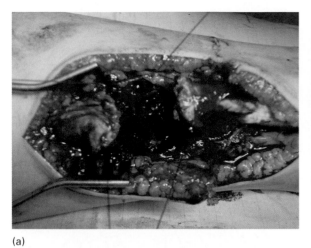

(a)

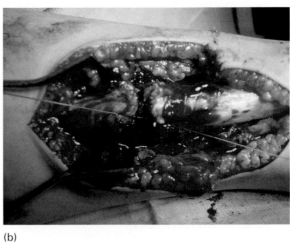

(b)

Fig. 16.5a,b Re-approximating of the tendon's ruptured ends.

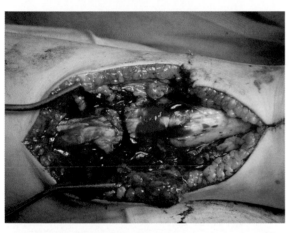

Fig. 16.6 With the foot plantarflexed up to 5°, the knee flexed at 30°, and whilst observing the contralateral limb, the sutures are tied, approximating the ruptured ends.

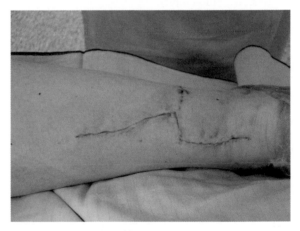

Fig. 16.8 Closure of the wound.

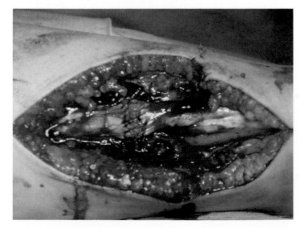

Fig. 16.7 The edges of the tendon repair are then made perfectly smooth by using a peripheral running suture which passes around the whole circumference of the tendon repair.

- The edges of the tendon repair are then made perfectly smooth by using a peripheral running suture which passes around the whole circumference of the tendon repair (Fig. 16.7).

Closure

- Close the defect in the gastrocnemius fascia and tendon sheath with 2.0 absorbable sutures.
- Close the skin with a running subcuticular 3.0 monofilament suture (Fig. 16.8).
- Apply non-adherent dressings.
- A short-leg plastic boot is applied, with the foot in gravity equinus.

Post-operative treatment

- Suture removal after 2 weeks.
- At 3 weeks the patient is allowed to increase weight bearing progressively.
- After 6 weeks the patient begins active and active-assisted range of motion exercises.
- After 2–4 weeks, initiation of isokinetic strengthening.
- Gain of full strength and full endurance achieved in 4 months after surgery.

16.2 REPAIR OF TENDON INJURIES IN THE HAND

Indications

Diagnosis of tendon injury:

- This is usually obvious and can be inferred by the position of the overlying laceration and the posture of the hand.
- Specific tests to get the patient to actively flex or extend the injured finger confirm the diagnosis (Fig. 16.9).

Associated injuries:

- Associated injuries to the median, ulnar, radial and digital nerves should be expected and specifically excluded.
- The vascular status of the finger and hand should be assessed.
- The condition of the overlying skin should be examined to ensure that viable skin is available over the tendon repair.

Competence:

- Flexor tendon repairs in Zone II (Table 16.1) are technically difficult and should only be undertaken by experienced surgeons.
- If you do not have the necessary experience, clean the wound, close it under local anaesthetic, prescribe the patient antibiotics, splint the hand and refer the patient to a centre that is used to dealing with these injuries.
- If the patient has neurovascular injuries or large skin defects and you do not have the necessary microsurgical or plastic surgical experience to deal with these, the patient should be transferred to a centre that can.

Table 16.1. Classification of tendon injuries

Zone I	Distal to flexor digitorum superficialis insertion
Zone II	Digital flexor sheath containing superficialis and profundus tendons – 'no man's land'
Zone III	Mid-palm
Zone IV	Within carpal tunnel
Zone V	Proximal to carpal tunnel

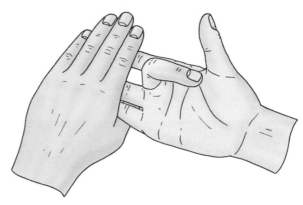

Fig. 16.9 Specific tests to get the patient to actively flex or extend the injured finger confirm the diagnosis.

- Injuries that present late, more than a few days post-injury, are also better dealt with by an experienced unit.

Operative treatment

Anaesthesia

- Single extensor tendon injuries over the back of the hand may be treated under local anaesthetic. Most tendon injuries, however, will require the use of a regional anaesthetic in order to allow the patient to tolerate the tourniquet for the necessary period of the repair.
- Occasionally a general anaesthetic may be necessary.
- A tourniquet is placed around the upper arm and inflated to approximately 100 mmHg above the systolic blood pressure. A pressure of 250 mmHg will suffice for most adult patients.
- The use of prophylactic antibiotics is recommended. The author uses a single dose of 1 g of flucloxacillin on induction. Alternatively, specific hospital protocols may be followed.

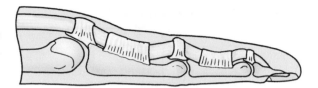

Table and equipment

- A tray of fine surgical operating instruments should be made available containing Adsen's toothed forceps and a fine needle holder capable of grasping 6.0 sutures.

Patient positioning

- The patient is draped in a supine position with the abducted arm on a large hand table.
- A lead hand or alternative to hold the digits and hand is required to assist operating.

Magnification

- Loope magnification is recommended for all tendon repairs. The use of the operating microscope is preferred for nerve repair and necessary for repair of associated vessels.

Flexor tendon injury

Skin incisions

- Incisions on the flexor surface of the fingers, hand and wrist have a tendency to contract as they mature. Every effort, therefore, should be made to convert open lacerations into Brunner-type incisions by extending them longitudinally in an intelligently planned zig-zag fashion.
- In the forearm the incision is deepened through the deep fascia to the flexor tendons. Over the wrist it may be necessary to divide the carpal ligament to find the injured tendons.
- Prior to dividing the carpal ligament, however, it is worthwhile flexing the fingers to see whether the severed ends of the tendons protrude into the wound. If they do not, the wound should be extended into the palm and the carpal tunnel opened.

Flexor pulley preservation

- In the fingers, the flexor tendons are encased by a fibrous flexor sheath containing 5 annular pulleys (Fig. 16.10). These pulleys should not be divided and every attempt must be made to preserve their integrity.
- The distal end of the severed tendons can usually be made to appear like toothpaste from a squeezed tube by simply flexing the interphalangeal joints (Fig. 16.11). It is occasionally possible to retrieve the proximal end of the severed tendons by flexing the wrist

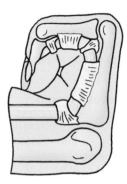

Fig. 16.10 In the fingers, the flexor tendons are encased by a fibrous flexor sheath containing five annular pulleys.

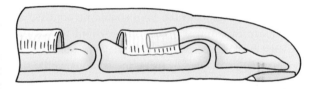

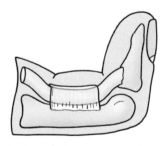

Fig. 16.11 The distal end of the severed tendons can usually be made to appear like toothpaste from a squeezed tube by simply flexing the interphalangeal joints.

and milking the flexor muscle belly in a proximal to distal direction.

- If the end of the tendon is still not visible, extend the incision into the palm of the hand, locate the severed flexor tendons, pass either a fine plastic catheter or a loop of 0 Prolene down the flexor sheath and suture it to the severed ends of the flexor tendon and railroad the tendons back through the flexor sheath.

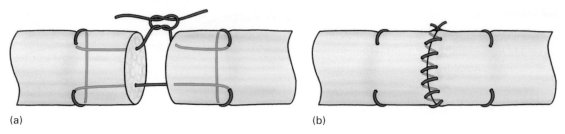

(a)   (b)

Fig. 16.12 (a) Each tendon is repaired individually using a kessler core suture of 3.0 or 4.0 Prolene or Ethibond on a round-bodied needle. (b) The edges of the tendon repair are then made perfectly smooth by using a peripheral running suture of 5.0 or 6.0 Prolene on a round-bodied needle which passes around the whole circumference of each of the tendon repairs.

Repair of the nerves and vessels

- Before embarking upon the repair of the flexor tendon, any associated injuries to the nerves and vessels should be repaired at this point.

Maintenance of the tendon position

- In order to repair the flexor tendon the ends of the tendon should be in gentle apposition. The posture of the joints of the limb should be adjusted to achieve this. You will need an assistant to flex the wrist and the interphalangeal joints. The position can then be maintained by fixing the tendons within the flexor sheath by transfixing them with hypodermic needles.
- Each tendon is repaired individually using a Kessler core suture of 3.0 or 4.0 Prolene or Ethibond on a round-bodied needle (Fig. 16.12a).
- The edges of the tendon repair are then made perfectly smooth by using a peripheral running suture of 5.0 or 6.0 Prolene on a round-bodied needle which passes around the whole circumference of each of the tendon repairs (Fig. 16.12b).
- If the injury has occurred distal to the decussation of the flexor digitorum superficialis, the tendon slips are flat and these slips should be repaired with simple mattress sutures.
- Flexor tendon repairs proximal to the mid-palm do not require the peripheral running suture and can be repaired by a single 3.0 non-absorbable Kessler core suture.
- Repair the flexor sheath: following the tendon repair the flexor sheath should be repaired with 6.0 Prolene.
- Ensure smooth excursion of the tendon repair.
- Once the repair is complete, the fingers should be flexed and extended 5–6 times to make certain that there is a full, smooth excursion of the repaired tendons.

Closure

- The skin is closed with either 4.0 Vicryl Rapide or 4.0 Prolene.
- Dress the wound with a non-adherent, absorbent dressing, ensuring the minimum amount of bulk in the hand to allow the fingers joints to be passively moved through a full range of movement during the convalescence.

Splintage

- Apply the splint to keep the tension on the tendon repairs to a minimum and to prevent accidental over-extension of the fingers.
- The splint extends from beyond the fingertips to the proximal forearm.
- The wrist is held in approximately 20° of flexion and the metacarpophalangeal joints at approximately 30° of flexion.
- The interphalangeal joints are allowed to extend fully (Fig. 16.13).

Special cases

Avulsion of the flexor digitorum profundus tendon from the distal interphalangeal joint is treated by railroading the flexor digitorum profundus (see above) along the flexor sheath and securing it to the distal phalanx with a core suture that is passed through a drill hole in the distal phalanx and secured by a button over the nail (Fig. 16.14).

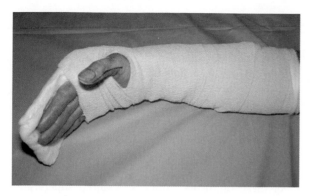

Fig. 16.13 The interphalangeal joints are allowed to extend fully.

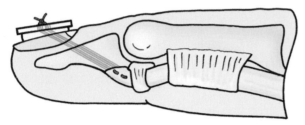

Fig. 16.14 A core suture that is passed through a drill hole in the distal phalanx and secured by a button over the nail.

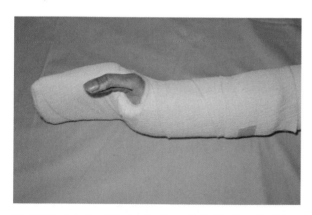

Fig. 16.15 A plaster of Paris splint is applied with the wrist fully extended, the metacarpophalangeal joints partially flexed to approximately 30° and inerphalangeal joints completely extended.

Extensor tendon injuries

Skin incision

Extensor tendons rarely retract far from the site of injury. Only a small extension of the wound is usually required to locate and repair the tendons.

Tendon repair

- The tendons over the finger and on the dorsum of the hand are flat and are repaired with a non-absorbable 4.0 mattress or figure-of-eight suture.
- In the forearm the tendons are large and round and should be repaired with a 3.0 non-absorbable Kessler core suture.

Extensor retinaculum

- Over the extensor surface of the wrist, part of the extensor retinaculum must be retained to prevent later bowstringing.
- If it is not possible to perform the repair without opening the extensor retinaculum, it should be opened through a stepped incision so that it can be repaired at the end of the procedure.

Closure

- The skin is sutured with 4.0 Vicryl Rapide or 5.0 Prolene.
- A non-adherent, absorbent dressing is placed over the wound.

Splintage

- A plaster of Paris splint is applied with the wrist fully extended, the metacarpophalangeal joints partially flexed to approximately 30° and interphalangeal joints completely extended. (Fig. 16.15).

Special cases

- Closed mallet injuries and closed boutonnière injuries can be treated conservatively by splintage.
- By contrast, open injuries over the insertion of the extensor tendon should be treated by K-wiring the distal interphalangeal joint in extension and repairing the extensor tendon.
- Open boutonnière injuries should be treated by K-wiring the proximal interphalangeal joint in extension and suturing the central slip of the extensor tendon.

Post-operative rehabilitation

Extensor tendons

- These are treated by static splintage or by dynamic splintage for 1 month depending on the local treatment protocol.
- Most patients require further physiotherapy to obtain a full range of movement.

Flexor tendon repairs in the forearm

- Flexor tendon repairs in the forearm are treated by static splintage for 1 month followed by a course of physiotherapy.

Flexor tendon repairs in the hand and wrist

- Flexor tendon repairs in the hand and wrist are treated by moving the repaired flexor tendons in a controlled fashion throughout the early post-operative period.
- A splint must be worn throughout this period of time.
- The controlled movement is achieved either by rubber band traction, passive mobilization or controlled active mobilization.
- All these protocols require specialized supervision from the physiotherapy services.

Part VI

Compartments

Decompression fasciotomies

Roderick Dunn and Simon Kay

17.1 FASCIOTOMY FOR ACUTE COMPARTMENT SYNDROMES OF THE UPPER AND LOWER LIMBS

Definition of compartment syndrome

A persistent rise in the pressure within a confined fibro-osseous compartment that leads to partial or complete infarction and fibrosis of the vital components of that compartment. (See p. 269 for fasciotomy for compartment syndrome of the foot.)

Aetiology

- Bleeding.
- Ischaemia and reperfusion.
- Crush.
- Electrical burns.
- Posture.
- Iatrogenic.
- Injection.

Indications

- Clinical suspicion is the main indicator.
- Raised compartment pressure measurements (see below under *Clinical assessment*).
  - 30 mmHg for 8 hours or for an unknown period.
  - 20 mmHg below diastolic pressure.
  - Clinical suspicion plus compartment pressure of 30 mmHg.
- Revascularization of a limb (always).

Clinical assessment

- Clinical suspicion is the main indicator.

- Pulses are NOT a useful sign – peripheral vascularity does NOT correlate with compartment status.
- The degree of distal ischaemia is VARIABLE with compartment syndrome.
- Compartment pressure measurement is the only useful investigation.
- Damage varies with pressure differential and time.

Symptoms

PAIN:
- Severe.
- Unrelieved by analgesia (look at drug chart).
- Persistent.
- Progressive.
- Passive stretch exacerbates.
- Unrelieved by immobilization.

Signs

- Limb feels tense.
- Pain on passive stretch.
- Reduced sensibility in distribution of nerves that pass *through* the compartment.
- Weakness of muscles in compartment.
- Presence of pulse does NOT exclude compartment syndrome.

Investigations

- Direct compartment pressure measurement is the most useful investigation. There is no place for any other imaging in the management of acute compartment syndrome.
- Instruments:

Practical Procedures in Orthopaedic Trauma Surgery: A Trainee's Companion, ed. Peter V. Giannoudis and Hans-Christoph Pape.
Published by Cambridge University Press. © Cambridge University Press 2006.

- Stryker® dedicated device (Stryker Pressure monitor and Quick pressure monitor system).
- Pressure transducer from CVP monitor and hypodermic needle (19 G or 21 G).
- Manometer.
- Measuring compartment pressure:
  - Calibrate instrument.
  - Insert needle or catheter into compartment and take pressure reading.
  - Take measurements from different sites in the compartment (compartments are not fluid, so pressure varies within compartment).
  - Measurements depend on technique and may vary between operators.
  - Look at the trend if a single measurements is equivocal.
  - Can compare with contralateral unaffected limb if unsure.
- When to intervene:
  - 30 mmHg for 8 hours or unknown period.
  - 20 mmHg below diastolic pressure.
  - Clinical suspicion plus pressure of 30 mmHg.
- Blood tests. Check creatine kinase (CK) and urea and electrolytes. A very high CK may indicate muscle necrosis. This may lead to acute renal failure, so monitor U & ES and consider early renal dialysis if indicated (speak to ITU and/or renal physicians).

Operative treatment

Fasciotomy of the upper and lower limbs: general principles

- General or regional anaesthesia
- Use tourniquet for safe initial exposure.
- Must be complete and full length.
- Incise the skin (dermotomy) and deep fascia (fasciotomy).
- Design incisions to avoid exposed nerves or tendons.
- Try to minimize cutaneous nerve damage and preserve longitudinal veins.
- Closed, subcutaneous fasciotomy is NOT indicated in trauma.
- Examine the epimysium of individual muscle bellies systematically and incise when tight (epimysiotomy).
- Excise obviously dead muscle with the tourniquet inflated, or prior to revascularization to reduce the risk of acute renal failure from myoglobinaemia. If in doubt, do not excise it, and look again after the tourniquet is deflated (dead muscle does not bleed, is soft and

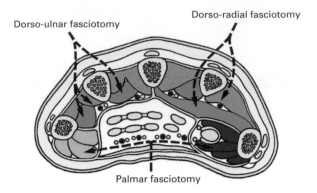

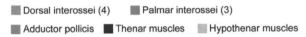

Fig. 17.1 Anatomy of the ten compartments of the hand in cross-section.

mushy, does not twitch, and is either dark or very pale (not pink)).
- Release the tourniquet to assess muscle viability.
- Perform a second look at 24 to 48 hours.

Fasciotomy of the upper limb

- Remove any rings from the digits.
- Position the patient supine on the operating table with the arm on a hand table.
- Apply a high tourniquet to the arm.
- Clean the arm to the axilla with surgical disinfectant.
- Drape the arm just below the tourniquet.

The hand

This is confusing unless you understand the anatomy of the 10 compartments of the hand in cross-section (Fig. 17.1). These are:

- Dorsal interossei (4).
- Palmar interossei (3).
- Adductor (often neglected).
- Thenar.
- Hypothenar.

Dorsal incisions (Fig. 17.2)

- The dorsal (4) and palmar (3) interosseous and adductor (1) compartments are all decompressed through 2 dorsal incisions between the 2nd and 3rd metacarpals

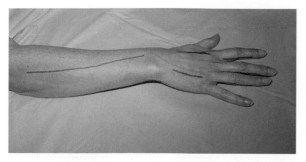

Fig. 17.2 Dorsal incisions.

and the 4th and 5th metacarpals. Incise the skin, preserving the dorsal veins where possible.

- Through the 2 dorsal incisions, incise the fascia over each of the 4 dorsal interosseous compartments, retracting the skin to gain access to the 1st and 3rd dorsal interossei, which are not directly under the incisions. Avoid damage to the superficial branch of the radial nerve when dividing the fascia over the 1st dorsal interosseous muscle.
- The 1st palmar interosseous and adductor compartments are reached through the radial incision by inserting tenotomy scissors perpendicularly along the ulnar border of the 2nd metacarpal, with the blades in the line of the metacarpal, and spreading them widely. You need to feel the dorsal fascia of the palmar interosseous compartment give way as you push the scissors into it.
- The 2nd and 3rd palmar interosseous compartments are reached similarly through the ulnar incision by inserting the scissors along the radial side of the 4th metacarpal (2nd palmar interosseous) and 5th metacarpal (3rd palmar interosseous).

Palmar incision

- The median and ulnar nerves, and the thenar and hypothenar muscles in the palm are decompressed using one incision (Fig. 17.3).
- Make a lazy S-incision from the distal wrist crease over the carpal tunnel in the midline, between thenar and hypothenar eminences to the proximal palmar crease. This may be continued into the palm in a zig-zag fashion as necessary.
- Deepen the incision through the flexor retinaculum to decompress the contents of the carpal tunnel, taking care to protect the median nerve branches, in particular the thenar motor branch of the median nerve passing radially into the thenar muscles in the distal part of the carpal tunnel.

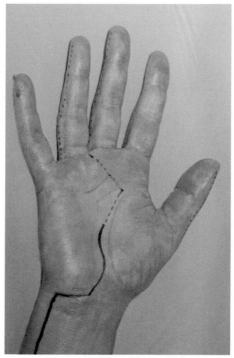

Fig. 17.3 Palmar incision.

- Incise the fascia over the thenar muscles to decompress the thenar compartment.
- Deepen the incision in an ulnar direction to decompress the ulnar nerve in Guyon's canal (superficial to the flexor retinaculum of the carpal tunnel, and more superficial than you think).
- Continue into the hypothenar muscles, preserving the deep motor branches of the ulnar nerve, and the ulnar artery as it divides into the superficial palmar arch and deep palmar branch.
- If the digits require decompressing, incise along the mid-axial line (see below) of the digits, on the non-dependent side (the ulnar side of the index, middle and ring fingers and the radial side of the thumb and little fingers).
- The mid-axial line is safe as it is dorsal to the neurovascular bundles (NVB) of the fingers. It is drawn by flexing the fingers into the palm, drawing a dot at the apex of the skin creases of the metacarpophalyngeal (MCP), proximal interphalyngeal (PIP) and distal interphalyngeal (DIP) joints, and then joining the dots with the finger in extension (Fig. 17.4a,b,c). The dissection is continued dorsal to the NVB, volar to the flexor tendon sheath, and then dorsal to the NVB on the opposite side (Fig. 17.5).

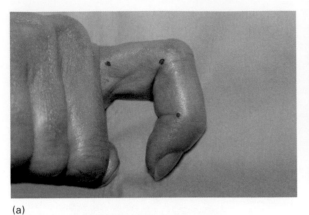

(a)

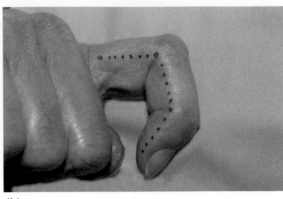

(b)

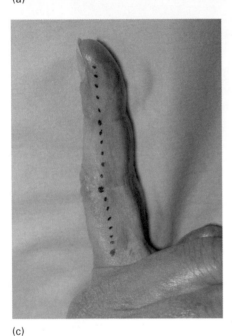

(c)

Fig. 17.4a,b,c Draw a dot at the apex of the skin creases of the MCP, PIP and DIP joints, and then join the dots with the finger in extension.

The forearm

Extensor mobile wad, common flexor mass, pronator quadratus.

Flexor incision (Fig. 17.6)

- Extend the midline incision in the palm ulna wards along the distal wrist crease (Fig. 17.7).
- Continue for 5 cm along the ulnar border of the forearm (providing a flap to cover the ulnar and median nerves) and then radially and proximally towards the radial side of the antecubital fossa.

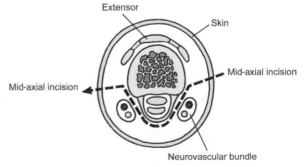

Fig. 17.5 The dissection is continued dorsal to the NVB, volar to the flexor tendon sheath, and then dorsal to the NVB on the opposite side.

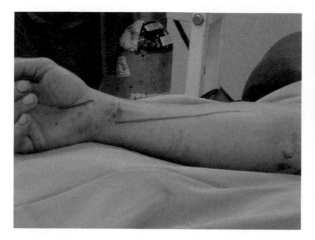

Fig. 17.6 Flexor incision.

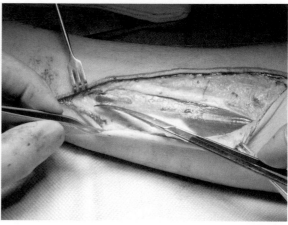

Fig. 17.7 Extend the midline incision in the palm ulna wards along the distal wrist crease.

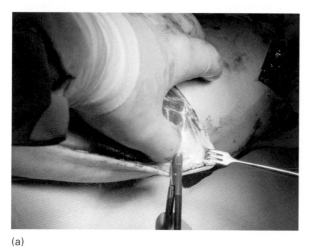

(a)

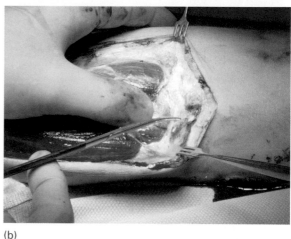

(b)

Fig. 17.8a,b Continue ulna wards across the antecubital fossa in the line of the flexion crease allowing extension into the upper arm as necessary.

- Continue ulna wards across the antecubital fossa in the line of the flexion crease allowing extension into the upper arm as necessary (Fig. 17.8).
- Examine the long flexors of the wrist and digits systematically.
- Examine the pronator quadratus deep to the long flexors.
- Explore the median and ulnar nerves in the wrist and forearm.
- Avoid the palmar cutaneous branch of the median nerve (arises 5 cm proximal to the wrist crease on the radial side and passes distally).
- Avoid the dorsal sensory branch of the ulnar nerve

(arises 5 cm proximal to the pisiform, passing dorsally and ulna wards).
- Explore the median nerve in the antecubital fossa to release constriction from the lacertus fibrosus next to the biceps aponeurosis, and the proximal edges of the flexor digitorum superficialis and the pronator teres (Fig. 17.9a,b,c).

Extensor incision (Fig. 17.10)

- Make a single longitudinal midline incision on the extensor aspect of the forearm.

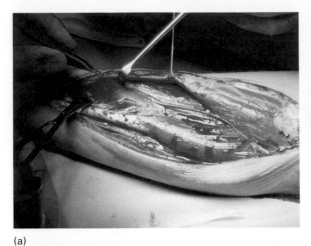

(a)

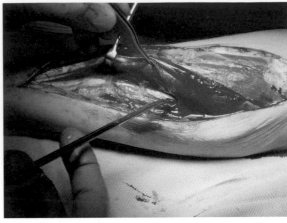

(b)

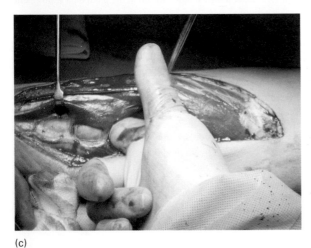

(c)

Fig. 17.9a,b,c Examine the long flexors of the wrist and digits systematically. Examine the pronator quadratus deep to the long flexors.

- Examine the extensor muscles systematically (Fig. 17.11a,b,c).

Upper arm

Flexor and extensor compartments

- Continue the incision proximally over the posteromedial aspect of the biceps brachii to decompress the biceps compartment, brachial artery and branches of the brachial plexus.
- The posterior triceps compartment can be reached through this incision if necessary, avoiding damage to the radial nerve.

Fasciotomy of the lower limb

- Position the patient supine on the operating table.
- Apply a tourniquet to the leg.

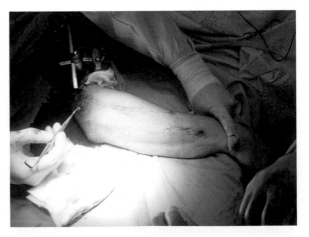

Fig. 17.10 Extensor incision.

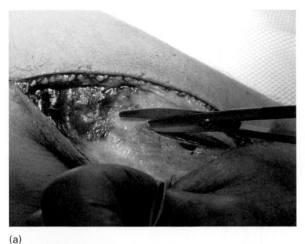

(a)

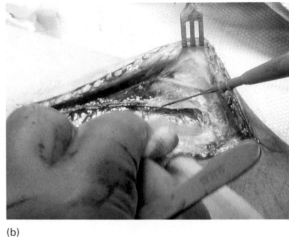

(b)

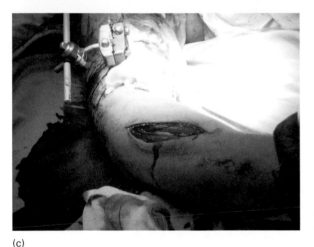

(c)

Fig. 17.11a,b,c Assessment and release of the extensor compartment of the forearm.

- Clean the leg to the thigh with surgical disinfectant.
- Drape the leg to just below the tourniquet.
- There are 4 compartments in the lower leg; anterior, peroneal, superficial posterior, deep posterior (often neglected) (Fig. 17.12 cross section of leg).
- Do NOT try and do it through a single incision.
- Do NOT remove the fibula.
- Fasciotomy is performed through 2 incisions, on the medial and lateral sides of the leg. These incisions should always be longitudinal and are designed to preserve fasciocutaneous perforator vessels to allow subsequent local flap closure if required.
- The medial incision (Fig. 17.13) follows a line 2 cm posterior to the medial subcutaneous border of the tibia, from the knee to the ankle. Incise the fascia of the superficial posterior compartment longitudinally, exposing the gastrocnemius and soleus muscles. Retract the gastrocnemius posteriorly from the tibia, exposing the fascia of the deep posterior compartment, and divide this fascia longitudinally. Examine the muscles of the deep posterior compartment and the posterior tibial neurovascular bundle.
- The lateral incision (Fig. 17.14) follows a line between the lateral subcutaneous border of the tibia and the fibula. Incise the deep fascia of the anterior compartment and examine the muscles of the anterior compartment. Follow the undersurface of the anterior compartment fascia laterally to find the vertical septum of the peroneal compartment and incise this to gain access to the peroneal compartment. Examine the muscles of the peroneal compartment (Fig. 17.15a,b,c).

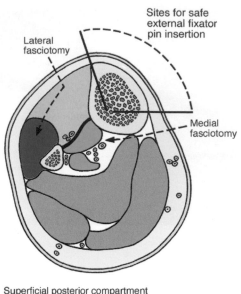

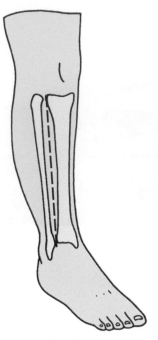

Superficial posterior compartment
(gastrocnemius, soleus)

Deep posterior compartment
(flexor hallucis longus, flexor digitorum longus, tibialis posterior)

Peroneal compartment
(peroneus longus, peroneus brevis)

Anterior compartment
(tibialis anterior, extensor hallucis longus,
extensor digitorum longus, peroneus tertius)

Fig. 17.12 Cross-section of the leg. There are four compartments in the lower leg; anterior, peroneal, superficial posterior, deep posterior (often neglected).

Lateral fasciotomy

Fig. 17.14 The lateral incision follows a line between the lateral subcutaneous border of the tibia and the fibula.

Wound closure

- Fasciotomy wounds cannot usually be closed directly. It may be possible to close them partially with sutures, or to close one side of the limb.
- Healing by secondary intention often produces over-granulating wounds and hypertrophic scars.
- Close open fasciotomy wounds with very thin split skin grafts (which will contract and facilitate later excision). Refer to plastic surgery or use a powered dermatome to minimize skin graft donor site morbidity.
- Splint the limb for 5 days after skin grafting to allow graft take.
- Leave the donor site dressing intact for 14 days.
- Avoid deep tension sutures or other methods of closure relying on tension, such as vascular slings looped between staples. These are slow and leave ugly, unstable scars.

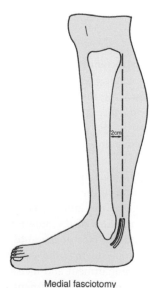

Medial fasciotomy

Fig. 17.13 The medial incision follows a line 2 cm posterior to the medial subcutaneous border of the tibia, from the knee to the ankle.

Post-operative rehabilitation

- Mobilize the limb under supervision of physiotherapists for 6–12 weeks to prevent adhesions and stiffness once wound is closed/skin graft stable.
- Night splints for 4–6 weeks to prevent contractures.

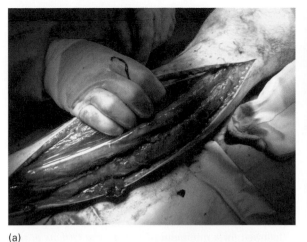

(a)

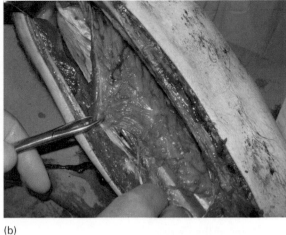

(b)

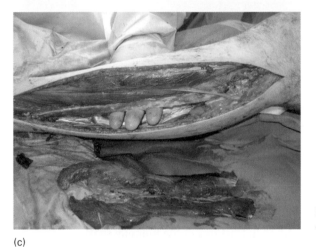

(c)

Fig. 17.15 a,b,c Medial and lateral incisions and excision of devitalized tissues.

- Upper limb in functional position (thumb abducted, 30° wrist extension, 60° MP (metaphalyngeal) joint flexion, 180° extension of PIP joint and DIP joint).
- Lower limb in ankle dorsiflexion.

Outpatient follow up

- See in dressing clinic until wounds are healed.
- Review at 6 weeks and 3 months.
- Consider excision of skin grafts or scar revision at 9–12 months.
- Consider tendon transfer or microvascular functional muscle transfer following significant loss of flexor or extensor compartment in upper limb (refer to plastic surgery).

Summary

- Acute compartment syndrome is common and dangerous.
- Adverse consequences can be prevented.
- Vigilance and suspicion are needed.
- Pressure measurement is the only useful investigation.
- Fasciotomy is the only useful treatment.

References

Part I Upper extremity
1 Fractures of the clavicle
1.1 Open reduction and internal fixation of midshaft fractures
Peter V. Giannoudis, B.Sc., M.B. B.S., M.D., E.E.C. (Orth.)

1. McKee, M. D., Wild, L. M., & Schemitsch, E. H. Midshaft malunions of the clavicle. Surgical technique. *J. Bone Joint Surg. Am.* 2004;**86-A** Suppl. **1**:37–43.
2. Hoe-Hansen, C. E. & Norlin, R. Intramedullary cancellous screw fixation for nonunion of midshaft clavicular fractures. *Acta Orthop. Scand.* 2003;**74**(3):361–4.
3. McKee, M. D., Wild, L. M., & Schemitsch, E. H. Midshaft malunions of the clavicle. *J. Bone Joint Surg. Am.* 2003;**85-A**(5):790–7.
4. Proubasta, I. R., Itarte, J. P., Caceres, E. P., *et al.* Biomechanical evaluation of fixation of clavicular fractures. *J. South. Orthop. Assoc.* 2002;**11**(3):148–52.
5. Zlowodzki, M., Zelle, B. A., Cole, P. A., Jeray, K., & McKee, M. D. Evidence-based orthopaedic trauma Working Group. Treatment of acute midshaft clavicle fractures: systematic review of 2144 fractures: on behalf of the Evidence-Based Orthopaedic Trauma Working Group. *J. Orthop. Trauma* 2005;**19**(7):504–7.

2 Section I: Fractures of the proximal humerus
2.1 General considerations
David Limb, B.Sc., F.R.C.S., Ed. (Orth.)

2.2 Tension band wiring for displaced greater tuberosity fractures
David Limb, B.Sc., F.R.C.S., Ed. (Orth.)

2.3 Open reduction and internal fixation of 3- and 4-part fractures (using a Philos plate)
David Limb, B.Sc., F.R.C.S., Ed. (Orth.)

2.4 Hemiarthroplasty for fracture dislocation
David Limb, B.Sc., F.R.C.S., Ed. (Orth.)

1. Bjorkenheim, J. M., Pajarinen, J., & Savolainen, V. Internal fixation of proximal humeral fractures with a locking compression plate: a retrospective evaluation of 72 patients followed for a minimum of 1 year. *Acta Orthop. Scand.* 2004;**75**(6):741–5.
2. Iannotti, J. P., Ramsey, M. L., Williams, G. R. Jr., & Warner, S. J. Nonprosthetic management of proximal humeral fractures. *Instruc. Course Lect.* 2004;**53**:405–16.
3. Kwon, Y. W. & Zuckerman, J. D. Outcomes after treatment of proximal humeral fractures with humeral head replacement. *Instruct. Course Lect.* 2005; **27**(3):232–7.
4. Mighell, M. A., Kolm, G. P., Collinge, C. A., & Frankle, M. A. Outcomes of hemiarthroplasty for fractures of the proximal humerus. *J. Shoulder Elbow Surg.* 2003;**12**(6):569–77.
5. Prakash, U., McGurty, D. W., & Dent, J. A. Hemiarthroplasty for severe fractures of the proximal humerus. *J. Shoulder Elbow Surg.* 2002;**11**(5):428–30.

Section II: Fractures of the humeral shaft
2.5 Open reduction and internal fixation: posterior approach
Peter V. Giannoudis, B.Sc., M.B. B.S., M.D., E.E.C. (Orth.)

1. Chao, T. C., Chou, W. Y., Chung, J. C., & Hsu, C. J. Humeral shaft fractures treated by dynamic compression plates, Ender nails and interlocking nails. *Int. Orthop.* 2005;**29**(2):88–91.
2. Crosby, L. A., Norris, B. L., Dao, K. D., & McGuire, M. H. Humeral shaft nonunions treated with fibular allograft and compression plating. *Am. J. Orthop.* 2000;**29**(1):45–7.
3. Gibbs, J. R., Pimple, M., & Ricketts, D. Bridge plate osteosynthesis of humeral shaft fractures. *Injury* 2005; **36**(4):576.
4. Schildhauer, T. A., Nork, S. E., Mills, W. J., & Henley, M. B. Extensor mechanism-sparing paratricipital posterior approach to the distal humerus. *J. Orthop. Trauma* 2003;**17**(5):374–8.
5. Ziran, B. H., Smith, W. R., Balk, M. L., Manning, C. M., & Agudelo, J. F. A true triceps-splitting approach for treatment of distal humerus fractures: a preliminary report. *J. Trauma* 2005;**58**(1):70–5.

2.6 Antegrade intramedullary nailing of the humerus
Paige T. Kendrick, B.A., Craig S. Roberts, M.D.,
David Seligson, M.D.

1. Ajmal, M., O'Sullivan, M., McCabe, J., & Curtin, W. Antegrade locked intramedullary nailing in humeral shaft fractures. *Injury* 2001;**32**(9):692–4.
2. Farragos, A. F., Schemitsch, E. H., & McKee, M. D. Complications of intramedullary nailing for fractures of the humeral shaft: a review. *J. Orthop. Trauma* 19.;**13**(4):258–67.
3. Lin, J. & Hou, S. M. Rotational alignment of humerus after closed locked nailing. *J. Trauma* 2000;**49**(5):854–9.
4. Lin, J., Hou, S. M., Inoue, N., Chao, E. Y., & Hang, Y. S. Anatomic considerations of locked humeral nailing. *Clin. Orthop. Rel. Res.* 1999;**368**:247–54.
5. Riemer, B. L. & D'Ambrosia, R. The risk of injury to the axillary nerve, artery, and vein from proximal locking screws of humeral intramedullary nails. *Orthopedics* 1992;**15**(6):697–9.

Section III: Fractures of the distal humerus
2.7 Open reduction and internal fixation of supracondylar fractures
Paige T. Kendrick, B.A., Craig S. Roberts, M.D.,
David Seligson, M.D.

1. Hausman, M. & Panozzo, A. Treatment of distal humerus fractures in the elderly. *Clin. Orthop. Rel. Res.* 2004;**425**:55–63.
2. Helfet, D. L. & Hotchkiss, R. N. Internal fixation of the distal humerus: a biomechanical comparison of methods. *J. Orthop. Trauma* 1990;**4**(3):260–4.
3. Jacobson, S. R., Glisson, R. R., & Urbaniak, J. R. Comparison of distal humerus fracture fixation: a biomechanical study. *J. South. Orthop. Assoc.* 1997;**6**(4):241–9.
4. Korner, J., Diederichs, G., Arzdorf, M., *et al.* A biomechanical evaluation of methods of distal humerus fracture fixation using locking compression plates versus conventional reconstruction plates. *J. Orthop. Trauma* 2004;**18**(5):286–93.
5. O'Driscoll, S. W. Optimizing stability in distal humeral fracture fixation. *J. Shoulder Elbow Surg.* 2005;**14**:186S–94S.

2.8 Open reduction internal fixation: capitellum
Paige T. Kendrick, B.A., Craig S. Roberts, M.D.,
David Seligson, M.D.

1. Poynton, A. R., Kelly, I. P., & O'Rourke, S. K. Fractures of the capitellum: a comparison of two fixation methods. *Injury* 1998;**29**(5):341–3.
2. Ring, D., Jupiter, J. B., & Gulotta, L. Articular fractures of the distal part of the humerus. *J. Bone Joint Surg.* 2003;**85-A**(2):232–8.
3. Sano, S., Rokkaku, T., Saito, S., Tokunaga, S., Abe, Y., & Moriya, H. Herbert screw fixation of capitellar fractures. *J. Shoulder Elbow Surg.* 2005;**14**(3):307–11.

2.9 Retrograde intramedullary nailing
Paige T. Kendrick, B.A., Craig S. Roberts, M.D.,
David Seligson, M.D.

1. Blum, J., Janzing, H., Gahr, R., Langendorff, H. S., & Rommens, P. M. Clinical performance of a new medullary humeral nail: antegrade versus retrograde insertion. *J. Orthop. Trauma* 2001;**15**(5):342–9.
2. Farragos, A. F., Schemitsch, E. H., & McKee, M. D. Complications of intramedullary nailing for fractures of the humeral shaft: a review. *J. Orthop. Trauma* 1999.;**13**(4): 258–67.
3. Kumta, S. M., Quintos, A. D., Griffin, J. F., Chow, L. T., & Wong, K. C. Closed retrograde nailing of pathological humeral fractures. *Int. Orthop.* 2002;**26**(1):17–19.
4. Lin, J., Hou, S. M., Inoue, N., Chao, E. Y., & Hang, Y. S. Anatomic considerations of locked humeral nailing. *Clin. Orthop. Rel. Res.* 19.;**368**:247–54.
5. Strothman, D., Templeman, D. C., Varecka, T., & Bechtold, J. Retrograde nailing of humeral shaft fractures: a biomechanical study of its effects on the strength of the distal humerus. *J. Orthop. Trauma* 2000;**14**(2):101–4.

2.10 Paediatric supracondylar fractures: MUA/percutaneous fixation of distal humerus fractures
Paige T. Kendrick, B.A., Craig S. Roberts, M.D.,
David Seligson, M.D.

1. Ay, S., Akinci, M., Kamiloglu, S., & Ercetin, O. Open reduction of displaced pediatric supracondylar humeral fractures through the anterior cubital approach. *J. Pediatr. Orthop.* 2005;**25**(2):149–53.
2. Mehlman, C. T., Strub, W. M., Roy, D. R., Wall, E. J., & Crawford, A. H. The effect of surgical timing on the perioperative complications of treatment of supracondylar humeral fractures in children. *J. Bone Joint Surg.* 2001;**83-A**(3):323–7.
3. Sabharwal, S., Tredwell, S. J., Beauchamp, R. D., *et al.* Management of pulseless pink hand in pediatric supracondylar fractures of the humerus. *J. Pediatr. Orthop.* 1997;**17**(3):303–10.

3 Section I: Fractures of the proximal ulna
3.1 Tension band wiring of olecranon fractures
Gregoris Kambouroglou, M.D.

3.2 Open reduction and internal fixation of olecranon fractures
Gregoris Kambouroglou, M.D.

1. Candal-Couto, J. J., Williams, J. R., & Sanderson, P. L. Impaired forearm rotation after tension-band-wiring fixation of olecranon fractures: evaluation of the transcortical K-wire technique. *J. Orthop. Trauma* 2005;**19**(7): 480–2.

2. Hutchinson, D. T., Horwitz, D. S., Ha, G., Thomas, C. W., & Bachus, K. N. Cyclic loading of olecranon fracture fixation constructs. *J. Bone Joint Surg. Am.* 2003;**85-A**(5):831–7.

3. Molloy, S., Jasper, L. E., Elliott, D. S., Brumback, R. J., & Belkoff, S. M. Biomechanical evaluation of intramedullary nail versus tension band fixation for transverse olecranon fractures. *J. Orthop. Trauma* 2004;**18**(3):170–4.

4. Rommens, P. M., Kuchle, R., Schneider, R. U., & Reuter, M. Olecranon fractures in adults: factors influencing outcome. *Injury* 2004;**35**(11):1149–57.

5. Wake, H., Hashizume, H., Nishida, K., Inoue, H., & Nagayama, N. Biomechanical analysis of the mechanism of elbow fracture-dislocations by compression force. *J. Orthop. Sci.* 2004;**9**(1):44–50.

Section II: Fractures of the ulnar shaft
3.3 Open reduction and internal fixation: plating
Gregoris Kambouroglou, M.D.

3.4 Elastic nails for ulnar shaft fractures
Gregoris Kambouroglou, M.D.

1. Henry, W. A., *Extensile Exposures*, 2nd edn. New York: Churchill Livingstone, 1973: p. 100.

2. Duncan, R., Geissler, W., Freeland, A. E., & Savoie, F. H. Immediate internal fixation of open fractures of the diaphysis of the forearm. *J. Orthop. Trauma* 1992; **6**:25–31.

3. Mittal, R., Hafez, M. A., & Templeton, P. A. "Failure" of forearm intramedullary elastic nails. *Injury* 2004;**35**(12):1319–21.

4. Myers, G. J., Gibbons, P. J., & Glithero, P. R. Nancy nailing of diaphyseal forearm fractures. Single bone fixation for fractures of both bones. *J. Bone Joint Surg. Br.* 2004;**86**(4):581–4.

Section III: Fractures of the distal ulna
3.5 Open reduction and internal fixation for distal ulnar fractures
Gregoris Kambouroglou, M.D.

1. Handoll, H. H. & Pearce, P. K. Interventions for isolated diaphyseal fractures of the ulna in adults. *Cochrane Database Syst. Rev.* 2004;(2):CD000523.

2. Mih, A. D., Cooney, W. P., Idler, R. S., & Lewallen, D. G. Long-term follow up of forearm bone diaphyseal plating. *Clin. Orthop.* 1994; **299**:256–8.

3. Schmittenbecher, P. P., State-of-the-art treatment of forearm shaft fractures. *Injury* 2005;**36** Suppl. 1:A25–34.

4 Section I: Fractures of the proximal radius
4.1 Open reduction and internal fixation of radial head fractures
Reinhard Meier, M.D.

4.2 Excision of radial head
Reinhard Meier, M.D.

1. Herbertsson, P., Josefsson, P. O., Hasserius, R., Besjakov, J., Nyqvist, F., & Karlsson, M. K. Fractures of the radial head and neck treated with radial head excision. *J. Bone Joint Surg. Am.* 2004;**86-A** (9):1925–30.

2. Ikeda, M., Yamashina, Y., Kamimoto, M., & Oka, Y. Open reduction and internal fixation of comminuted fractures of the radial head using low-profile mini-plates. *J. Bone Joint Surg. Br.* 2003;**85**(7):1040–4.

3. McKee, M. D., Pugh, D. M., Wild, L. M., Schemitsch, E. H., & King, G. J. Standard surgical protocol to treat elbow dislocations with radial head and coronoid fractures. Surgical technique. *J. Bone Joint Surg. Am.* 2005;**87** Suppl. 1(Pt 1):22–32.

4. Ring, D. Open reduction and internal fixation of fractures of the radial head. *Hand Clin.* 2004;**20**(4):415–27.

5. Ring, D., Quintero, J., & Jupiter, J. B. Open reduction and internal fixation of fractures of the radial head. *J. Bone Joint Surg. Am.* 2002;**84-A**(10):1811–15.

Section II: Fractures of the radial shaft
4.3 Open reduction and internal fixation: anterior approach
Christopher C. Tzioupis, M.D., Trauma Fellow, Peter V. Giannoudis, B.Sc., M.B. B.S., M.D., E.E.C. (Orth.)

1. Eglseder, W. A., Jasper, L. E., Davis, C. W., & Belkoff, S. M. A biomechanical evaluation of lateral plating of distal radial shaft fractures. *J. Hand Surg. [Am.]* 2003;**28**(6):959–63.

2. Fernandez Dell' Oca, A. A. & Masliah Galante, R. Osteosynthesis of diaphyseal fractures of the radius and ulna using an internal fixator (PC-Fix). A prospective study. *Injury* 2001;**32** Suppl. 2:B44–50.

3. Murray, P. M. Diagnosis and treatment of longitudinal instability of the forearm. *Tech. Hand Up. Extrem. Surg.* 2005;**9**(1):29–34.

4. Schmittenbecher, P. P. State-of-the-art treatment of forearm shaft fractures. *Injury* 2005;**36** Suppl. 1:A25–34.

4.4 Elastic intramedullary nailing for diaphyseal forearm fractures in children
Brian W. Scott, F.R.C.S., Orth.

1. Calder, P. R., Achan, P., & Barry, M. Diaphyseal forearm fractures in children treated with intramedullary fixation: outcome of K-wire versus elastic stable intramedullary nail. *Injury* 2003;**34**(4):278–82.

2. Jubel, A., Andermahr, J., Isenberg, J., *et al.* Outcomes and complications of elastic stable intramedullary nailing for forearm fractures in children. *J. Pediatr. Orthop. B* 2005;**14**(5):375–80.

3. Lee, S., Nicol, R. O., & Stott, N. S. Intramedullary fixation for pediatric unstable forearm fractures. *Clin. Orthop. Rel. Res.* 2002;**402**:245–50.

4. Rodriguez-Merchan, E. C. Pediatric fractures of the forearm. *Clin. Orthop. Rel. Res.* 2005;**432**:65–72.

5. Yung, P. S., Lam, C. Y., Ng, B. K., Lam, T. P., & Cheng, J. C. Percutaneous transphyseal intramedullary Kirschner wire pinning: a safe and effective procedure for treatment of displaced diaphyseal forearm fracture in children. *J. Pediatr. Orthop.* 2004;**24**(1):7–12.

Section III: Fractures of the distal radius

4.5 Open reduction and internal fixation for distal radius fractures: volar approach

Peter V. Giannoudis, B.Sc., M.B. B.S, M.D., E.E.C. (Orth.)

1. Drobetz, H. & Kutscha-Lissberg, E. Osteosynthesis of distal radial fractures with a volar locking screw plate system. *Int. Orthop.* 2003;**27**(1):1–6.

2. Orbay, J. L. & Fernandez, D. L. Volar fixation for dorsally displaced fractures of the distal radius: a preliminary report. *J. Hand Surg. [Am.]* 2002;**27**(2):205–15.

3. Orbay, J. L. The treatment of unstable distal radius fractures with volar fixation. *Hand Surg.* 2000;**5**(2):103–12.

4. Smith, D. W. & Henry, M. H. Volar fixed-angle plating of the distal radius. *J. Am. Acad. Orthop. Surg.* 2005;**13**(1):28–36.

5. Wright, T. W., Horodyski, M., & Smith, D. W. Functional outcome of unstable distal radius fractures: ORIF with a volar fixed-angle tine plate versus external fixation. *J. Hand Surg. [Am.]* 2005;**30**(2):289–99.

4.6 Open reduction and internal fixation for distal radius fractures: dorsal approach

Doug Campbell, F.R.C.S., Orth.

1. Ruch, D. S., Ginn, T. A., Yang, C. C., *et al.* Use of a distraction plate for distal radial fractures with metaphyseal and diaphyseal comminution. *J. Bone Joint Surg. Am.* 2005;**87**(5):945–54.

2. Ruch, D. S., Weiland, A. J., Wolfe, S. W., Geissler, W. B., Cohen, M. S., & Jupiter, J. B. Current concepts in the treatment of distal radial fractures. *Instruc. Course Lect.* 2004;**53**:389–401.

3. Sanchez, T., Jakubietz, M., Jakubietz, R., *et al.* Complications after Pi Plate osteosynthesis. *Plast. Reconstr. Surg.* 2005;**116**(1):153–8.

4. Trease, C., McIff, T., & Toby, E. B. Locking versus nonlocking T-plates for dorsal and volar fixation of dorsally comminuted distal radius fractures: a biomechanical study. *J. Hand Surg. [Am.]* 2005;**30**(4):756–63.

5. Trumble, T. E., Culp, R. W., Hanel, D. P., Geissler, W. B., & Berger, R. A. Intra-articular fractures of the distal aspect of the radius. *Instruc. Course Lect.* 1999.;**48**:465–80.

4.7 Closed reduction and K-wire fixation of distal radius fractures

Reinhard Meier, M.D.

1. Azzopardi, T., Ehrendorfer, S., Coulton, T., & Abela, M. Unstable extra-articular fractures of the distal radius: a prospective, randomised study of immobilisation in a cast versus supplementary percutaneous pinning. *J. Bone Joint Surg. Br.* 2005;**87**(6):837–40.

2. Lindemann-Sperfeld, L., Pilz, F., Marintschev, I., & Otto, W. Fractures of the distal radius. Minimally invasive pin fixation: indications and results. *Chirurgie* 2003;**74**(11):1000–8.

3. Singh, S., Trikha, P., & Twyman, R. Superficial radial nerve damage due to Kirschner wiring of the radius. *Injury* 2005;**36**(2):330–2.

4. Strohm, P. C., Muller, C. A., Boll, T., & Pfister, U. Two procedures for Kirschner wire osteosynthesis of distal radial fractures. A randomized trial. *J. Bone Joint Surg. Am.* 2004;**86-A**(12):2621–8.

5. Willcox, N., Kurta, I., & Menez, D. Treatment of distal radial fractures with grafting and K-wiring. *Acta Orthop. Belg.* 2005;**71**(1):36–40.

4.8 Closed reduction and application of an external fixator in distal radius fractures

Reinhard Meier, M.D.

1. Bednar, D. A. & Al-Harran, H. Nonbridging external fixation for fractures of the distal radius. *Can. J. Surg.* 2004;**47**(6):426–30.

2. Dicpinigaitis, P., Wolinsky, P., Hiebert, R., *et al.* Can external fixation maintain reduction after distal radius fractures? *J. Trauma* 2004;**57**(4):845–50.

3. Grewal, R., Perey, B., Wilmink, M., & Stothers, K. A randomized prospective study on the treatment of intra-articular distal radius fractures: open reduction and internal fixation with dorsal plating versus mini open reduction, percutaneous fixation, and external fixation. *J. Hand Surg. [Am.]* 2005;**30**(4):764–72.

4. Harley, B. J., Scharfenberger, A., Beaupre, L. A., Jomha, N., & Weber, D. W. Augmented external fixation versus percutaneous pinning and casting for unstable fractures of the distal radius–a prospective randomized trial. *J. Hand Surg. [Am.]* 2004;**29**(5):815–24.

5. Hegeman, J. H., Oskam, J., Vierhout, P. A., & Ten Duis, H. J. External fixation for unstable intra-articular distal radial fractures in women older than 55 years. Acceptable functional end results in the majority of the patients despite significant secondary displacement. *Injury* 2005;**36**(2):339–44.

6. Krishnan, J., Wigg, A. E., Walker, R. W., & Slavotinek, J. Intra-articular fractures of the distal radius: a prospective randomised controlled trial comparing static bridging and

dynamic non-bridging external fixation. *J. Hand Surg. [Br.]* 2003;**28**(5):417–21.

5 Fractures of wrist

5.1 Percutaneous fixation of scaphoid fractures
Doug Campbell, F.R.C.S. (Orth.)

1. Chen, A. C., Chao, E. K., Hung, S. S., Lee, M. S., & Ueng, S. W. Percutaneous screw fixation for unstable scaphoid fractures. *J. Trauma* 2005;**59**(1):184–7.
2. Cooney, W. P. 3rd. Scaphoid fractures: current treatments and techniques. *Instruc. Course Lect.* 2003;**52**:197–208.
3. Jeon, I. H., Oh, C. W., Park, B. C., Ihn, J. C., & Kim, P. T. Minimal invasive percutaneous Herbert screw fixation in acute unstable scaphoid fracture. *Hand Surg.* 2003;**8**(2):213–18.
4. Wu, W. C. Percutaneous cannulated screw fixation of acute scaphoid fractures. *Hand Surg.* 2002;**7**(2):271–8.
5. Yip, H. S., Wu, W. C., Chang, R. Y., & So, T. Y. Percutaneous cannulated screw fixation of acute scaphoid waist fracture. *J. Hand Surg. [Br.]* 2002;**27**(1):42–6.

5.2 Open reduction and internal fixation of acute scapholunate dissociation
Doug Campbell, F.R.C.S. (Orth.)

1. Bloom, H. T., Freeland, A. E., Bowen, V., & Mrkonjic, L. The treatment of chronic scapholunate dissociation: an evidence-based assessment of the literature. *Orthopedics* 2003;**26**(2):195–203.
2. Moran, S. L., Cooney, W. P., Berger, R. A., & Strickland, J. Capsulodesis for the treatment of chronic scapholunate instability. *J. Hand Surg. [Am.]* 2005;**30**(1):16–23.
3. Minami, A., Kato, H., & Iwasaki, N. Treatment of scapholunate dissociation: ligamentous repair associated with modified dorsal capsulodesis. *Hand Surg.* 2003;**8**(1):1–6.
4. Shih, J. T., Lee, H. M., Hou, Y. T., Horng, S. T., & Tan, C. M. Dorsal capsulodesis and ligamentoplasty for chronic pre-dynamic and dynamic scapholunate dissociation. *Hand Surg.* 2003;**8**(2):173–8.
5. Tomaino, M. M., Preliminary lunate reduction and pinning facilitates restoration of carpal height when treating perilunate dislocation, scaphoid fracture and nonunion, and scapholunate dissociation. *Am. J. Orthop.* 2004;**33**(3):153–4.

6 Section I: Fractures of the first metacarpal

6.1 K-wire fixation of basal fractures of the first metacarpal
Reinhard Meier, M.D.

1. Cullen, J. P., Parentis, M. A., Chinchilli, V. M., & Pellegrini, V. D. Simulated Bennett fracture treated with closed reduction and percutaneous pinning. *J. Bone Joint Surg.* 1997; **79-A**: 413–20.
2. Lutz, M., Angermann, P., Sailer, R., Kathrein, A., Gabl, M., & Pechlaner, S. Closed reduction and percutaneous K-wire fixation of Bennett's fracture dislocation. *Handchir. Mikrochir. Plast. Chir.* 2002;**34**(1):41–8.
3. Sawaizumi, T., Nanno, M., Nanbu, A., & Ito, H. Percutaneous leverage pinning in the treatment of Bennett's fracture. *J. Orthop. Sci.* 2005;**10**(1):27–31.
4. Soyer, A. D. Fractures of the base of the first metacarpal: current treatment options. *J. Am. Acad. Orthop. Surg.* 1999.;**7**(6):403–12.

6.2 Open reduction and internal fixation of basal fractures of the first metacarpal
Reinhard Meier, M.D.

1. Bruske, J., Bednarski, M., Niedzwiedz, Z., Zyluk, A., & Grzeszewski, S. The results of operative treatment of fractures of the thumb metacarpal base. *Acta Orthop. Belg.* 2001;**67**(4):368–73.
2. Meyer, C., Hartmann, B., Bohringer, G., Horas, U., & Schnettler, R. Minimal invasive cannulated screw osteosynthesis of Bennett's fractures. *Zentralbl. Chir.* 2003;**128**(6):529–33.
3. Rolando, S. Fracture of the base of the first metacarpal and a variation that has not yet been described. *Clin. Orthop. Rel. Res.* 1996;**327**:4–8.

6.3 Ulnar collateral ligament repair
Reinhard Meier, M.D.

1. Draganich, L. F., Greenspahn, S., & Mass, D. P. Effects of the adductor pollicis and abductor pollicis brevis on thumb metacarpophalangeal joint laxity before and after ulnar collateral ligament reconstruction. *J. Hand Surg. [Am.]* 2004;**29**(3):481–8.
2. Firoozbakhsh, K., Yi, I. S., Moneim, M. S., & Umada, Y. A study of ulnar collateral ligament of the thumb metacarpophalangeal joint. *Clin. Orthop. Rel. Res.* 2002;**403**:240–7.
3. Harley, B. J., Werner, F. W., & Green, J. K. A biomechanical modeling of injury, repair, and rehabilitation of ulnar collateral ligament injuries of the thumb. *J. Hand Surg. [Am.]* 2004;**29**(5):915–20.
4. Oka, Y., Harayama, H., & Ikeda, M. Reconstructive procedure to repair chronic injuries to the collateral ligament of metacarpophalangeal joints of the hand. *Hand Surg.* 2003;**8**(1):81–5.

Section II: Fractures of the metacarpals II–V

6.4 Open reduction and internal fixation of midshaft fractures of the metacarpals
Reinhard Meier, M.D.

1. Dona, E., Gillies, R. M., Gianoutsos, M. P., & Walsh, W. R. Plating of metacarpal fractures: unicortical or bicortical screws? *J. Hand Surg. [Br.]* 2004;**29**(3):218–21.

2. Freeland, A. E., Geissler, W. B., & Weiss, A. P. Surgical treatment of common displaced and unstable fractures of the hand. *Instruc. Course Lect*. 2002;**51**:185–201.

3. McNemar, T. B., Howell, J. W., & Chang, E. Management of metacarpal fractures. *J. Hand Ther*. 2003;**16**(2):143–51.

4. Ouellette, E. A., Dennis, J. J., Milne, E. L., Latta, L. L., & Makowski, A. L. Role of soft tissues in metacarpal fracture fixation. *Clin. Orthop. Rel. Res*. 2003;**412**:169–75.

5. Roth, J. J. & Auerbach, D. M. Fixation of hand fractures with bicortical screws. *J. Hand Surg. [Am.]* 2005;**30**(1):151–3.

6.5 Closed reduction and intramedullary fixation of distal third fractures of the metacarpals II–V
Reinhard Meier, M.D.

1. Black, D. M., Mann, R. J., Constine, R., & Daniels, A. U. Comparison of internal fixation techniques in metacarpal fracture. *J. Hand Surg. [Am.]* 1985; **10**:466–72.

2. Foucher, G., "Bouquet" osteosynthesis in metacarpal neck fractures: a series of 66 patients. *J. Hand Surg. [Am.]* 1995;**20**:S86–90.

3. Greene, T. L., Metacarpal fractures. In *American Society for the Surgery of the Hand*, ed. Hand Surgery Update. Rosemont, IL: American Academy of Orthopaedic Surgery, 1996: 11–15.

4. Kozin, S. H., Thoder, J. J., & Lieberman, G. Operative treatment of metacarpal and phalangeal shaft fractures. *J. Am. Acad. Orthop. Surg*. 2000;**8**(2):111–21.

Section III: Fractures of the phalanx
6.6 Open reduction and internal fixation of condylar fractures
Reinhard Meier, M.D.

6.7 Open reduction and internal fixation of midshaft fractures
Reinhard Meier, M.D.

1. Badia, A. & Riano, F. A simple fixation method for unstable bony mallet finger. *J. Hand Surg. [Am.]* 2004;**29**(6):1051–5.

2. Freeland, A. E. & Benoist, L.A. Open reduction and internal fixation method for fractures at the proximal interphalangeal joint. *Hand Clin*.1994; **10**:239–50.

3. Horton, T. C., Hatton, M., & Davis, T. R. A prospective randomized controlled study of fixation of long oblique and spiral shaft fractures of the proximal phalanx: closed reduction and percutaneous Kirschner wiring versus open reduction and lag screw fixation. *J. Hand Surg. [Br.]* 2003;**28**(1):5–9.

4. Lahav, A., Teplitz, G. A., & McCormack, R. R. Jr. Percutaneous reduction and Kirschner-wire fixation of impacted intra-articular fractures and volar lip fractures of the proximal interphalangeal joint. *Am. J. Orthop*. 2005;**34**(2): 62–5.

5. Ouellette, E. A., Dennis, J. J., Latta, L. L., Milne, E. L., & Makowski, A. L. The role of soft tissues in plate fixation of proximal phalanx fractures. *Clin. Orthop. Rel. Res*. 2004;**418**:213–18.

Part II Pelvis and acetabulum
7 Fractures of the pelvic ring
7.1 Application of anterior frame
Peter V. Giannoudis, B.Sc., M.B. B.S., M.D., E.E.C. (Orth.)

1. Chiu, F. Y., Chuang, T. Y., & Lo, W. H. Treatment of unstable pelvic fractures: use of a transiliac sacral rod for posterior lesions and an external fixator for anterior lesions. *J. Trauma* 2004;**57**(1):141–4.

2. Galois, L., Pfeffer, F., Mainard, D., & Delagoutte, J. P. The value of external fixation for unstable pelvic ring injuries. *Acta Orthop. Belg*. 2003;**69**(4):321–7.

3. Haidukewych, G. J., Kumar, S., & Prpa, B. Placement of half-pins for supra-acetabular external fixation: an anatomic study. *Clin. Orthop. Rel. Res*. 2003;**411**:269–73.

4. Mason, W. T., Khan, S. N., James, C. L., Chesser, T. J., & Ward, A. J. Complications of temporary and definitive external fixation of pelvic ring injuries. *Injury* 2005;**36**(5):599–604.

5. Ponsen, K. J., Hoek van Dijke, G. A., Joosse, P., & Snijders, C. J. External fixators for pelvic fractures: comparison of the stiffness of current systems. *Acta Orthop. Scand*. 2003;**74**(2):165–71.

7.2 Plating of the pubic symphysis
Peter V. Giannoudis, B.Sc., M.B. B.S., M.D., E.E.C. (Orth.)

1. Phieffer, L. S., Lundberg, W. P., & Templeman, D. C. Instability of the posterior pelvic ring associated with disruption of the pubic symphysis. *Orthop. Clin. North Am*. 2004;**35**(4):445–9.

2. Raman, R., Roberts, C. S., Pape, H. C., & Giannoudis, P. V. Implant retention and removal after internal fixation of the symphysis pubis. *Injury* 2005;**36**(7):827–31.

3. Sagi, H. C., Ordway, N. R., & DiPasquale, T. Biomechanical analysis of fixation for vertically unstable sacroiliac dislocations with iliosacral screws and symphyseal plating. *J. Orthop. Trauma* 2004;**18**(3):138–43.

4. Templeman, D. C., Simpson, T., & Matta, J. M. Surgical management of pelvic ring injuries. *Instruc. Course Lect*. 2005;**54**:395–400.

7.3 Sacroiliac screw insertion
Peter V. Giannoudis, B.Sc., M.B. B.S., M.D., E.E.C. (Orth.)

1. Hinsche, A. F., Giannoudis, P. V., & Smith, R. M. Fluoroscopy-based multiplanar image guidance for insertion of sacroiliac screws. *Clin. Orthop. Rel. Res*. 2002;**395**:135–44.

2. Sagi, H. C. & Lindvall, E. M. Inadvertent intraforaminal iliosacral screw placement despite apparent appropriate

positioning on intraoperative fluoroscopy. *J. Orthop. Trauma* 2005;**19**(2):130–3.

3. Routt, M., Simonian, P., & Inaba, J. Iliosacral screw fixation of the disrupted sacroiliac joint. *Tech. Orthop.* 1994; **9**:300–14.

4. Simonian, P. T., Routt, M. L. C., Harrington, R. M., & Tencerr, A. F. Internal fixation of the transforaminal sacral fracture. *Clin. Orthop.* 1996; **323**:202–9.

5. van den Bosch, E. W., van Zwienen, C. M., & van Vugt, A. B. Fluoroscopic positioning of sacroiliac screws in 88 patients. *J. Trauma* 2002;**53**(1):44–8.

7.4 Open reduction and internal fixation of Sacro-iliac joint anteriorly

Peter V. Giannoudis, B.Sc., M.B. B.S., M.D., E.E.C. (Orth.)

1. Latenser, B., Gentilello, L., & Tarver, A. Improved outcome with early fixation of skeletally unstable pelvic fractures. *J. Trauma* 1991; **31**:28–31.

2. Leighton, R. K. & Waddell, J. P. Techniques for reduction and posterior fixation through the anterior approach. *Clin. Orthop. Rel. Res.* 1996;**329**:115–20.

3. Matta, J. & Saucedo, T. Internal fixation of pelvic ring fractures. *Clin. Orthop.* 1989; **242**:83–7.

4. Yinger, K., Scalise, J., Olson, S. A., Bay, B. K., & Finkemeier, C. G. Biomechanical comparison of posterior pelvic ring fixation. *J. Orthop. Trauma* 2003;**17**(7):481–7.

8 Fractures of the acetabulum

8.1 Open reduction and internal fixation of posterior wall fractures

Peter V. Giannoudis, B.Sc., M.B. B.S., M.D., E.E.C. (Orth.)

1. Giannoudis, P. V., Grotz, M. R., Papakostidis, C., & Dinopoulos, H. Operative treatment of displaced fractures of the acetabulum. A meta-analysis. *J. Bone Joint Surg. Br.* 2005;**87**(1):2–9.

2. Morgan, S. J., Jeray, K., & Kellam, J. F. Treatment of acetabular fractures. *J. South. Orthop. Assoc.* 2000;**9**(1):55–64.

3. Richter, H., Hutson, J. J., & Zych, G. The use of spring plates in the internal fixation of acetabular fractures. *J. Orthop. Trauma* 2004;**18**(3):179–81.

4. Tornetta, P. 3rd. Displaced acetabular fractures: indications for operative and nonoperative management. *J. Am. Acad. Orthop. Surg.* 2001;**9**(1):18–28.

5. Wiss, D. A., What's new in orthopaedic trauma. *J. Bone Joint Surg. Am.* 2002;**84**-A(11):2111–19.

8.2 Open reduction and internal fixation via the ilioinguinal approach

Peter V. Giannoudis, B.Sc., M.B. B.S., M.D., E.E.C. (Orth.)

1. Karunakar, M. A., Le, T. T., & Bosse, M. J. The modified ilioinguinal approach. *J. Orthop. Trauma* 2004;**18**(6):379–83.

2. Kloen, P., Siebenrock, K. A., & Ganz, R. Modification of the ilioinguinal approach. *J. Orthop. Trauma* 2002;**16**(8):586–93.

3. Matta, J. M. Operative treatment of acetabular fractures through the ilioinguinal approach. *Clin. Orthop.* 1994; **305**:10–19.

4. Qureshi, A. A., Archdeacon, M. T., Jenkins, M. A., Infante, A., DiPasquale, T., & Bolhofner, B. R. Infrapectineal plating for acetabular fractures: a technical adjunct to internal fixation. *J. Orthop. Trauma* 2004;**18**(3):175–8.

5. Stockle, U., Hoffmann, R., Nittinger, M., Sudkamp, N. P., & Haas, N. P. Screw fixation of acetabular fractures. *Int. Orthop.* 2000;**24**(3):143–7.

Part III: Lower extremity
9 Section I: Extracapsular fractures of the hip
9.1 Dynamic compression hip screw

Raghu Raman, M.R.C.S., Specialist Registrar Peter V. Giannoudis, B.Sc., M.B. B.S., M.D., E.E.C. (Orth.)

1. Lorich, D. G., Geller, D. S., & Nielson, J. H. Osteoporotic pertrochanteric hip fractures: management and current controversies. *Instruc. Course Lect.* 2004;**53**:441–54.

2. Moroni, A., Faldini, C., Pegreffi F., *et al.* Dynamic hip screw compared with external fixation for treatment of osteoporotic pertrochanteric fractures. A prospective, randomized study. *J. Bone Joint Surg. Am.* 2005;**87**(4):753–9.

3. Pajarinen, J., Lindahl, J., Michelsson, O., Savolainen, V., & Hirvensalo, E. Pertrochanteric femoral fractures treated with a dynamic hip screw or a proximal femoral nail. A randomised study comparing post-operative rehabilitation. *J. Bone Joint Surg. Br.* 2005;**87**(1):76–81.

4. Parker, M. J. & Handoll, H. H. Gamma and other cephalocondylic intramedullary nails versus extramedullary implants for extracapsular hip fractures. *Cochrane Database Syst. Rev.* 2004;**1**:CD000093.

Section II: Intracapsular fractures of the hip
9.2 Cannulated screw fixation

Christopher C. Tzioupis, M.D., Trauma Fellow, Peter V. Giannoudis, B.Sc., M.B. B.S., M.D., E.E.C. (Orth.)

1. Chen, W. C., Yu, S. W., Tseng, I. C., Su, J. Y., Tu, Y. K., & Chen, W. J. Treatment of undisplaced femoral neck fractures in the elderly. *J. Trauma* 2005;**58**(5):1035–9.

2. Gardner, M. J., Lorich, D. G., & Lane, J. M. Osteoporotic femoral neck fractures: management and current controversies. *Instruc. Course Lect.* 2004;**53**:427–39.

3. Maurer, S. G., Wright, K. E., Kummer, F. J., Zuckerman, J. D., & Koval, K. J. Two or three screws for fixation of femoral neck fractures? *Am. J. Orthop.* 2003;**32**(9):438–42.

4. Parker, M. J. & Tagg, C. E. Internal fixation of intracapsular fractures. *J. Roy. Coll. Surg. Edin.* 2002;**47**(3):541–7.

5. Selvan, V. T., Oakley, M. J., Rangan, A., & Al-Lami, M. K. Optimum configuration of cannulated hip screws for the fixation of intracapsular hip fractures: a biomechanical study. *Injury* 2004;**35**(2):136–41.

9.3 Hemiarthroplasty for intracapsular hip fractures: Austin Moore uncemented arthroplasty and Thompson's cemented arthroplasty
David A. Macdonald, F.R.C.S. (Orth.)

1. Dixon, S. & Bannister, G. Cemented bipolar hemiarthroplasty for displaced intracapsular fracture in the mobile active elderly patient. *Injury* 2004;**35**(2):152–6.
2. Khan, R. J., MacDowell, A., Crossman, P. *et al.* Hip fractures in Hungary and Sweden - differences in treatment and rehabilitation. *Int. Orthop.* 2002;**26**(4):222–8.
3. Parker, M. J., Khan, R. J., Crawford, J., & Pryor, G. A. Hemiarthroplasty versus internal fixation for displaced intracapsular hip fractures in the elderly. A randomised trial of 455 patients. *J. Bone Joint Surg. Br.* 2002;**84**(8):1150–5.
4. Rodriguez-Merchan, E. C., Displaced intracapsular hip fractures: hemiarthroplasty or total arthroplasty? *Clin. Orthop. Rel. Res.* 2002;**399**:72–7.
5. Sharif, K. M. & Parker, M. J. Austin Moore hemiarthroplasty: technical aspects and their effects on outcome, in patients with fractures of the neck of femur. *Injury* 2002;**33**(5):419–22.

10 Section I: Subtrochanteric fractures of the femur

10.1 Intramedullary fixation for subtrochanteric fractures using a proximal femoral nail
Peter V. Giannoudis, B.Sc., M.B. B.S, M.D., E.E.C. (Orth.)

1. Bedi, A. & Toan, Le T. Subtrochanteric femur fractures. *Orthop. Clin. North Am.* 2004;**35**(4):473–83.
2. Bredbenner, T. L., Snyder, S. A., Mazloomi, F. R., Le, T., & Wilber, R. G. Subtrochanteric fixation stability depends on discrete fracture surface points. *Clin. Orthop. Rel. Res.* 2005;**432**:217–25.
3. Haidukewych, G. J. & Berry, D. J. Nonunion of fractures of the subtrochanteric region of the femur. *Clin. Orthop. Rel. Res.* 2004;**419**:185–8.
4. Kakkar, R., Kumar, S., & Singh, A. K. Cephalomedullary nailing for proximal femoral fractures. *Int. Orthop.* 2005;**29**(1):21–4.

Section II: Fractures of the femoral shaft

10.2 General aspects
Hans-Christoph Pape, M.D., Stefan Hankemeier, M.D., Thomas Gosling, M.D.

10.3 Open reduction and internal fixation: plating
Stefan Hankemeier, M.D., Thomas Gosling, M.D., Hans-Christoph Pape, M.D.

10.4 Intramedullary nailing
Stefan Hankemeier, M.D., Thomas Gosling, M.D., Hans-Christoph Pape, M.D.

10.5 Flexible intramedullary nails in children
Brian W. Scott, F.R.C.S. (Orth.)

1. Barry, M. & Paterson, J. M. A flexible intramedullary nails for fractures in children. *J. Bone Joint Surg. Br.* 2004;**86**(7):947–53.
2. Cummings, R. J. Paediatric femoral fracture. *Lancet* 2005; **26**;365(9465):1116–17.
3. Flynn, J. M. & Schwend, R. M. Management of pediatric femoral shaft fractures. *J. Am. Acad. Orthop. Surg.* 2004;**12**(5):347–59.
4. Metaizeau, J. P. Stable elastic intramedullary nailing for fractures of the femur in children. *J. Bone Joint Surg. Br.* 2004;**86**(7):954–7.

10.6 Application of an external fixator
Stefan Hankemeier, M.D., Thomas Gosling, M.D., Hans-Christoph Pape, M.D.

1. Giannoudis, P. V., Pape, H. C., Cohen, A. P., Krettek, C., & Smith, R. M. Review: systemic effects of femoral nailing: from Kuntscher to the immune reactivity era. *Clin. Orthop. Rel. Res.* 2002;**404**:378–86.
2. Malik, Z. U., Hanif, M. S., Safdar, A., & Masood, T. Planned external fixation to locked intramedullary nailing conversion for open fractures of shaft of femur and tibia. *J. Coll. Physi. Surg. Pak.* 2005;**15**(3):133–6.
3. Noumi, T., Yokoyama, K., Ohtsuka, H., Nakamura, K., & Itoman, M. Intramedullary nailing for open fractures of the femoral shaft: evaluation of contributing factors on deep infection and nonunion using multivariate analysis. *Injury* 2005;**36**(9):1085–93.
4. Seligson, D., Mulier, T., Keirsbilck, S., & Been, J. Plating of femoral shaft fractures. A review of 15 cases. *Acta Orthop. Belg.* 2001;**67**(1):24–31.
5. Tigani, D., Fravisini, M., Stagni, C., Pascarella, R., Boriani, S. Interlocking nail for femoral shaft fractures: is dynamization always necessary? *Int. Orthop.* 2005;**29**(2):101–4.
6. Wolinsky, P., Tejwani, N., Richmond, J. H., Koval, K. J., Egol, K., & Stephen, D. J. Controversies in intramedullary nailing of femoral shaft fractures. *Instruc. Course Lect.* 2002;**51**:291–303.

Section III: Fractures of the distal femur

10.7 General aspects
Stefan Hankemeier, M.D., Thomas Gosling, M.D., Hans-Christoph Pape, M.D.

10.8 Minimally invasive plate osteosynthesis
Stefan Hankemeier, M.D., Thomas Gosling, M.D., Hans-Christoph Pape, M.D.

10.9 Retrograde nailing
Stefan Hankemeier, M.D., Thomas Gosling, M.D.,
Hans-Christoph Pape, M.D.

1. Kregor, P. J., Stannard, J. A., Zlowodzki, M., & Cole, P. A. Treatment of distal femur fractures using the less invasive stabilization system: surgical experience and early clinical results in 103 fractures. *J. Orthop. Trauma* 2004;**18**(8):509–20.
2. Krupp, R. J., Malkani, A. L., Goodin, R. A., & Voor, M. J. Optimal entry point for retrograde femoral nailing. *J. Orthop. Trauma* 2003; **17**: 100–5.
3. Markmiller, M., Konrad, G., & Sudkamp, N. Femur-LISS and distal femoral nail for fixation of distal femoral fractures: are there differences in outcome and complications? *Clin. Orthop. Rel. Res.* 2004;**426**: 252–7.
4. Ricci, A. R., Yue, J. J., Taffet, R., Catalano, J. B., DeFalco, R. A., & Wilkens, K. J. Less invasive stabilization system for treatment of distal femur fractures. *Am. J. Orthop.* 2004;**33**(5):250–5.
5. Seifert, J., Stengel, D., Matthes, G., Hinz, P., Ekkernkamp, A., & Ostermann, P. A. Retrograde fixation of distal femoral fractures: results using a new nail system. *J. Orthop. Trauma* 2003;**17**: 488–95.
6. Wong, M. K., Leung, F., & Chow, S. P. Treatment of distal femoral fractures in the elderly using a less-invasive plating technique. *Int. Orthop.* 2005;**29**(2):117–20.

11 Fractures of the patella
11.1 Tension band wiring
Stefan Hankemeier, M.D., Thomas Gosling, M.D.,
Hans-Christoph Pape, M.D.

1. Gardner, M. J., Griffith, M. H., Lawrence, B. D., & Lorich, D. G. Complete exposure of the articular surface for fixation of patellar fractures. *J. Orthop. Trauma* 2005;**19**(2):118–23.
2. Mehdi, M., Husson, J. L., Polard, J. L., Ouahmed, A., Poncer, R., & Lombard, J. Treatment results of fractures of the patella using pre-patellar tension wiring. Analysis of a series of 203 cases. *Acta Orthop. Belg.* 19.;**65**(2):188–96.
3. Patel, V. R., Parks, B. G., Wang, Y., Ebert, F. R., & Jinnah, R. H. Fixation of patella fractures with braided polyester suture: a biomechanical study. *Injury* 2000;**31**(1):1–6.
4. Wu, C. C., Tai, C. L., & Chen, W. J. Patellar tension band wiring: a revised technique. *Arch. Orthop. Trauma Surg.* 2001;**121**(1–2):12–16.

12 Section I: Fractures of the proximal tibia
12.1 Open reduction and internal fixation of a lateral tibial plateau fracture
John F. Keating, M. Phil., F.R.C.S. (Orth.)

12.2 Open reduction and internal fixation of a bicondylar tibial plateau fracture
John F. Keating, M. Phil., F.R.C.S. (Orth.)

12.3 External fixation of bicondylar tibial plateau fractures
John F. Keating, M. Phil., F.R.C.S. (Orth.)

1. Dirschl, D. R. & Dawson, P. A. Injury severity assessment in tibial plateau fractures. *Clin. Orthop. Rel. Res.* 2004;**423**:85–92.
2. Ebraheim, N. A., Sabry, F. F., & Haman, S. P. Open reduction and internal fixation of 117 tibial plateau fractures. *Orthopedics* 2004;**27**(12):1281–7.
3. El Barbary, H., Abdel, Ghani, H., Misbah, H., & Salem, K. Complex tibial plateau fractures treated with Ilizarov external fixator with or without minimal internal fixation. *Int. Orthop.* 2005;**29**(3):182–5.
4. Mills, W. J., & Nork, S. E. Open reduction and internal fixation of high-energy tibial plateau fractures. *Orthop. Clin. North Am.* 2002;**33**(1):177–98.
5. Keating, J. F., Re: Outcome of the tibial plateau fractures managed with calcium phosphate cement. *Injury* 2005;**36**(8):986.
6. Sirkin, M. S., Bono, C. M., Reilly, M. C., & Behrens, F. F. Percutaneous methods of tibial plateau fixation. *Clin. Orthop. Rel. Res.* 2000;**375**:60–8.
7. Su, E. P., Westrich, G. H., Rana, A. J., Kapoor, K., & Helfet, D. L. Operative treatment of tibial plateau fractures in patients older than 55 years. *Clin. Orthop. Rel. Res.* 2004;**421**:240–8.
8. Watson, J. T. & Hybrid external fixation for tibial plateau fractures. *Am. J. Knee Surg.* 2001;**14**(2):135–40.

12.4 Open reduction and internal fixation of anterior tibial spine fractures
John F. Keating, M. Phil., F.R.C.S. (Orth.)

1. Janarv, P. M., Westblad, P., Johansson, C., & Hirsch, G. Long-term follow-up of anterior tibial spine fractures in children. *J. Pediatr. Orthop.* 1995;**15**(1):63–8.
2. Kocher, M. S., Mandiga, R., Klingele, K., Bley, L., & Micheli, L. J. Anterior cruciate ligament injury versus tibial spine fracture in the skeletally immature knee: a comparison of skeletal maturation and notch width index. *J. Pediatr. Orthop.* 2004;**24**(2):185–8.
3. Schmitgen, G. F. & Utukuri, M. M. Arthroscopic treatment of tibial spine fractures in children: a review of three cases. *Knee* 2000;**7**(2):115–19.
4. Wessel, L. M., Scholz, S., Rusch, M. *et al.* Hemarthrosis after trauma to the pediatric knee joint: what is the value of magnetic resonance imaging in the diagnostic algorithm? *J. Pediatr. Orthop.* 2001;**21**(3):338–42.

Section II: Fractures of the tibial shaft
12.5 Intramedullary nailing
Charles M. Court-Brown, M.D., F.R.C.S., Ed. (Orth.)

12.6 Open reduction and internal fixation: plating
Charles M. Court-Brown, M.D., F.R.C.S., Ed. (Orth.)

1. Court-Brown, C. M., Will, E., Christie, J., & McQueen, M. M. Reamed or unreamed nailing for closed tibial fractures. *J. Bone Joint Surg. Br.* 1996; **78B**: 580–3.
2. Dunbar, R. P., Nork, S. E., Barei, D. P., & Mills, W. J. Provisional plating of Type III open tibia fractures prior to intramedullary nailing. *J. Orthop. Trauma* 2005;**19**(6):412–14.
3. Larsen, L. B., Madsen, J. E., Hoiness, P. R., & Ovre, S. Should insertion of intramedullary nails for tibial fractures be with or without reaming? A prospective, randomized study with 3.8 years' follow-up. *J. Orthop. Trauma* 2004;**18**(3):144–9.
4. Nork, S. E., Schwartz, A. K., Agel, J., Holt, S. K., Schrick, J. L., & Winquist, R. A. Intramedullary nailing of distal metaphyseal tibial fractures. *J. Bone Joint Surg. Am.* 2005;**87**(6):1213–21.
5. Ricci, W. M., Rudzki, J. R., & Borrelli, J. Jr. Treatment of complex proximal tibia fractures with the less invasive skeletal stabilization system. *J. Orthop. Trauma* 2004;**18**(8):521–7.
6. Ziran, B. H., Darowish, M., Klatt, B. A., Agudelo, J. F., & Smith, W. R. Intramedullary nailing in open tibia fractures: a comparison of two techniques. *Int. Orthop.* 2004;**28**(4):235–8.

Section III: Fractures of the distal tibia
12.7 Open reduction and internal fixation: plating pilon
Peter V. Giannoudis, B.Sc., M.B. B.S., M.D., E.E.C. (Orth.)

1. Borrelli, J. Jr & Ellis, E. Pilon fractures: assessment and treatment. *Orthop. Clin. North Am.* 2002;**33**(1):231–45.
2. Conroy, J., Agarwal, M., Giannoudis, P. V., & Matthews, S. J. Early internal fixation and soft tissue cover of severe open tibial pilon fractures. *Int. Orthop.* 2003;**27**(6):343–7.
3. Pollak, A. N., McCarthy, M. L., Bess, R. S., Agel, J., & Swiontkowski, M. F. Outcomes after treatment of high-energy tibial plafond fractures. *J. Bone Joint Surg. Am.* 2003;**85-A**(10):1893–900.
4. Sirkin, M., Sanders, R., DiPasquale, T., & Herscovici, D. Jr. A staged protocol for soft tissue management in the treatment of complex pilon fractures. *J. Orthop. Trauma* 2004;**18**(8 Suppl.):S32–8.
5. Topliss, C. J., Jackson, M., & Atkins, R. M. Anatomy of pilon fractures of the distal tibia. *J. Bone Joint Surg. Br.* 2005;**87**(5):692–7.

12.8 Circular frame fixation for distal tibial fractures
Toby Branfoot, M.B. B.S., F.R.C.S., Ed. (Tr. & Orth.), M.Sc.

1. Blauth, M., Bastian, L., Krettek, C., Knop, C., & Evans, S. Surgical options for the treatment of severe tibial pilon fractures: a study of three techniques. *J. Orthop. Trauma* 2001;**15**(3):153–60.
2. Bone, L., Stegemann, P., McNamara, K., & Seibel, R. External fixation of severely comminuted and open tib-

ial pilon fractures. *Clin. Orthop. Rel. Res.* 1993;**292**: 101–7.
3. Leung, F., Kwok, H. Y., Pun, T. S., & Chow, S. P. Limited open reduction and Ilizarov external fixation in the treatment of distal tibial fractures. *Injury* 2004;**35**(3):278–83.
4. Marsh, J. L., Bonar, S., Nepola, J. V., Decoster, T. A., & Hurwitz, S. R. Use of an articulated external fixator for fractures of the tibial plafond. *J. Bone Joint Surg. Am.* 1995;**77**(10):1498–509.

13 Fractures of the ankle
13.1 Open reduction and internal fixation of bimalleolar ankle fractures
Christopher C. Tzioupis, M.D, Trauma Fellow, Peter V. Giannoudis, B.Sc., M.B. B.S., M.D., E.E.C. (Orth.)

1. Day, G. A., Swanson, C. E., & Hulcombe, B. G. Operative treatment of ankle fractures: a minimum ten-year follow-up. *Foot Ankle Int.* 2001;**22**(2):102–6.
2. Konrath, G., Karges, D., Watson, J. T., *et al.* Early vrs delayed treatment of severe ankle fractures: a comparison of results. *J. Orthop. Trauma* 1995; **9**: 377–80.
3. Michelson, J. D. Ankle fractures resulting from rotational injuries. *J. Am. Acad. Orthop. Surg.* 2003;**11**(6):403–12.
4. Wissing, J. C., van Laarhoven, C. J., & van der Werken C. The posterior antiglide plate for fixation of fractures of the lateral malleolus. *Injury* 1992; **23**:94–6.

14 Fractures of the foot
14.1 Open reduction and internal screw fixation for talar neck fractures
Martinus Richter, M.D.

14.2 Open reduction and internal plate fixation for os calcis fractures
Martinus Richter, M.D.

14.3 Open reduction and internal screw and K-wire fixation for Lisfranc fracture dislocations
Martinus Richter, M.D.

1. Adelaar, R. S., Complex fractures of the talus. *Instruc. Course Lect.* 1997; **46**:323–38.
2. Coughlin, M. J. Calcaneal fractures in the industrial patient. *Foot Ankle Int.* 2000; **21**(11):896–905.
3. Essex-Lopresti, P. The mechanism, reduction technique, and results in fractures of the os calcis, 1951–52. *Clin. Orthop.* 1993;**290**:3–16.
4. Grob, D., Simpson, L. A., Weber, B. G., & Bray, T. Operative treatment of displaced talus fractures. *Clin. Orthop.* 1985;**199**:88–96.
5. Hardcastle, P. H., Reschauer, R., Kutscha-Lissberg, E., & Schoffmann, W. Injuries to the tarsometatarsal joint. Incidence, classification and treatment. *J. Bone Joint Surg. Br.* 1982; **64**(3):349–56.

6. Hawkins, L. G. Fractures of the neck of the talus. *J. Bone Joint Surg. Am.* 1970;**52**(5):991–1002.

7. Richter, M., Thermann, H., Hufner, T., & Krettek C. Aetiology, treatment and outcome in lisfranc joint dislocations and fracture dislocations. *Foot Ankle Surg.* 2002;**8**: 21–32.

8. Squires, B., Allen, P. E., Livingstone, J., & Atkins, R. M. Fractures of the tuberosity of the calcaneus. *J. Bone Joint Surg. Br.* 2001;**83**(1):55–61.

Part IV: Spine
15 Fractures of the cerrical spine

15.1 Application of a halo and halo-vest for cervical spine trauma
Peter Millner, F.R.C.S. (Orth.)

15.2 Operative posterior stabilization of thoraco-lumbar burst fractures
Peter Millner, F.R.C.S. (Orth.)

15.3 Anterior stabilization of complex thoraco-lumbar burst fractures
Peter Millner, F.R.C.S. (Orth.)

1. British Trauma Society. Guidelines for the initial management and assessment of spinal injury. British Trauma Society, 2002. *Injury* 2003;**34**(6):405–25.

2. Hsu, J. M., Joseph, T., & Ellis, A. M. Thoracolumbar fracture in blunt trauma patients: guidelines for diagnosis and imaging. *Injury* 2003;**34**(6):426–33.

3. Kossmann, T., Trease, L., Freedman, I., & Malham, G. Damage control surgery for spine trauma. *Injury* 2004;**35**(7):661–70.

Part V: Tendon injuries
16 Reconstruction of tendons

16.1 Achilles tendon repair
Peter V. Giannoudis, B.Sc., M.B. B.S., M.D., E.E.C. (Orth.)

16.2 Repair of tendon injuries in the hand
Caroline McGuiness F.R.C.S. (Plas Surg), Simon Knight, M.B. B.S., F.R.C.S.

1. Bulstrode, N. W., Burr, N., Pratt, A. L., & Grobbelaar, A. O. Extensor tendon rehabilitation a prospective trial comparing three rehabilitation regimes. *J. Hand Surg. [Br.]* 2005;**30**(2):175–9.

2. Chu, M. M. Splinting programmes for tendon injuries. *Hand Surg.* 2002;**7**(2):243–9.

3. Scott, S. C. Closed injuries to the extension mechanism of the digits. *Hand Clin.* 2000;**16**(3):367–73.

4. Groth, G. N. Current practice patterns of flexor tendon rehabilitation. *J. Hand. Ther.* 2005;**18**(2):169–74.

5. Luo, J., Mass, D. P., Phillips, C. S., & He, T. C. The future of flexor tendon surgery. *Hand Clin.* 2005;**21**(2):267–73.

6. Mehta, V., Phillips, C. S. Flexor tendon pulley reconstruction. *Hand Clin.* 2005;**21**(2):245–51.

7. Movin, T., Ryberg, A., McBride, D. J., & Maffulli, N. Acute rupture of the Achilles tendon. *Foot Ankle Clin.* 2005;**10**(2):331–56.

8. Stamos, B. D. & Leddy, J. P. Closed flexor tendon disruption in athletes. *Hand Clin.* 2000;**16**(3):359–65.

9. Strickland, J. W., The scientific basis for advances in flexor tendon surgery. *J. Hand. Ther.* 2005;**18**(2):94–110.

10. Young, J. S., Kumta, S. M., & Maffulli, N. Achilles tendon rupture and tendinopathy: management of complications. *Foot Ankle Clin.* 2005;**10**(2):371–82.

Part VI: Compartments
17 Decompression fasciotomies

17.1 Fasciotomy for acute compartment syndromes of the upper and lower limbs
Roderick Dunn, M.B. B.S., D.M.C.C., F.R.C.S. (Plast.), Simon Kay, F.R.C.S., F.R.C.S. (Plast.), F.R.C.S.E.

1. Alford, J. W., Palumbo, M. A., & Barnum, M. J. Compartment syndrome of the arm: a complication of noninvasive blood pressure monitoring during thrombolytic therapy for myocardial infarction. *J. Clin. Monit. Comput.* 2002;**17**(3–4):163–6.

2. Del Pinal, F., Herrero, F., Jado, E., Garcia-Bernal, F. J., & Cerezal, L. Acute hand compartment syndromes after closed crush: a reappraisal. *Plast. Reconstr. Surg.* 2002;**110**(5):1232–9.

3. Kies, S. J., Danielson, D. R., Dennison, D. G., Warner, M. E., & Warner, M. A. Perioperative compartment syndrome of the hand. *Anesthesiology* 2004;**101**(5):1232–4.

4. Leigh, W. & Pai, V. Beware: compartment syndrome of the hand. *N Z Med. J.* 2005; **11**:118(1209):U1300.

5. Ozkayin, N. & Aktuglu, K. Absolute compartment pressure versus differential pressure for the diagnosis of compartment syndrome in tibial fractures. *Int. Orthop.* 2005;**10**; 1–6.

6. Ronel, D. N., Mtui, E., Nolan, W. B. 3rd. Forearm compartment syndrome: anatomical analysis of surgical approaches to the deep space. *Plast. Reconstr. Surg.* 2004;**114**(3):697–705.

7. Touliopolous, S. & Hershman, E. B. Lower leg pain. Diagnosis and treatment of compartment syndromes and other pain syndromes of the leg. *Sports Med.* 19.;**27**(3):193–204.

Index

acetabulum
  ilioinguinal approach 143–50
  posterior approach 135–43
Achilles tendon 289–90
Acutrak screws 37, 260
adductor compartment of the
      hand 300–1
adductor muscles (leg) 180
anatomic plates, precontoured 31
ankle
  bimalleolar fracture 249–56
  distal tibial fracture
      external fixation 241–8
      nailing 229
      plating 239–41
  talar neck fracture 257–61
anterior cruciate ligament 221
anticoagulants 125, 131, 143, 144, 150,
      165, 278
AO classification of fracture
      geometry 180
AO small fragment set 36, 66, 78
AO USS Fixator Interne screw set 279,
      280–1
arthritis see osteoarthritis
arthrodesis, foot 267
arthroplasty
  elbow 62
  hip 165–9, 200, 205
  knee 200, 205
  shoulder 14, 17–21
aspirin 143, 150, 165
Austin Moore hemiarthroplasty 165–9
avascular necrosis
  capitellum 38
  femoral capital epiphyses
      (paediatric) 191
  humeral head 8, 16, 17
  talus 259
axillary nerve 9, 11, 26, 40

ball-tipped guide wires 27
Bennett's fracture 100–3
biceps, fasciotomy 304
bladder catheterization 122, 283
Boehler's angle 263, 264
bone grafts
  humerus 19, 32

metacarpal I 102
olecranon 46
radius 71
spine 281, 283, 285
tibia 232
ulna 46
boutonnière injuries 295
bowels 283, 285
Boyd approach 49
brachial artery 39, 304
brachial plexus 3, 22, 304
brachioradialis muscle 68
bridging plates 49, 231, 234
Broden's view 261, 265
burst fractures of the spine 276–86
buttress plates 37, 200

cable technique 181, 203, 207
cages, telescopic 282, 283, 285
calcaneus 261–5
calcaneus plates 264
cannulated screws 128
  hip 160–5
  pelvis 129
  tibia 223
capitellum 35–8
carpal bones
  scaphoid 92–5
  scapho-lunate dissociation 95–9
carpal tunnel
  decompression 301
  tendon repair 292, 293, 296
catheterization, bladder 122, 283
cement use
  hip hemiarthroplasty 167–8
  shoulder hemiarthroplasty 17, 19
  tibial fracture 213, 219
central venous lines 283, 286
cephalic vein 10
cerclage wiring of the patella 210
cervical spine 273–6
chest drains 285, 286
children see paediatric fractures
chylothorax 286
circular frames 220–1, 241–8
CK (creatine kinase) 300
clavicle 3–7
clover-leaf plates 239

compartment syndrome
  description 299–300, 307
  fasciotomy 269, 300–7
  foot 257, 261, 266, 269
  forearm 48, 51, 67, 302–4
  hand 300–2
  lower leg 304–6
      distal tibia 239
      proximal tibia 212, 216, 220
      tibial shaft 224, 231, 237
  pressure measurement 269, 299–300
  upper arm 41, 304
  upper leg 170, 179
compression screws see lag screws
computerised tomography (CT) scans
  calcaneus 262
  pelvis 123, 127, 135, 144
  shoulder 8
  spine 277, 281
  talus 258
  tibia 212, 216, 239, 242
  wrist 87, 90
condylar screw plates 200
corona mortis 147
coronoid process of the ulna 49
corpectomy 284–5
cortical step sign 181
creatine kinase (CK) 300
cruciate ligaments 200, 221
CT scans see computerised tomography
      scans
curved awls 27

damage control surgery
  femur 180, 185, 198–9, 200
  pelvis 119–22
  spine 276–7
DCP plates see dynamic compression
      plates
deep vein thrombosis 125, 134, 144, 150
deltoid ligament 259
deltoid muscle 9–10, 11, 14, 29
DFN (distal femoral nail) 204–7
DHS instrumentation set 154
diameter difference sign 181
diaphragm 284, 285
digital nerves 291, 301
digits see fingers

dislocation
  cervical spine 273, 275
  elbow 49
  hip 135, 169
  metacarpal I 100, 101
  phalanges 111–12
  shoulder 8, 11
  tarso-metatarsal joint (Lisfranc) 265–9
Distal femoral nail (DFN) 204–7
distal radio-ulnar joint (DRUJ) 48, 58, 64,
    82, 85
dorsalis pedis artery 267
dynamic compression hip screws 153–9
dynamic compression plates (DCP) 4
  clavicle 4
  femur 182–5
  humerus 22, 24–5
  radius 69–70
  sacro-iliac joint 133
  tibia 231, 233, 235
  ulna 52, 57
  see also low-contact dynamic
      compression plates
dynamic reconstruction plates 33

elastic nails
  femur 191–8
  forearm 53–5, 71–6
elbow
  arthroplasty 62
  dislocation 49
  distal humerus
    nailing 38–40
    plating 30–5
    screw fixation (capitellum) 35–8
    supracondylar fracture 30–5,
        40–4
  olecranon
    plating 48–50
    TBW (tension band wiring) 45–8
  paediatric fracture 40–4
  proximal radius
    radial head excision 62–4
    screw fixation 60–2
emergency surgery
  fasciotomy 269
  femur 160, 180, 185, 198–9, 200
  pelvis 119–22
  spine 276–7
epidural haematoma 277, 278
epimysiotomy 300
extensor pollicis longus (EPL) 83, 85,
    104
extensor retinaculum 295
extensors of the hand/forearm
  fasciotomy 303–4
  tendon repair 292, 295–6
external fixation
  cervical spine stabilization 273–6
  femur 180, 185, 191, 198–9, 200
  pelvis 119–22
  radius 56, 90–1
  tibia 220–1, 239, 241–8
external iliac artery 148
external oblique muscle 147, 284
eye, closure while fitting halo device 275

Farabeuf clamps 150
fasciotomy 300, 306–7
  foot 257, 261, 266, 269
  lower limb 304–6
  upper limb 300–4
  wound closure 306
fat embolism 180
fat pad sign 40, 41
FCR (flexor carpi radialis) 68, 78–9
FDS (flexor digitorum sublimes) 68
femoral distractors 188
femoral nerve 147, 148
femoral vessels 147
femur
  distal 200
    MIPPO 200–4
    nailing 200, 204–7
  hip
    arthroplasty 165–9, 200, 205
    cannulated screw fixation 160–5
    dislocation 135, 169
    dynamic compression screw
        fixation 153–9
  shaft 179–81
    external fixation 180, 185, 191, 198–9
    nailing 180, 185–98
    open fracture 179–80, 180–1
    paediatric fracture 191–8
    plating 182–5, 191
    subtrochanteric fracture, PFN
        fixation 170–8
fibula
  in ankle fracture 251, 253
  in fasciotomy 305
fingers
  condylar fracture 111–12
  fasciotomy 301–2
  midshaft fracture 112–15
  tendon repair 293–4
flexible intramedullary nailing
  femur 191–8
  forearm 53–5, 71–6
flexor carpi radialis muscle (FCR) 68,
    78–9
flexor digitorum profundis tendon 294
flexor digitorum sublimes muscle
    (FDS) 68
flexor digitorum superficialis muscle 303
flexor policis longus muscle (FPL) 68,
    79
flexors of the hand/forearm
  fasciotomy 302–3
  tendon repair 291–2, 293–5, 296
floating knee 225
Foley catheters 122
foot
  Achilles tendon 289–90
  calcaneus 261–5
  Lisfranc fracture 265–9
  talus 257–61
forearm
  compartment syndrome 48, 51, 67,
      302–4, 306–7
  tendon repair 296
  see also radius; ulna
FPL (flexor policis longus) 68, 79

fracture tables 186, 192
'free-hand technique' 189, 228

Galeazzi fractures 73
Gallows traction 191
gastrocnemius muscle 180, 202, 206, 305
gastrointestinal tract 283, 285
gemeli muscles 139
genitourinary system in pelvic
    injuries 119, 122, 127
glenoid fossa 8, 19
gluteus maximus muscle 137, 180
gluteus medius tendon 166
grafts see bone grafts
Gustilo classification of femoral shaft
    fractures 179–80
Guyon's canal 301

halo and halo-vest devices 273–6
hand
  fasciotomy 300–2, 306–7
  metacarpal I 100–5
  metacarpals II-V 106–10
  phalanges 111–15
  tendon repair 290–6
  ulnar collateral ligament 103–5
Hawkins classification of talar neck
    fractures 258
heel
  Achilles tendon 289–90
  calcaneus 261–5
hemiarthroplasty
  hip 165–9
  shoulder 14, 17–21
heparin 125, 143, 150, 278
Herbert screws 37, 60, 201, 260
hip
  acetabulum
    ilioinguinal approach 143–50
    posterior approach 135–43
  dislocation 135, 169
  femur
    arthroplasty 165–9, 200, 205
    cannulated screw fixation 160–5
    dynamic compression screw
        fixation 153–9
Hoffa fracture 201
Hoffmann II external fixator pelvic
    tray 119
humerus
  dislocation 8, 11
  distal
    nailing 38–40
    paediatric fracture 40–4
    plating 30–5
    screw insertion (capitellum) 35–8
    supracondylar fracture 30–5, 40–4
  proximal 8–10
    hemiarthroplasty 14, 17–21
    plating 14–17
    tension band wiring (TBW) of
        greater tuberosity 10–14
  shaft
    nailing 26–9
    plating 22–6
hypothenar muscles 300, 301

ileus 285
iliac crest 120, 146, 150, 283
iliac vessels 147, 148
iliacus muscle 146
ilioinguinal approach
    to acetabulum 145–50
    to sacroiliac joint 133–4
ilioinguinal nerve 147
iliopectineal fascia 147
iliopsoas muscle 147, 148, 180
ilium
    acetabulum
        ilioinguinal approach 143–50
        posterior approach 135–43
    external fixation of the pelvic
        ring 119–22
    iliac crest 120, 146, 150, 283
impotence 127
infection
    femoral shaft fractures 180–1
    hip hemiarthroplasty 169
    pin sites 248
    tibial fractures 224, 231
inguinal hernia 150
inguinal ligament 147, 150
Insall index 208
interfragmentary screw and
    neutralization plates 232–3
interosseus compartments of the
    hand 300–1
interosseus nerves
    anterior 41
    posterior 30
intramedullary nailing
    for fractures of
        femur 170–8, 180, 185–98, 200, 204–7
        humerus 26–9, 38–40
        radius 71–6
        tibia 224–30
        ulna 53–5, 71–6
    nail types
        distal femoral nail (DFN) 204–7
        flexible 53–5, 71–6, 191–8
        locked nailing set 226
        proximal femoral nail (PFN) 170–8
intramedullary wiring of
    metacarpals 108–10
ischaemia
    in compartment syndrome 299
    talar fracture repair 259
    see also avascular necrosis

Judet views of the pelvis 126, 144, 145, 149

K-wires see Kirschner wires
Kapandji pinning of distal radius 88–9
Kessler sutures 290, 294
kidney failure 300
Kirschner wires
    Lisfranc fracture 267
    metacarpals 100–1, 108–10
    radius 87–90
    scapho-lunate dissociation 97–8
    tendon repair 295
    ulna 46–7, 58

knee
    arthroplasty 200, 205
    distal femur
        MIPPO 200–4
        nailing 204–7
    external fixation 198–9, 220–1
    patella 208–11
    proximal tibia
        anterior tibial spine 221–3
        bicondylar tibial plateau 216–21
        lateral tibial plateau 212–16
knee brace 216, 223
kyphosis, correction of 280, 283

lacertus fibrosus 303
lag screws
    acetabulum 141
    femur
        dynamic compression hip screw
            fixation 153–9
        metaphyseal/diaphyseal
            fractures 201, 205
        plating of shaft 183
    hand 102, 104–5, 107, 112, 113
    humerus 24
    malleolus 250, 253
    olecranon 49
    patella 208, 211
    sacro-iliac joint 129
lateral femoral cutaneous nerve 147
lateral geniculate nerve 225
LC-DCP (low-contact dynamic
    compression plates) 182–5, 231,
    233–4, 235, 239
see also dynamic compression plates
LCP (locking compression plates) 216,
    219, 231, 235, 237
lead gowns 279
Less Invasive Stabilization System
    (LISS) 201–4, 231, 237
lesser trochanter shape sign/
    method 181, 187, 203,
    207
linea alba 124, 125
Lisfranc fracture 265–9
Lister's tubercle 83
load-sharing classification of spinal
    fractures 277
locked screw plates 200
locking compression plates (LCP) 216,
    219, 231, 235, 237
lordosis, correction of 280
low-contact dynamic compression plates
    (LC-DCP) 182–5, 231, 233–4, 235,
    239
see also dynamic compression plates
lower limb
    Achilles tendon 289–90
    fasciotomy 300, 304–7
    see also individual bones and joints
lumbar nerve roots 131, 133
lumbar spine see thoraco-lumbar burst
    fracture
lunate, scapho-lunate dissociation 95–9
lung 284, 286

MacDonald's elevators 46, 54
magnetic resonance imaging (MRI) 259,
    277, 289
malleolus 249–56
mallet injuries 295
malunion 73; see also non-union
Mason–Johnson classification of radial
    fractures 60, 61, 62
Matta plating system 123, 124–5, 141, 150
median nerve
    fasciotomy 301, 303
    radial fracture 79, 81
    supracondylar fracture 41
    tendon repair 291
    wrist fracture 92, 95, 98
metacarpals
    I 100–5
    II–V 106–10
    ulnar collateral ligament 103–5
metatarsals, Lisfranc fracture 267
mini-plates 102, 105, 107, 113
minimally invasive percutaneous plate
    osteosynthesis (MIPPO) 182, 184,
    200–4
minor trochanter technique (lesser
    trochanter shape sign) 181, 187,
    203, 207
MIPPO (minimally invasive
    percutaneous plate
    osteosynthesis) 182, 184, 200–4
Monteggia fractures 51–3, 73
MRI (magnetic resonance imaging) 259,
    277, 289
musculocutaneous nerve 39

nailing see Intramedullary nailing
nailing table 224–5
nasogastric tubes 283, 285
neck 273–6
neutralization plates 183, 232–3, 251
nightstick injury 51
non-union
    humerus 38
    radius 73
    spine 282
    tibia 237

obturator artery 147
obturator internus tendon 139, 141
olecranon
    osteotomy 32
    plating 48–50
    TBW (tension band wiring) 45–8
olecranon fossa 39
open fractures
    femur 179–80, 180–1, 200
    humerus 22, 27, 30, 35
    tibia 224, 229, 239
open reduction and internal fixation see
    ORIF
operating microscopes 293
orbicularis muscle 275
ORIF (open reduction and internal
    fixation)
    acetabulum 135–50
    calcaneus 261–5

ORIF (*cont.*)
  capitellum 35–8
  clavicle 3–7
  femur 182–5
  humerus
    proximal 14–17
    shaft 22–6
    supracondylar 30–5
  Lisfranc injury 265–9
  malleolus 249–56
  metacarpal I 101–3
  metacarpals II-V 106–7
  phalanges (upper limb) 111–15
  pubic symphysis 122–7
  radius 72
    distal 77–86
    proximal 60–2
    shaft 65–71
  sacro-iliac joint 131–4
  scapho-lunate dissociation 95–9
  talar neck 257–61
  tibia
    distal 239–41
    proximal 212–20, 221–3
    shaft 230–8
  ulna
    distal 56–9
    olecranon 48–50
    shaft 51–3
os calcis 261–5
osteoarthritis
  hip 143, 150
  knee 210, 213, 220, 221
osteopaenia 48, 200, 207, 231,
    237
osteoporosis 167, 170
osteosynthesis set 66, 171
osteotomy
  olecranon 32
  radial head 62–4

paediatric fractures
  femur 191–8
  humerus (supracondylar) 40–4
  radius 60, 63, 71–6
  tibia 223
  ulna 53–5, 71–6
palm
  fasciotomy 301
  see also metacarpals
patella 208–11
patellar tendon 208
pectoralis major muscle 10
pedicle screws 279, 280–1
pelvic reconstruction plates 123, 124–5,
    141, 150
pelvis
  acetabulum
    ilioinguinal approach 143–50
    posterior approach 135–43
  external fixation 119–22
  pubic symphysis 122–7
  sacro-iliac joint
    plating 131–4
    screw fixation 127–31
Penrose drains 147

percutaneous fixation
  MIPPO 182, 184, 200–4
  paediatric supracondylar fracture 40–4
  paediatric ulnar fracture 54
  scaphoid 92–5
peritoneal sac 284
peroneal compartment 305, 306
peroneal nerve 212, 216, 220, 221, 250
peroneal tendons 262
Pfaennestiel incision 123
PFN (proximal femoral nailing) 170–8
phalanx (upper limb)
  condylar fracture 111–12
  midshaft fracture 112–15
Philos® plates 14–17
phrenic nerve 8
pilon fracture 239–48
pins
  care of 247, 248, 275
  distal radius 87–90
  external fixation
    halo devices 274–5
    pelvis 120–1
    tibia 246–7
  metacarpals 100–1, 108–10
  paediatric supracondylar fracture 40–4
  scapho-lunate dissociation 97–8
piriformis tendon 138, 139, 141
plates *see individual types*
pneumothorax 3, 8
'poller screws' 185, 189, 205, 229
polylactic acid bioabsorbable screws 260
posterior cruciate ligament 200
profunda branchii artery 23
profunda femoris artery 137
pronator quadratus muscle 68, 79,
    303
pronator teres muscle 303
prostheses
  hip 165–9
  shoulder 17–21
proximal femoral nailing (PFN) 170–8
psoas major muscle 284, 285
pubic symphysis 122–7
pulmonary embolism 134, 144, 150
pulses
  in compartment syndrome 299
  radial pulse in upper limb injuries 41,
    71

quadriceps muscle 209, 211
Quenu and Küss classification of Lisfranc
    fractures 266

radial artery 92
radial nerve
  fasciotomy 301, 304
  humeral fracture 22, 23, 24, 26, 35, 39
  radial shaft fracture 68
  supracondylar fracture 30, 32, 33, 41
  tendon repair 291
radial pulse 41, 71
radiocarpal joint 82, 85
radiography, before and after shots
  ankle 250, 256
  clavicle 4, 6

femur
  distal 203, 205
  hip 154, 158, 161, 164
  shaft 183, 184, 188, 196, 197
  subtrochanter 171, 177
foot 258, 260, 262, 265, 268
humerus
  distal 31, 34, 36, 37, 38, 40, 41
  proximal 8, 11, 14, 15, 17, 18, 21
  shaft 23, 26, 27, 29
metacarpals 100, 101, 103, 107, 108,
    109
patella 209, 210
pelvis 122, 126, 127, 132, 136, 144, 149
phalanges 112, 113, 114
radius
  distal 78, 83, 86, 87, 88, 90
  proximal 61, 62, 63
  shaft 65, 72, 75
spine 278, 280, 281, 282
tibia
  distal 240, 244, 247
  proximal 213, 216, 217, 218, 219,
    222
  shaft 224, 225, 233, 234, 237
ulna
  distal 57, 58
  proximal 46, 47, 48, 49
  shaft 53, 72, 75
wrist 95, 96, 97
see also CT scans
radiography, general considerations
  distal femoral fractures 200
  femoral shaft fractures 180
radius
  combined radial and ulnar fracture 49,
    51–3, 56
  distal
    external fixation 56, 90–1
    K-wire fixation 87–90
    plating 77–86
  paediatric fracture 60, 63, 71–6
  proximal
    osteotomy 62–4
    screw fixation 60–2
  shaft
    intramedullary nailing 71–6
    plating 65–71
reamers 39
reconstruction plates 4, 31
  clavicle 4
  humerus 33
  olecranon 49
  pelvis 123, 124–5, 141, 150
rectus abdominis muscle 123, 124, 125,
    147
reduction clamps 201
removal of implants
  femur 178, 191, 198, 207
  halo pins 276
  humerus 29, 35, 38, 44
  pelvic external fixators 122
  radius 86, 91
  spine 282
  tibia 213, 220, 221, 223, 238, 248
  ulna 55

renal failure 300
Retzius' space 147
rib, removal during spinal surgery 283–4
Richards compression screws 157
Rolando fracture 101, 102
rotator cuff
    humeral shaft fracture 29
    shoulder fracture 12, 13, 15

sacral nerve roots 131, 133
sacro-iliac joint
    plating 131–4
    screw fixation 127–31
Sanders classification of calcaneus
        fractures 261
saphenous nerve 209
scalene block 8
scaphoid 92–5
scapho-lunate dissociation 95–9
scaphotrapezial joint (STJ) 93
Schanz screws 188, 198, 202, 206, 263,
    280
sciatic nerve 135, 136, 138, 139
sciatic notch 139
screws, use in
    hip fixation
        cannulated screws 160–5
        dynamic compression screws 153–9
    humeral fracture 35–8
    Lisfranc fracture 267
    radial head fracture 60–2
    sacro-iliac fixation 127–31
    scaphoid fracture 92–5
    spinal fracture 276–82
    talar neck fracture 257–61
    tibial spine fracture 221–3
    see also cannulated screws; lag screws;
        self-compressing screws
self-compressing screws 36
    Acutrak 37, 260
    Herbert 37, 60, 201, 260
shoulder
    dislocation 8, 11
    fracture 8–10
        hemiarthroplasty 14, 17–21
        plating 14–17
        TBW (tension band wiring) of greater
            tuberosity 10–14
spermatic cord 147
spinal cord monitoring 278, 283
spine
    cervical fractures 273–6
    thoraco-lumbar burst fracture
        anterior stabilization 277, 281,
            282–6
        posterior stabilization 276–82
    see also sacro-iliac joint
splanchic nerve 284
Stecher's view of the wrist 87,
        90
steel wire sutures 11
Stener lesion 103–5
STJ (scaphotrapezial joint) 93
stomach 283
superficial veins of forearm 68

supracondylar fracture
    adult 30–5
    paediatric 40–4
sural nerve 250, 262, 289
suturing
    lower leg 244
    tendons 290, 294, 295
    tension band fixation of humeral
        tuberosities 12–13, 15, 18, 20–1
    ulnar collateral ligament 104

t-handle chucks 27
T-plate 79
talus 257–61
tarsometatarsal joint 265–9
TBW see tension band wiring
telescopic fusion cages 282, 283, 285
tendon repair
    Achilles 289–90
    hand/forearm 290–6
tenosynovitis 86
tension band wiring (TBW)
    humerus
        distal 33
        tuberosities 10–14, 15, 18, 20–1
    patella 208–11
    ulna
        distal 58
        olecranon 45–8
THA (total hip arthroplasty) 200, 205
thenar muscles 300, 301
Theraband loops 247
Thomas splints 191
Thompson's hemiarthroplasty 165–9
thoracic duct 286
thoraco-lumbar burst fracture
    anterior stabilization 277, 281, 282–6
    posterior stabilization 276–82
thromboprophylaxis 125, 131, 143, 144,
        150, 166, 278
thumb
    decompression of thenar
        compartment 301
    metacarpal I fracture 100–3
    ulnar collateral ligament repair 103–5
tibia
    distal
        external fixation 239, 241–8
        plating 239–41
    proximal
        anterior tibial spine 221–3
        bicondylar tibial plateau 216–21
        lateral tibial plateau 212–16
    shaft
        nailing 224–30
        plating 230–8
tibialis anterior tendon 240
titanium nails/screws 72, 259
total hip arthroplasty (THA) 200, 205
    see also hemiarthroplasty, hip
total knee arthroplasty (TKA) 200, 205
tourniquets
    lower limb 212, 257
    upper limb 45, 67, 82, 292
Trethowan spike 167

triceps compartment 304
triceps muscle 23, 32
triceps tendon 23, 33, 40
trochanter
    inter-trochanter fracture 153–9
    lesser trochanter shape
        sign/method 181, 187, 203, 207
Tscherne classification of femoral shaft
        fractures 179
'tube-to-tube' technique 199
tubular plates 239, 251

U&Es 300
ulna
    distal 56–9
    proximal
        plating 48–50
        TBW (tension band wiring) 45–8
    shaft
        elastic nails 53–5, 71–6
        plating 51–3
ulnar artery 301
ulnar collateral ligament 103–5
ulnar nerve
    fasciotomy 301, 303
    supracondylar fracture 30, 32, 33, 41,
        43–4
    tendon repair 291
    ulnar fracture 45, 56
ultrasound
    Stener lesion 104
    tendons 289
upper limb
    fasciotomy 300–4, 306–7
    tendon repair 290–6
    see also individual bones and joints
urea & electrolytes 300
urethra 122
urinary tract in pelvic injuries 119, 122,
        127

varus/valgus alignment 181, 203, 207,
        225, 229, 259
vastus lateralis muscle/tendon 155, 161,
        166, 216
vertebral column see spine
vests (halo-vest devices) 273, 275

Watson–Cheyne elevators 46
Wilson frames 279, 280
wires see Kirschner wires; tension band
        wiring
wrist
    distal radius
        external fixation 90–1
        plating 77–86
        wiring 87–90
    scaphoid 92–5
    scapho-lunate dissociation 95–9
    tendon repair 292, 293, 295, 296

X-rays see radiography

Young's classification of pelvic
        fractures 120

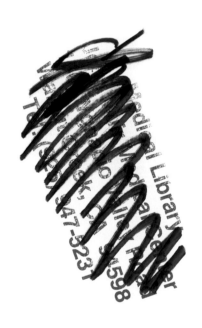